KW-064-228

INVASIVE ULTRASOUND

For my wife, Caroline
WRL

For my wife, Harriet
EAL

WN 420

3280
ATOK

WITHDRAWN

SINGLETON HOSPITAL
STAFF LIBRARY

INVASIVE ULTRASOUND

EDITED BY

William R Lees, FRCR, FRACR (Hon)

Professor, Department of Medical Imaging and
Director, Academic Department of Imaging
University College London

Consultant Radiologist
The Middlesex Hospital
London, UK

Edward A Lyons, FRCP(C), FACR

Professor of Radiology and Obstetrics & Gynecology
Chairman and Head, Department of Radiology
Health Sciences Centre and University of Manitoba
Winnipeg, Manitoba, Canada

MARTIN DUNITZ

SINGLETON HOSPITAL
STAFF LIBRARY

© Martin Dunitz 1996

First published in the United Kingdom in 1996 by
Martin Dunitz Ltd, 7–9 Pratt Street, London NW1 OAE

All rights reserved. No part of this publication may
be reproduced, stored in a retrieval system, or transmitted
in any form or by any means, without the prior permission
of the publisher.

A CIP catalogue record of this book is
available from the British Library.

ISBN: 1-85317-133-6

Composition by Scribe Design, Gillingham, Kent, UK
Origination by Imago Publishing Ltd
Manufactured by Imago Publishing Ltd
Printed and bound in Hong Kong

Contents

Contributors

Paul Allan FRCR, FRCP (Ed)
Senior Lecturer and Honorary Consultant Radiologist
The University of Edinburgh
Edinburgh, UK

Clive I Bartram FRCP, FRCR
Consultant Radiologist
St Mark's Hospital
Northwick Park, Harrow, UK

John Beynon MS, FRCS
Consultant General and Colorectal Surgeon
Singleton Hospital
Swansea, UK

Roger Chisholm MA, MRCP, FRCR
Consultant in Diagnostic Radiology
Hope Hospital (University of Manchester)
Salford, UK

Wui K Chong MRCP (UK), FRCR
Assistant Professor of Radiology
  and Radiological Sciences
Vanderbilt University Medical Center
Nashville, USA

Sidney M Dashefsky MD, FRCP(C)
Assistant Professor
Department of Radiology
Health Sciences Centre
University of Manitoba
Winnipeg, Manitoba, Canada

O James Garden FRCS (Ed & Glas)
Senior Lecturer and Honorary Consultant Surgeon
The University of Edinburgh
Edinburgh, UK

John E Gardener MSc, PhD
Consultant Clinical Scientist
Department of Medical Physics and Bioengineering
University College London Hospitals
London, UK

Jonathan R Glover MA, FRCS, FRCR
Consultant Radiologist
Department of Radiology
St Peter's Hospital
Chertsey, UK

Barry B Goldberg MD
Professor of Radiology
Director, Division of Diagnostic Ultrasound and
  Jefferson Ultrasound Research and Education Institute
Thomas Jefferson University Hospital
Philadelphia, USA

Adrian R W Hatfield MD, FRCP
Consultant Gastroenterologist
Gastroenterology Unit
University College London Hospitals
The Middlesex Hospital
London, UK

Timothy G John FRCS (Ed)
Lecturer in Surgery
The University of Edinburgh
Edinburgh, UK

Ian M G Kelly MRCPI, FRCR
Consultant Radiologist
Department of Radiology
Royal Victoria Hospital
Belfast, UK

Fotini Laoudi MD
Consultant Gastroenterologist
Department of Ultrasound
Athens Medical Centre
Athens, Greece

Clifford S Levi MD, FRCP(C)
Professor
Department of Radiology
Health Sciences Centre
University of Manitoba
Winnipeg, Manitoba, Canada

Ji-Bin Liu MD
Research Assistant Professor of Radiology
Division of Diagnostic Ultrasound
Thomas Jefferson University Hospital
Philadelphia, USA

W Norman McDicken BSc, PhD
Professor of Medical Physics and Medical
    Engineering
Department of Medical Physics and Medical
    Engineering
University of Edinburgh
Edinburgh, UK

A Roger Morgan BSc, FRCS (Ed)
Senior Surgical Registrar
Department of Colorectal Surgery
Singleton Hospital
Swansea, UK

Andreas Müller MD
Consultant Gastroenterologist
Gastroenterologie-Zentrum
Hirslanden
Zürich, Switzerland

David Rickards FRCR
Consultant Uroradiologist
Department of Radiology
University College London Hospitals
The Middlesex Hospital
London, UK

Preface

Ultrasonography is an evolutionary medium and consequently there has been gradual optimization of probe design to fit a particular target. Direct application of a transducer to the area of interest allows the use of the highest frequencies without beam degradation and clutter caused by overlying tissues. This has led to invasion of every conceivable body cavity and to highly invasive techniques such as intraoperative and laparoscopic ultrasound. Invasive ultrasound probes vary from 1 mm to 50 mm in size and operate at frequencies up to 30 MHz with sub-millimetric resolution. These probes are used by radiologists, surgeons and physicians across the whole spectrum of medical imaging.

Invasive ultrasound in all its forms is now mature, robust and remarkably economical compared with other scanning techniques such as CT and MRI. Instruments can be taken anywhere within the hospital or clinic environment, even to the bedside in the intensive care unit. As experience has improved, so have diagnostic capabilities and it is now surprising that many of these techniques took so long to become established. The scientific validity of invasive ultrasound is beyond question. Wider use will come with improvements in transducer technology together with reductions in price as a result of mass production.

There are many technical improvements still to come. Duplex and colour Doppler imaging are still not available on many invasive transducers, particularly the mechanically-driven type. Pulse-shaping and optimization, signal-processing and three-dimensional reconstruction all will lead to significant improvements in resolution and display of invasive ultrasound images.

Invasive ultrasound will persist long after externally-applied ultrasound is displaced by advances in CT and MRI.

The Editors wish to acknowledge the indefatigable energy and patience of Alan Burgess and Jacky Alderson at Martin Dunitz Ltd in readying this book for publication.

Chapter 1 **Invasive Ultrasound Transducers**

W Norman McDicken

INTRODUCTION

One of the attractions of working in medical ultrasonics is the versatility of the techniques due to the wide range of transducers (probes) which are available. It is even possible to collaborate at moderate expense with a manufacturer or local Biomedical Engineering department in the design of a transducer for a novel application. During invasive procedures the ultrasound beam is required to penetrate less tissue than with percutaneous scanning since the transducer is placed nearer to the structures of interest. Higher ultrasound frequencies are therefore employed with a resulting improvement in image resolution.[1] Typically, percutaneous methods utilize ultrasound frequencies in the range 3–10 MHz, in contrast to the 5–30 MHz used invasively. Research projects are in hand to extend the upper limit of application towards 100 MHz for imaging tissues on a histological scale.[2]

In the past, manufacture of high-frequency transducers has been difficult since thin crystal elements were brittle; however, the development of new piezoelectric materials is helping to solve this problem. It is worth emphasizing that, where their use is justified, invasive techniques overcome in one step the three main problems associated with ultrasonic imaging, i.e. beam degradation due to gas, bone and fat. On the other hand, the flexibility familiar with external scanning is restricted when the transducer is within the body. Multiplane scanning transducers and three-dimensional imaging are at least partially overcoming this restriction. With invasive Doppler methods, higher ultrasonic frequency of operation can result in more aliasing artifacts in the measurement of high blood velocity.

At present only a few catheter transducers can realistically be considered as disposable items and even those are relatively expensive. If the demand were to grow, a reasonably large range of transducers could be manufactured as disposables for invasive procedures.

TRANSDUCER CLASSIFICATION AND TYPES

The basic principles of real-time transducer assemblies used invasively for pulse-echo and Doppler imaging may be classified as follows:

- Mechanical sector oscillator.
- Mechanical rotator.
- Moving mirror.
- Electronic linear array.
- Electronic curved array.
- Electronic sector scanner (phased array).
- Water-bath (liquid-filled balloon) scanner.
- Catheter scanner.

Fig. 1.1 illustrates these principles in invasive systems.

The physical principles of the transducers are identical to those of transducers used externally.[3] To date, no new scanning principles have been introduced for invasive imaging; however, specific designs[4] and dramatic miniaturization are often evident. In many invasive applications where static or only slowly moving structures are to be imaged, the frame rate can be quite low, e.g. 5/s, with a resulting improvement in line density in the image.

PIEZOELECTRIC ELEMENTS

Transducers operating at frequencies below 10 MHz usually use piezoelectric ceramic elements (crystals) of a solid solution of lead zirconate titanate, e.g. PZT5A, the trade name of Vernitron Ltd, England.[5,6] Above 10 MHz, electrical and mechanical problems associated with thin crystals result in poor performance. Indeed, many transducers labelled 10 MHz by manufacturers actually operate at lower frequencies. The development of piezoelectric plastics such as the polymer polyvinylidene difluoride (PVDF), permits easier manufacture of high-frequency devices. Its acoustic impedance is less than that of ceramics,

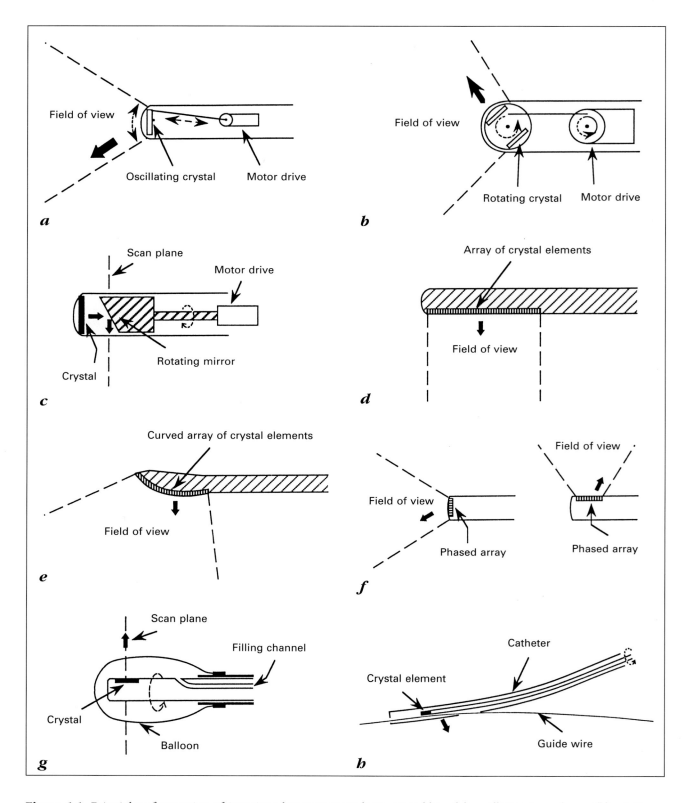

Figure 1.1 *Principles of operation of invasive ultrasonic transducer assemblies: (a) oscillating transducer; (b) rotating transducer; (c) moving mirror transducer; (d) linear array; (e) curved array; (f) phased array; (g) water-bath transducer; (h) catheter transducer.*

making it better matched to soft tissue and resulting in more efficient transmission and reception of ultrasound.

When a pulsed wave transducer is labelled with a particular frequency, this is in fact its central frequency of operation. It will actually operate over a range of neighbouring frequencies, referred to as its frequency bandwidth. For example, a transducer with a central frequency of 5 MHz might have a bandwidth from 2.5 to 7.5 MHz. Recently, wide-bandwidth transducers have become available which are sensitive over a wider range of frequency, e.g. 2–12 MHz.[7] The piezoelectric element in these devices is a composite of materials such as PZT and PVDF. Rods or particles of ceramic are imbedded in the plastic. It is possible with wide-band transducers to change the central ultrasonic frequency during a scan without changing the transducer, e.g. from 4–8 MHz. Apart from reducing the number of transducers which need to be purchased, this capability has obvious convenience for invasive scanning.

MECHANICAL SECTOR OSCILLATOR

This is the simplest type of real-time transducer assembly and can readily be designed as an invasive probe. The crystal is driven by a mechanism to oscillate about an axis close to and parallel to its front face. It is contained in a small, thin-walled plastic chamber which is normally filled with an oil of suitable viscosity (Fig. 1.1a). The ultrasonic pulses travel through the oil and plastic wall with little degradation. The angular measurement information may be derived directly from the motor drive or from a separate sensor.

The transducer is normally a single crystal with a fixed focus. Annular arrays can be fitted into this type of assembly to bring the benefit of swept focusing with true axial symmetry.[8] It is easier to fabricate high-frequency transducers, above 10 MHz, as single-crystal devices rather than as arrays. All mechanical systems need to be very well made, as otherwise they are prone to breakdown. Inevitably, bubbles due to degassing arise in the oil within the plastic chamber, and therefore a simple means of replacing the oil should be part of the design.

Oscillating sector scanners normally have a scan plane (field of view) pointing forwards and symmetrical about the central axis of the transducer assembly (Fig. 1.1a). The sector angle of the field can be in excess of 180° but is typically less than 120°. The line density in the image or the frame rate may be increased by reducing the angle. Multiplane scanning is discussed below in which the crystal element is moved to change the plane of scan.

MECHANICAL ROTATOR

The mechanical rotator design is similar in many ways to that of the oscillator except that typically one, two, three or four transducers are mounted on a rotating wheel (Fig. 1.1b). Only the crystal adjacent to the plastic window is activated at any particular time. In some units the crystals operate at different frequencies, permitting the frequency to be changed without removing the assembly from within the patient. The electrical connections to continuously rotating transducers are more complex than to a single oscillating one, and as a result the option of altering the direction of the plane of scan is not usually available in this type of scanner. Invasive probes based on a rotating transducer are also designed such that the plane of scan is perpendicular to the longitudinal axis of the transducer assembly (see Fig. 1.1g).

MOVING MIRROR

Electrical connections to moving transducers require small slip-rings or rotating transformers. While these are often small, elegant devices, their use can be avoided by a design in which the crystal is held static and the ultrasound beam is swept by reflecting it off a moving mirror (Fig. 1.1c). This approach has been used commercially but it has not found extensive application. Multiple reflections in the oil between the crystal and the mirror may produce artifact echoes. This design has also been used in catheter scanners. One way of making a very efficient light-weight mirror is to seal a thin air film between two sheets of metal foil.

ELECTRONIC LINEAR ARRAY

A diagram of the structure of a linear array is shown in Fig. 1.1d. The transducer assembly is made of a line of piezoelectric strip elements placed side by side. Material between the elements is selected to provide electrical and ultrasonic insulation so that the elements function independently. In a transducer designed for internal use, 128 elements operating at 10 MHz is typical. To generate a pulse of ultrasound which will produce a scan line of echoes, a group of neighbouring elements is activated. The number of elements being used at any time is not fixed and could, for example, be 32 or 64. Computer-controlled machines are very versatile in the way in which they use elements. To focus the transmitted field at depth, 128 elements may be employed, while for more superficial focusing it may be 32. Similarly, during reception of echoes, the number of elements will vary depending on the depth from which echoes are being received at each instant. Considerable engineering design effort is put into making the electronic focusing on transmission and reception as effective as possible.[3]

To step the beam rapidly across the plane of scan, different groups of elements are employed. The beam is therefore swept without any physical movement of the whole transducer assembly. This is one of the main attractions of electronic arrays. The shape of the field of view from a linear array is rectangular, its width being determined by the length of the array. Since the length of the array is inevitably limited in an internal scanner, the field of view is often smaller than might be desired. The use of such a device is usually restricted to intraoperative or rectal scanning.

ELECTRONIC CURVED ARRAY

A scanner which functions by the activation of neighbouring groups of piezoelectric elements need not be of a linear construction. The field of view can be increased by curving the array (Fig. 1.1e). Obviously the beam directions in the scan plane must be exactly known to permit an accurate image to be constructed. The degree of curvature of arrays may vary from slight to very marked which enables them to be tailored to the application. For example, both forward-scanning strongly curved devices with a field of view of 120° and gently curved side-viewing ones find application in obstetrics and gynaecology, depending on the region of the pelvis to be imaged. Since small curved arrays can have relatively large fields of view, this type of transducer assembly is popular in invasive imaging.

ELECTRONIC SECTOR SCANNER (PHASED ARRAY)

The electronic sector scanner is attractive from an invasive probe point of view, since it can be made

small and the beam is swept without physical movement. In this case the array of parallel elements is substantially smaller than a linear array of the same frequency (Fig. 1.1f). A rapid beam sector scanning action is achieved by applying different electronic delays to both the excitation pulses and subsequent echo signals at each transducer element for different beam directions. The number of elements in phased arrays ranges from 32 to 128. Phased arrays are more complex than linear or curved arrays and often have less well-defined beams. However, for internal scanning their small size may more than compensate for the slight degradation in image quality.[9] The small size of this type of transducer has permitted two arrays to be mounted on the same transducer assembly in such a way that two perpendicular scan planes can be used. Biplane transducers are of value in transoesophageal heart imaging.

WATER-BATH (LIQUID-FILLED BALLOON) SCANNER

Water-bath scanners for invasive use take the form of a liquid-filled balloon around a transducer (Fig. 1.1g). The balloon serves two functions: to make good contact between the transducer and the tissue by removing gas; and to push the tissue away from the transducer face, where the beam is rather wide, and move it nearer to the focal region.

The transducer face may often be parallel to the surface of the balloon and hence multiple reflection artifacts are common with such devices. It may not be possible to eliminate this artifact, say by angling the transducer, and therefore it has to be clearly identified. The regular spacing of the artifact echo usually makes this possible but with liquid-filled structures reflected ultrasound can reach the transducer by indirect routes, since the attenuation in most liquids is low.

CATHETER SCANNER

Miniature real-time imaging catheter transducers have been developed over many years; however, their recent commercial availability has greatly increased interest in applications. In principle, they could be used repeatedly in several patients, but the fear of HIV infection rules this out. As a result the technique is expensive and is primarily being used as a research tool at present. Commonly known as IVUS (intravascular ultrasound), it is providing information on the

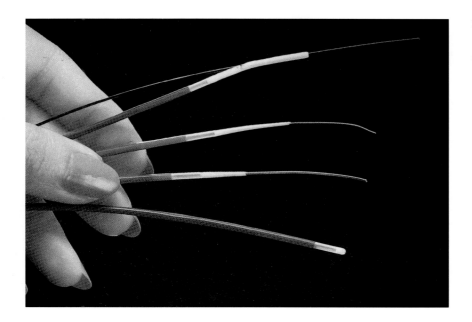

Figure 1.2 *Examples of miniature catheters. (Courtesy of Hewlett Packard.)*

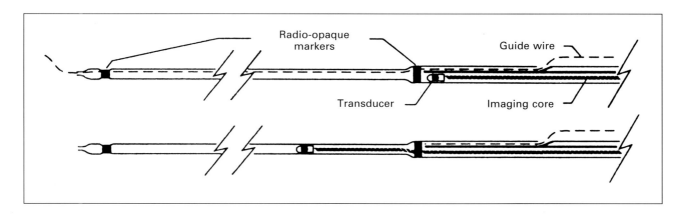

Figure 1.3 *Structure of catheter transducer. (Courtesy of Hewlett Packard.)*

disease processes associated with artery walls. Since this type of probe is newer than those described above, it will be considered in more detail.

The most common design of catheter transducer assembly involves a single transducer element rotating in water in a thin plastic tube to give a 360° field of view (Fig. 1.1h). It is essentially a scaled-down version of a mechanical scanner in which the transducer rotates in an oil-filled plastic cylinder. Rotation of the transducer is by a long flexible cable attached to an external motor. The miniaturization with good ultrasonic performance which has been achieved is

quite remarkable, overall sizes down to 3.5 French gauge (1.1 mm diameter) being available (Fig. 1.2). To date, catheters operate at frequencies up to 30 MHz, but higher frequency devices are being developed in research laboratories. At 30 MHz the depth of penetration in tissue is around 5 mm.

Within a blood vessel, the catheter is moved along a guide wire which has been passed previously to the site of interest under X-ray screening control. The relative positions of the ultrasonic transducer, the guide wire and the thin plastic catheter are shown in Fig. 1.3. The guide wire acts as a monorail for the

SINGLETON HOSPITAL
STAFF LIBRARY

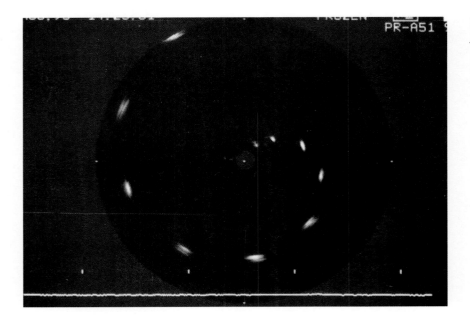

Figure 1.4 *Images of thin nylon filament targets at increasing distances from the transducer. Axial and lateral resolution were measured from the image spots.*

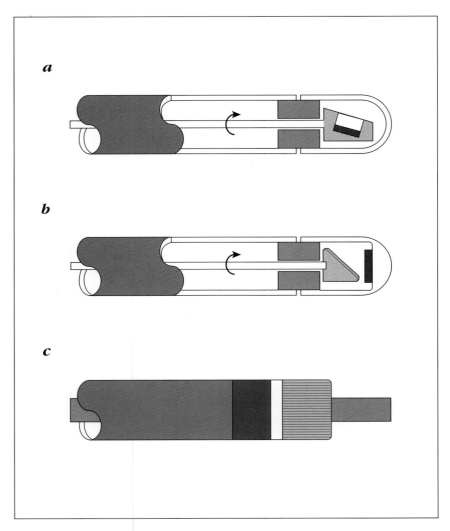

Figure 1.5 *(a) Rotating transducer catheter. (b) Rotating mirror catheter. (c) Cylindrical array catheter. (Courtesy of N. Bom, Rotterdam.)*

catheter and transducer. To perform a scan, the guide wire is partially withdrawn and this allows the transducer to be passed into the end portion of the catheter.

The use of high-frequency PVDF transducers and the limited space available for transducer backing material raise questions about the ultrasonic performance of these new types of device. Assessments with miniature test objects have shown that the ultrasonic performance of catheter transducers is quite good. For example, results with a 3.5 French gauge IVUS catheter[10] show that the axial resolution at 30 MHz is always better than 0.3 mm when assessed with a thin nylon filament target in water. The lateral resolution increases with distance from the transducer but is still less than 1 mm at a range of 5 mm. There is no clear indication of any focusing (Fig. 1.4). The catheter scanner may be operated at 20 and 12 MHz but in the latter case increased penetration is obtained at the expense of significant beam side lobes. Sharp bending of the catheter causes the scanning to become uneven as the cable sticks at parts of its rotation. This results in image distortion of which the user may be unaware.

Miniature catheter transducers may also be made based on a cylindrical curved array, in which the parallel array elements lie round the surface of a small cylinder, and also on the rotating mirror principle shown in Fig. 1.5.[11] Catheter scanners can also be located within heart chambers to produce intracardiac images.[12]

Simple Doppler devices are available which perform in a pulsed or continuous wave mode by having one or two crystals mounted on the end of a catheter. The ultrasound beams point forward in the direction of the catheter axis. In theory it is possible to make colour flow Doppler imagers with their field of view pointing ahead of the catheter tip. However, this is much more difficult than the manufacture of the rotating transducer catheter discussed earlier, for which the mechanism and electronics are quite simple. In some situations pulsed wave and colour Doppler units may suffer readily from aliasing problems, since they operate at high ultrasonic frequencies and since their beams are directed almost parallel to the direction of flow so that high-velocity components are encountered.

MULTIPLANE (OMNIPLANE) SCANNER

The flexibility normally associated with hand-held transducers in external scanning is compromised

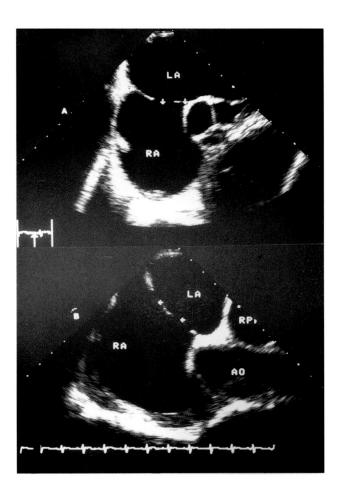

Figure 1.6 *Images from two orthogonal scan planes through the heart produced by two phased arrays on the same transoesophageal scanner (biplane scanner). (Courtesy of G.R. Sutherland, Edinburgh.)*

when transducers are employed internally. Some of this loss of flexibility can be compensated by designing each transducer to suit the intended application. This is normally a process of selecting an appropriate size, shape and direction for the field of view. Another approach is to have two phased arrays in the transducer assembly which scan in planes at 90° to each other. This makes quick switching between transverse and longitudinal sections easy (Fig. 1.6). Flexibility is further improved by enabling the transducer elements to be moved within the transducer assembly. For example, an oscillating transducer can be rotated through 180° about the central axis of the

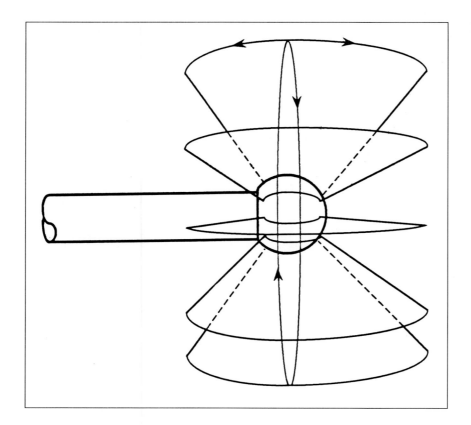

Figure 1.7 *Example of scan planes of an omniplane scanner.*

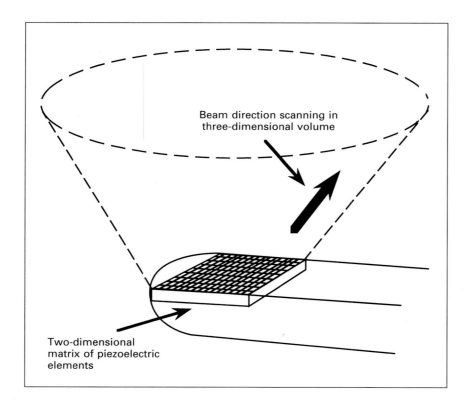

Beam direction scanning in three-dimensional volume

Two-dimensional matrix of piezoelectric elements

Figure 1.8 *Diagrammatic representation of an omniplane scanner based on a two-dimensional array of crystal elements.*

field of view to provide a succession of images from neighbouring scan planes (Fig. 1.7). This smooth alteration of the field of view to select the scan plane of most value is greatly appreciated. For example, in transoesophageal cardiac scanning the best image of a heart valve region can be selected first for B-scan imaging and then for colour Doppler imaging. Electronic sector scanners have also been developed in which a phased array transducer can be rotated through 180°. This reduces the amount of mechanical motion compared to rotating an oscillating single crystal, but there are still some difficulties to be solved with regard to the size of the whole assembly and the electrical connections to a large number of elements.

We noted earlier that a single line of piezoelectric elements, i.e. a one-dimensional phased array, can direct an ultrasound beam in different directions in the scan plane when the delays associated with excitation and reception at the elements are varied. If a two-dimensional array of elements (a matrix) is employed rather than a single line of elements, it is possible to direct the beam in different directions throughout a three-dimensional volume in front of the transducer (Fig. 1.8). The plane of scan can therefore be varied without moving the matrix array, allowing the operator to perform omniplane scanning. So far, only prototypes of omniplane matrix scanners have been reported. Techniques for constructing two-dimensional matrix arrays of elements are at an early stage of development; work continues to improve sensitivity.

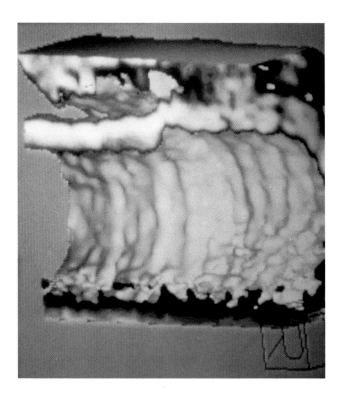

Figure 1.9 *One view of a three-dimensional ultrasonic image of an artery. (Courtesy of J. Gardener, London.)*

THREE-DIMENSIONAL SCANNER

We are very familiar with the idea that an ultrasonic beam can be swept through a two-dimensional plane and an image produced provided both the echo signals and the direction of the beam are continually stored. In a similar fashion, a beam can be swept through a three-dimensional volume and a three-dimensional image can be produced, provided the echo and beam information are stored. Two-dimensional images are readily displayed on a television screen; the display of three-dimensional images is more problematic and will be discussed later.

All of the transducer assembly technologies described above for invasive two-dimensional imaging can be used for three-dimensional imaging. It is only necessary to add a means of moving the two-dimensional scan plane through the three-dimensional volume. Indeed, multiplane transducers already perform this action. In the case of catheter

scanners, the third dimension in the scanning process is usually achieved by systematically moving the whole catheter along the blood vessel, although in theory only the elements within the catheter need be moved.

Once the echo information has been collected, it can be displayed on a television screen as a particular view of a three-dimensional structure (Fig. 1.9). It is usually also possible to rotate the three-dimensional image to assist the viewer in appreciating the shape of the structures presented. A three-dimensional image presented as a very large number of echoes can be difficult to interpret, since the external echoes may obscure the internal ones. Computer processing programs can be employed to peel off overlying echo layers or to smooth echo patterns to present more complete surfaces. However, the full presentation of a three-dimensional set of echo data is fundamentally difficult. Manufacturers often ease

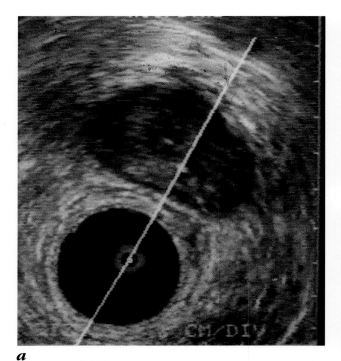

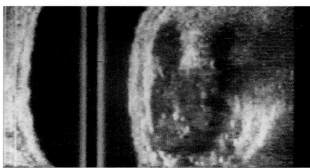

b

Figure 1.10 *Prostate scan using a transrectal scanner. (a) transverse image; (b) longitudinal image constructed from echo data gathered from consecutive transverse scans. (Courtesy of M. Halliwell, Bristol.)*

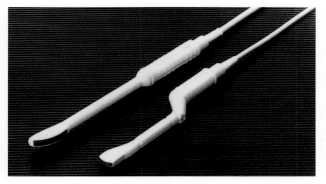

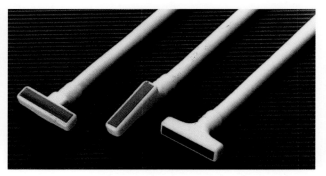

Figure 1.11 *Examples of intraoperative transducers. (Courtesy of Aloka.)*

access problems from gas and bone or from restricted transducer motion within the body (Fig. 1.10).

From our knowledge of real-time two-dimensional imaging, we know that it is just possible to gather a sufficient number of scan lines to produce 20–30 frames per second. At present, sufficient echo data cannot be acquired quickly enough to produce real-time three-dimensional images. Means are being sought to overcome this problem, e.g. by using a number of beams simultaneously in different directions into the body.[14]

INTRAOPERATIVE TRANSDUCERS

Transducers for use during surgery are similar to the devices described above.[15] Small linear or curved arrays are most commonly encountered but phased arrays and mechanical scanners are also used. They scan internal anatomy as they are passed over the

this problem by displaying a slab of echo information of limited thickness. Perhaps the most useful way of using three-dimensional scan data is to enable the operator to view an image of any plane through scanned volume.[13] Very many images are available with this type of facility, including those from planes which cannot be scanned directly due to ultrasound

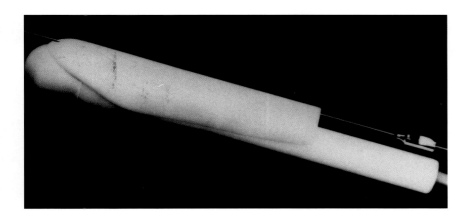

Figure 1.12 *Transvaginal transducer with biopsy needle attachment. (Courtesy of Philips.)*

surface of the structure or over one close to it. They are shaped to be easily held in the hand, perhaps by only two fingers or even by attachment to a single finger (Fig. 1.11). The transducers are watertight and smooth so that they can be easily cleaned.

Transducers for minimal invasive surgery also utilize the established technologies but are mounted on the end of a rod and have diameters up to 1 cm, which allows them to be passed through a small incision or laparoscopic port. Omnidirectional scanners could play an increasing role in this growing field. Selection of an appropriate technology often involves a choice between ultrasonic imaging and optical endoscopy.

COMBINATIONS OF TECHNIQUE

Invasive ultrasonic transducers can be combined with other medical instruments. The clinical value of most of these combinations is still being determined. Many manufacturers offer the combination of invasive probe and needle guidance attachment (Fig. 1.12). The latter finds widespread application, e.g. tumour cell biopsy, blood sampling, and chorion villus or follicle collection. This combination of devices can also be used in the reverse procedure of injecting liquid or contrast agents.[16]

Optical endoscopes and ultrasonic transducers have been combined to utilize the ability of the endoscopic methods to identify abnormal structures and tissue appearances and the ultrasonic methods to scan within the tissue of interest (Fig. 1.13). As minimal invasive surgery and therapy develop, we may see the use of invasive ultrasonic techniques with lasers for coagulating blood or vaporizing tissue and with optical (or acoustic) shock wave devices for disintegrating it.

There is strong interest in the combined use of angioplasty catheters and ultrasonic B–scanners, since this would allow immediate checks of the treatment of the diseased artery.[17] Doppler transducers could also be linked to angioplasty catheters. In the first instance this could be done with a simple continuous or pulsed wave device. As noted above in the discussion on catheters, forward-viewing Doppler imaging techniques are confronted with difficulties in manufacturing small scanning transducers and also aliasing problems in the measurement of high blood velocities.

STERILIZATION

Since transducers are fragile and expensive, the only practical sterilization techniques are immersion in a suitable liquid such as gluteraldehyde or exposure to ethylene oxide gas. Time delay may make this latter approach inconvenient. Autoclaving at high temperature guarantees sterility but damages both plastic materials and adhesive bonds. Aseptic procedures can be carried out by covering the transducer

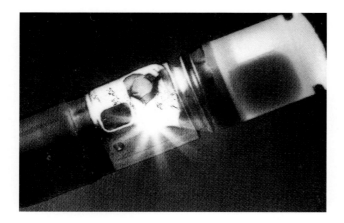

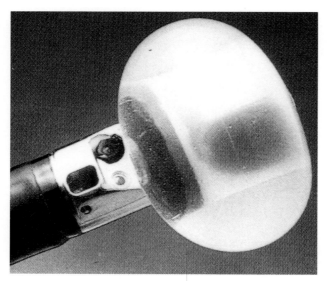

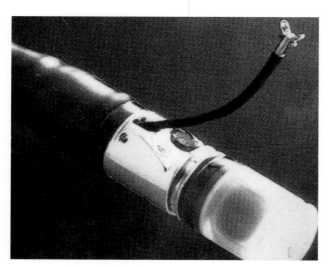

Figure 1.13 *Combination of rotating transducer scanner, optical endoscope and biopsy attachment. (Courtesy of Olympus.)*

assemblies with a thin rubber sheath or plastic bag. Provided that the coupling liquid excludes air both inside and outside the cover, the ultrasonic pulses will pass undistorted through the thin cover and liquid layers.

SAFETY

Considerations of safety from an ultrasonic exposure point of view are the same for invasive transducers as for externally applied ones.[18,19] Protection of sensitive structures, such as fetal ovaries, given by beam attenuation in overlying tissues is usually reduced in invasive techniques. The safety margins allowed for in safety recommendations do not depend on the attenuation of overlying layers. Regular safety statements are issued by organizations such as the European Federation for Ultrasound in Medicine and Biology and the American Institute for Ultrasound in Medicine. To date no confirmed harmful biological effects have been identified at ultrasonic intensity levels recommended for diagnostic use. When Doppler transducers are operated at a high pulse repetition rate, they have been observed on occasion to rise to temperatures in excess of 50°C. This is potentially harmful and the temperature of transducers should be checked.

Electrical instruments should always be tested for electrical safety. When several different instruments are connected to the patient, precautions such as checking that they have a common earth should be taken. Trained staff are available to most hospitals for electrical safety testing. Ultrasonic instruments present no special electrical safety problems, but any which might arise are particularly serious when the devices are used within the body. Catheter and transoesophageal systems need to be carefully tested by personnel with an accurate knowledge of the safety requirements.

Ultrasonic transducers are rarely checked for mechanical defects and there are no recommended methods for doing so. Perhaps the best practical approach is to carefully inspect the transducer prior to use, both visually and by listening. In this way structural integrity and the proper mode of operation will become well known. If planned preventative maintenance procedures are specified by the manufacturer they should obviously be adhered to.

REFERENCES

1. Fornage B, *Ultrasound of the Prostate* (Wiley: New York, 1988) 11–25.

2. Foster FS, Ryan LK, Lockwood GR, High frequency ultrasound scanning of the arterial wall. In: Roelandt, J. Gussenhoven EJ, Bom, N (eds.), *Intravascular Ultrasound* (Kluwer Academic Publishers: Dordrecht, 1993) 91–108.

3. McDicken WN, *Diagnostic Ultrasonics: Principles and Use of Instruments*, 3rd edn (Churchill Livingstone: Edinburgh, 1991) 79–86.

4. Papachrysostomou M, Pye SD, Wild SR, Smith AN, Anal endosonography: which probe? *Br J Radiol* (1992) **65**:715.

5. Hunt JW, Arditi M , Foster FS, Ultrasound transducers for pulse-echo medical imaging, *IEEE Trans Biomed Eng* (1983) **30**:453.

6. Silk MG, *Ultrasonic Transducers for Nondestructive Testing* (Adam Hilger: Bristol, 1984).

7. Gururaja TR, Schulze WA, Cross LE, Newnham RE, Piezoelectric composite materials for ultrasonic transducer applications. Part II: Evaluation of ultrasonic medical applications, *IEEE Trans Sonics Ultrason* (1985) **32**:566.

8. Angelsen BAJ, Dorum S, Hoem J, Brubakk AO, Skjaerpe T, Torp HG, Olstad B, Maehle J, Fehske W, Schipper K, Annular array multiplanar TEE probe allowing 3D reconstruction of cineloops of the heart. In: Hanrath P, Uebis R, Krebs W, eds, *Cardiovascular Imaging by Ultrasound* (Kluwer Academic Publishers; Dordrecht, 1993) 287–305.

9. Souquet J, Hanrath P, Zitelli L, Kremer R, Langenstein RA, Schluter M, Transesophageal phased array for imaging the heart, *IEEE Trans Biomed Eng* (1982) **29**:707.

10. Hoskins PR, McDicken WN, Techniques for the assessment of the imaging characteristics of intravascular ultrasound scanners, *Br J Radiol* (1994) **67**:695–700.

11. Bom N, ten Hoff H, Lancee CT, Gussenhoven WJ, Bosch JG, Early and recent intraluminal ultrasound devices, *Int J Card Imaging* (1989) **4**:79.

12. Pandian NG, Schwartz SL, Weintraub AR, Hsu TL, Konstam MA, Salem DN, Intracardiac echography: current developments, *Int J Card Imaging* (1991) **6**:207.

13. Halliwell M, Key H, Jenkins D, Jackson PC, Wells PNT, New scans from old: digital reformatting of ultrasound images, *Br J Radiol* (1989) **62**:824.

14. von Ramm OT, Smith SW, Pavy HG, High-speed ultrasound volumetric imaging systems. Parts I and II, *IEEE Trans, Ultrasons Ferroelect Freq Contr* (1991) **38**:100.

15. Sigel B, *Operative Ultrasonography*, 2nd edn (Raven Press: New York, 1988).

16. McDicken WN, Needle guidance techniques In: Wells PNT, ed., *Advances in Ultrasound Techniques and Instrumentation* (Churchill Livingstone: New York, 1993) Chapter 7.

17. Honye J, Mahon DJ, Jain A, White CJ, Ramee SR, Wallis JB, Al-Zarka A, Tobis JM, Morphological effects of coronary balloon angioplasty in vivo assessed by intravascular ultrasound imaging, *Circulation* (1992) **85**:1012.

18. AIUM, *The Bioeffects and Safety of Diagnostic Ultrasound* (American Institute of Ultrasound in Medicine: Rockville Maryland, 1993).

19. Docker MF, Duck FA (eds.) *The Safe Use of Diagnostic Ultrasound* (British Medical Ultrasound Society/British Institute of Radiology: London, 1991).

Chapter 2 **Transrectal Ultrasound**

David Rickards
Ian Kelly

IMAGING TECHNIQUES

There is no single probe configuration that can image the prostate in all planes; hence the variety of designs from different ultrasound manufacturers. For optimal diagnostic imaging, sections of the prostate need to be obtained in two planes, preferably true transverse axial and sagittal. For rectal guided biopsy, an end-viewing sagittal section is needed, whilst for perineal biopsy, imaging in the true sagittal plane is required. The decision as to which probe configuration is best suited to a particular unit depends upon the clinical requirement, what ultrasound machines are already in place and the cost involved. The options are as follows.

SINGLE PLANE PROBES

For complete imaging of the prostate, three probes will be needed. Linear array probes operating at 7 MHz and on 128 lines give sagittal images ideal for urethral and genital imaging as well as measurements of the length of the prostate, important in the insertion of permanent prostate stents and capable of guiding perineal biopsy. Curved array probes, again operating at 7 MHz and on 128 lines, but also capable of colour Doppler, give true transverse axial images and end-viewing images for rectal guided biopsy (Fig. 2.1). Although for complete imaging this option means

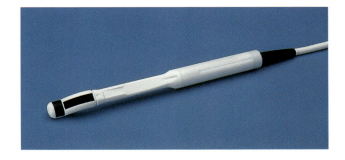

Figure 2.2 *Biplane probe. Two transducers set at right angles to each other will give true transverse axial and true sagittal images of the prostate. This probe cannot be used for rectal guided biopsy, but is ideal for perineal guided biopsy.*

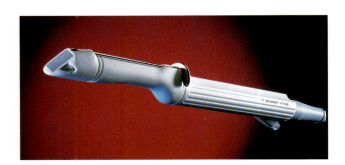

Figure 2.1 *Single-plane end-fire probe which will give elongated sagittal images of the prostate. The biopsy guide is in place.*

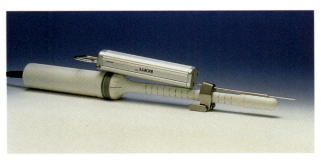

Figure 2.3 *Multiplane probe. A single transducer plane of scanning can be altered electronically. The biopsy guide, needle and triggering device are in place for rectal guided biopsy.*

changing probes within the rectum and is expensive, it does offer the best possible imaging and must be considered the preferred option.

Another option is the single-plane curved array probe that operates at 7 MHz on 128 lines and provides images in many planes by rotating the housing of the probe within the rectum. Such probes are ideal for rectal guided biopsy, but cannot be used for perineal biopsy easily. Images are obtained in the slightly forward-looking sagittal plane and not in the true transverse axial plane. If a unit can have only a single probe, this is the best configuration to obtain.

BIPLANE PROBES (FIG. 2.2)

Two transducers, one linear array and one curved array, set at right angles to each other are mounted on the same probe housing. This probe design is not ideal because the footprint of the linear array transducer will be short, and although it works at 7 MHz, the curved array probe works at 5 MHz. Images in the true transverse axial and true sagittal planes are obtained, but the probe cannot be used for rectal guided biopsy.

MULTIPLANE PROBES (FIG. 2.3)

Many designs are available, but the principle of them is that a single transducer is either mechanically or electronically orientated within a single probe housing to give images in any plane from the transverse axial to the sagittal. Such probes are capable of guiding both transrectal and perineal biopsy and work at 7 MHz or at varying frequencies from 5 to 7 MHz. They are not capable of colour Doppler imaging.

Irrespective of the probe used, the patient can be examined in either the lithotomy or the lateral decubitus position. The advantage of the decubitus position is that if a water bath is used, any air trapped within the bath will not degrade the image, whilst the lithotomy position demands that all air is carefully aspirated. The probes must be well lubricated and insertion should be preceded by the operator doing a digital rectal examination (DRE). This will tend to dilate the anal sphincter, making probe insertion easier, and will, of course, provide essential clinical information. Should faeces degrade the image, a low rectal wash-out has to be performed.

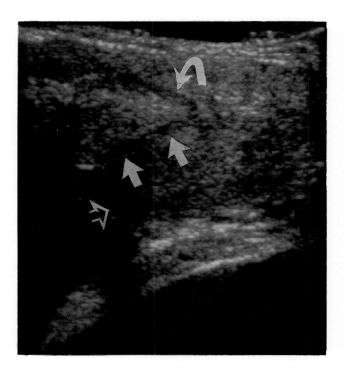

Figure 2.4 *Normal sagittal section of the prostate gland. The bladder neck appears slightly beaked and the urethra walls can be identified (arrows) as can one of the ejaculatory ducts (curved arrow). A small amount of anterior fibromuscular stroma is anterior to the urethra (open arrow).*

ANATOMY OF THE PROSTATE GLAND

Lowsley's[1] description of the prostate gland of five lobes has been replaced by McNeal's[2] concept of zonal anatomy. The prostate is divided into three areas, the transitional, central and peripheral zones. The transitional zone is not composed of prostatic tissue, but is fibromuscular stroma which is continuous with the prostatic capsule that extends laterally and posteriorly. The central zone includes the periurethral glandular tissue and extends from the base of the prostate at the bladder neck down to the level of the verumontanum (Fig. 2.4). The transitional part of the central zone of the gland is a small bilobed structure that lies either side of the urethra just superior to the verumontanum. The peripheral zone of the prostate is composed of

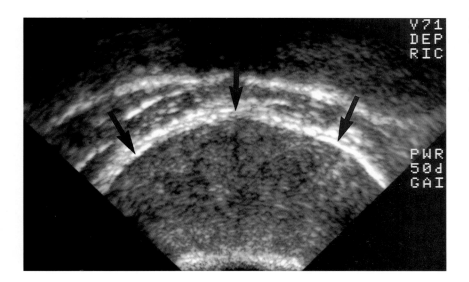

Figure 2.5 *Normal transverse axial section of the mid-prostatic area in a 25 year old. The entire gland is homogeneous as it comprises peripheral zone only at this level. The capsule of the gland (arrows) is the interface between the prostate and the periprostatic fat and is not the true capsule of the gland.*

acinar tissue and accounts for 75 per cent of the volume of the normal prostate in young males (Fig. 2.5). It extends posteriorly and laterally.

Benign prostatic hypertrophy (BPH) originates in the central part of the gland, whereas most cancers develop in the peripheral zone. None of these zones can be differentiated from each other by computed tomography (CT), but transrectal ultrasound (TRUS) and magnetic resonance imaging (MRI) can differentiate them. TRUS clearly defines the peripheral zone of the gland from the rest of the gland. The peripheral zone appears as a homogeneous, echogenic structure in which the ejaculatory ducts can be seen as echo-poor structures. The capsule of the gland cannot be imaged, but the ultrasound boundaries of the prostate are formed by periprostatic fat which forms a brightly echogenic interface. The neurovascular bundles enter the prostate laterally and can produce an echo-poor area within the peripheral zones that can mimic the TRUS appearances of cancer. Between the peripheral zone and the rest of the gland run ducts within which calcification of proteinaceous material can occur (Fig. 2.6). This forms the corpora amylacea and was considered to form the capsule of the gland by early endoscopists, who resected down to this calcification in the false belief that they had then resected the entire prostate gland. When prominent, such calcification can make imaging structures anterior to it impossible. Normal

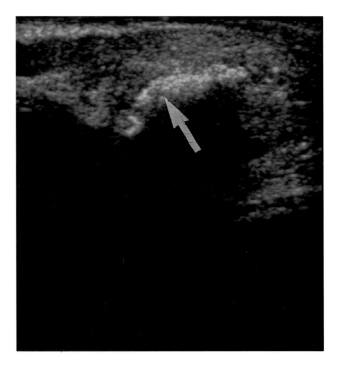

Figure 2.6 *Sagittal section of the prostate in which there is a heavy deposition of corpora amylacea (arrow) which attenuates the ultrasound beam to such an extent that the central and transitional parts of the gland cannot be imaged.*

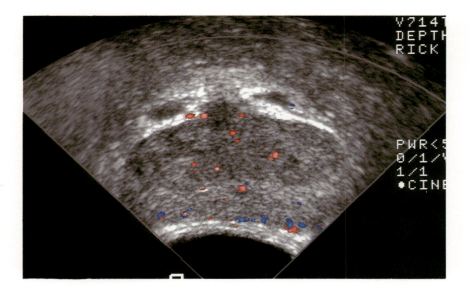

Figure 2.7 *Tranverse axial colour Doppler section of the normal prostate in a 27 year old. There is a little flow seen within the prostate.*

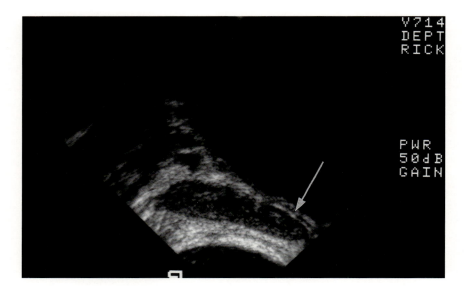

Figure 2.8 *Transverse axial section of a normal right seminal vesicle. The vas deferens can be seen between the seminal vesicle and the posterior aspect of the bladder (arrow).*

colour Doppler imaging (CDI) of the prostate shows flow in capsular vessels with virtually no flow within the prostate itself (Fig. 2.7). Doppler settings must be at the lowest flow rates for maximum sensitivity.

The urethra is best seen in the sagittal plane and appears as an echogenic line coursing through the prostate from bladder neck to distal sphincter. The normal bladder neck is usually surrounded by a small echo-poor area which anteriorly is the anterior fibro-muscular stroma, but posteriorly represents the muscle of the bladder neck mechanism, a sphincter of genital importance rather than a sphincter of urinary continence. A normal bladder neck is needed for antegrade ejaculation.

The ejaculatory ducts are imaged with linear array probes in the sagittal plane. They are seen running from the medial aspects of both seminal vesicles on a curved course to enter the urethra just at the verumontanum. The normal seminal vesicles tend to be the same size and appear either as homogeneous structures of middle-range echogenicity or with echo-free areas within them (Fig. 2.8).

Table 2.1 Methods of obtaining prostate tissue.

Technique	Zone of prostate biopsied
Transurethral resection	Central and transitional zones
Retropubic prostatectomy	Central and transitional zones
Total prostatectomy	All zones
During cystoscopy	Central and transitional zones
Digital guided rectal biopsy	Mainly peripheral zone
Ultrasound guided perineal biopsy	All zones
Ultrasound guided rectal biopsy	All zones

PROSTATE BIOPSY

Prostate tissue for histological analysis can be obtained by many different routes (Table 2.1).

Tissue obtained during transurethral resection (TURP), retropubic prostatectomy and cystoscopy will derive mainly from the central and transitional zones of the prostate. These methods are not site-specific and ignore the peripheral zone of the gland where most tumours originate. Digital guided biopsy can be performed either perineally or transrectally while the examining finger delineates the area of abnormality. The success of such a biopsy is very operator dependent; even in experienced hands, small lesions will be missed, and the technique ignores lesions that are not palpable. Ultrasound guided puncture is now the technique of choice and can be performed either perineally or transrectally. Guidance with other imaging techniques is not in wide use. CT cannot identify specific intraprostatic lesions and is of no value. MRI can define intraprostatic lesions, and with the advent of interventional MRI units, biopsy guidance becomes a possibility.

INDICATIONS FOR PROSTATE BIOPSY

Prostate tissue is most commonly needed to prove the diagnosis of cancer, but benign lesions also need to be confirmed in a small number of cases, and tissue is often required to substantiate the diagnosis of inflammatory disease or to obtain tissue for culture.

Biopsy for Prostate Cancer

There are well-defined indications for biopsy in prostate cancer and some rather ill-defined ones:

- Palpable lesion on DRE.
- Abnormal prostate-specific antigen (PSA).
- Abnormal area on TRUS.
- In the follow-up after treatment for prostate cancer.

The decision as to whether to biopsy or not depends upon the findings at clinical examination, the level of PSA the findings on TRUS and the knowledge of what treatment the patient may have had to the prostate gland. Biopsy by radiologist or urologist without such information is likely to be less effective.

Palpable lesion
The finding on DRE of an indurated area in the posterior aspect of the prostate gland associated with a nodule is likely to represent malignancy. Irrespective of what is found on TRUS or what the level of PSA is, the area in which the palpable abnormality was felt needs to be biopsied under TRUS control. Benign lesions can mimic such changes and these include inflammatory disease, calculi, areas of BPH and malakoplakia. Clearly, where doubt exists as to the nature of the lesions, a biopsy is necessary, but where TRUS shows an undeniably benign lesion, i.e. calculus, and the PSA is within normal limits, biopsy can be postponed.

Where the indication for biopsy is a palpable lesion, other areas within the gland should be biopsied at the same time.

Table 2.2 Indications for prostate biopsy – PSA levels.

Level of PSA (ng/ml)	Findings on DRE	Findings on TRUS	Biopsy
Below 4	Normal	Normal	No biopsy
Below 4	Positive	Normal	Biopsy
Below 4	Normal	Positive	Follow-up
4–6	Normal	Normal	No biopsy
4–6	Positive	Normal	Biopsy
4–6	Normal	Positive	Follow-up
Above 6	Normal	Normal	Biopsy
Above 6	Normal	Positive	Biopsy
Above 6	Positive	Normal	Biopsy

Abnormal prostate-specific antigen

PSA was first identified by Papsidero.[3] It is a glyco-protein with a molecular weight of 33 000 and origi-nates in the cytoplasm of the prostate epithelial cells. The levels of PSA that suggest malignancy depend upon the method of assay. Commercial packs are available; levels above 6 ng/ml obtained by using the Hybritech (Tandem-R PSA) are highly suspicious and demand biopsy (Table 2.2). Table 2.2 is an oversim-plification of prostate cancer and the need for biopsy, but forms a basis upon which to make decisions.

Approximately 20 per cent of early cancers have a PSA <4 ng/ml,[4] and, providing the DRE and TRUS are within normal limits, no biopsy and no further action is required.[5] Values of PSA between 4 and 6 ng/ml are to be regarded as suspicious for malig-nancy, because mildly raised levels can be expected with increasing age and BPH and attempts have been made to correct levels of PSA depending upon prostate volume.[6] Where there is no suspicion of malignancy on DRE or TRUS, such patients can be followed up in 6 months' time. Where PSA values are >6 ng/ml, 70 per cent of patients will have prostate cancer and biopsy must be performed.[7] Whether the decision to biopsy should be based on the PSA alone is open to question. It is a simple, noninvasive test that is independent of operator error, unlike DRE or TRUS. However, it must be borne in mind that a single focus of prostate cancer is a common pathological finding and patients are more likely to die with their prostate cancer than because of it.[8]

Abnormal area on TRUS

The appearances of prostate cancer on TRUS are well described, but the classic echo-poor lesion in the peripheral zone of the gland has only a 20 per cent chance of being malignant.[9] To biopsy on the TRUS appearances alone with no rise in PSA levels or no suspicion of malignancy on DRE is not indicated.

Follow-up of prostate cancer

Where prostate cancer has been treated by non-surgical means, i.e. with radiotherapy, hormone manipulation or chemotherapy, biopsy is often indicated to assess whether treatment has been effective or whether there is recurrent disease. Rising PSA levels may also indicate such problems. TRUS is inaccurate, especially in the gland treated with radio-therapy.

Indications for Prostate Biopsy in Benign Disease

There are few indications for prostate biopsy in benign disease:

- To obtain tissue for cytology and bacteriology in patients with clinical prostatic inflammatory disease.
- To confirm a suspected abnormality as benign, e.g. malakoplakia.

Neither of these indications is often invoked as a need for biopsy, but where prostatitis has been particularly resistant to antibiotic therapy, it may be indicated to get tissue from all zones of the prostate for culture so that the appropriate antibiotic might be prescribed. Such biopsies should be performed transperineally to reduce the potential to infect a potentially sterile field.

TECHNIQUE OF PROSTATE BIOPSY

Two routes are possible, transrectal and transperineal. The route chosen depends upon the indication for biopsy and the equipment available. As described above, not all probes allow for transrectal guided biopsy, the current method of choice.[10] Core biopsy or aspiration cytology can be performed, or both.

Core Biopsy

Many commercially available needles are in production. Pre-packed, one-time needles complete with their own triggering devices are available. The choice of needle is a personal one, but for diagnostic work, 18 gauge should be selected. Reusable triggering devices (Biopty) are quite heavy to hold, but are powerful, an important consideration when going through perineal skin, intervening soft tissues and the prostate itself, which if infiltrated with cancer can be hard. Most triggering devices have a 2-cm throw.

Aspiration Cytology

This is obtained by inserting into a suspicious lesion a 22–23 gauge needle and, whilst applying suction, oscillating the needle within the lesion and aspirating cells. Such a biopsy may provide only a few cells, which makes the histologist's task more difficult and grading of prostate cancer is often not possible. The complications of both types of biopsy are the same. Core biopsy is the method of choice.

Perineal Biopsy (Fig. 2.9)

Perineal biopsy is performed under sagittal TRUS control using a linear array probe. This can be performed free-hand or by using a biopsy guide attached to the TRUS probe. Free-hand guidance is recommended, as with experience all parts of the

prostate can be biopsied through the same skin entry site, which is not possible if a fixed guide is used. The steps involved are as follows:

1. The patient is placed in the left lateral position and a diagnostic TRUS is performed.
2. The perineum anterior to the probe is prepared with an antiseptic solution, e.g. Betadine.
3. Using a 22 gauge spinal needle which is 10 cm in length, the skin 3 cm directly anterior to the probe and exactly in the midline is punctured and infiltrated with 2 per cent lignocaine. Under continuous sagittal TRUS control, the needle is then advanced whilst scanning down to the prostatic capsule, being careful not to infiltrate within the prostate itself. Once the needle is at the capsule of the gland, the rest of the anaesthetic is injected (usually about 10 ml). The anaesthetic will be seen to disperse around the capsule of the gland. There is no need to withdraw the needle and redirect it laterally in order to anaesthetize those areas the needle will pass through for biopsy of the lateral aspects of the peripheral lobes of the gland. No more than 15 ml of lignocaine should be used, to guard against lignocaine intoxication. Care must be taken that no air is injected, as this will degrade further imaging. The needle is withdrawn, but not removed, so that it marks the exact entry site of anaesthetic. Once the anaesthetic is given, the operator should allow 5 min for it to take effect. This time can usefully be employed by filling in pathology forms etc.
4. The biopsy needle already deployed within its triggering device is inserted adjacent to the spinal needle. A small incision with a blade to facilitate this is not recommended, as perineal wounds tend to bleed a lot. The biopsy needle can always be pushed through the skin without pain as long as the anaesthetic has had sufficient time to take effect. Under TRUS control, the needle is then advanced into the area that is to be biopsied. Should a lesion be in the lateral aspects of the peripheral zone of the prostate, this is imaged by rotating the probe within the rectum and directing the needle to either side of the midline. To biopsy any part of the central part of the gland, the needle is directed more anteriorly. It is important to avoid the urethra, as failure to do this will inevitably result in post-biopsy haematuria.
5. Once all the biopsies have been taken, the biopsy and infiltration needle are removed and the perineum wiped clean.

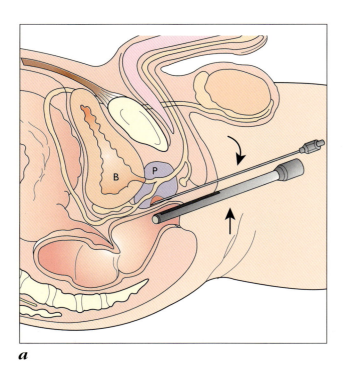

a

Figure 2.9 *(a) Diagram showing how a perineal biopsy is performed. The linear array transducer within the rectum continuously monitors the position of both local anaesthetic and biopsy needle down to a lesion within the prostate. (P, prostate; B, bladder). (b) Sagittal section of the prostate gland showing an echo-poor lesion (arrow) in the peripheral zone in a gland considerably enlarged by benign BPH. (c) Under continuous TRUS control, a 22 gauge needle is directed down to the apex of the prostate (arrow) and local anaesthetic instilled around the prostate. (d) The biopsy needle is directed down to the apex of the gland. (e) The biopsy triggering device is fired and the needle can be seen to pass directly through the echo-poor lesion (arrows), but not going into the anterior rectal wall.*

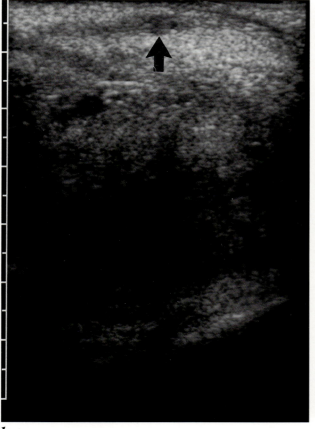

b

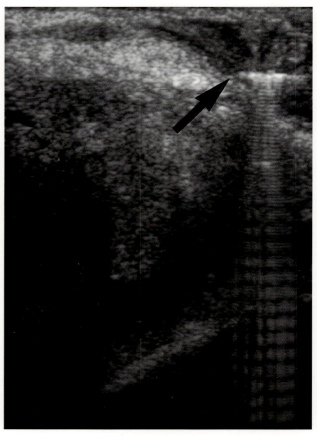

c

Transrectal Guided Biopsy (Fig. 2.10)

The development of end-fire transducers allows for biopsies of the prostate to be taken through the anterior rectal wall. This approach has become the preferred method. The steps involved are as follows:

1. Once a decision has been made to biopsy, intravenous antibiotics are given, e.g. gentamicin 80 mg and amoxicillin 500 mg.
2. If the rectum is obviously loaded with faeces, evident on DRE before the probe is inserted, a cleansing enema should be performed. In practice, this is rarely required.
3. The guide is attached to the biopsy probe and the probe is inserted into the rectum. Most guides come in the form of a hollow stainless steel tube down which the biopsy needle passes. Once used, they must be cleaned and resterilized using a gas autoclave. To attempt to sterilize such guides in sterilizing fluids is useless.
4. On all commercially available machines, a biopsy guide line can be displayed on the screen. Once this line passes through the part of the prostate to be biopsied, the biopsy needle is inserted through the guide and pushed under TRUS control through the anterior rectal wall. This will ensure that a biopsy of the anterior rectal wall is not taken. The triggering device is then used to take a 2 cm core

Figure 2.9 *(continued)*

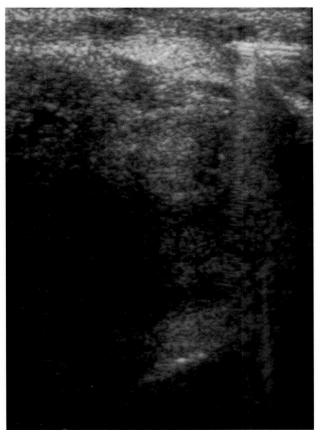

d

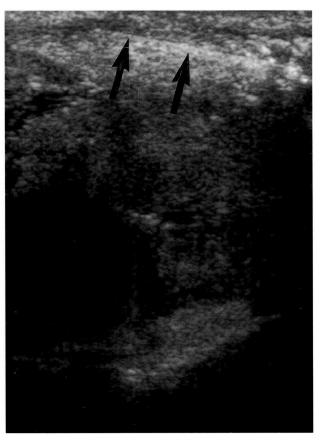

e

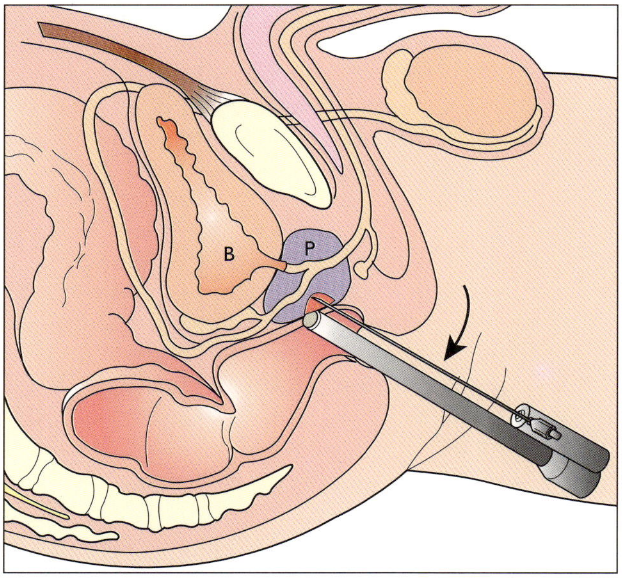

a

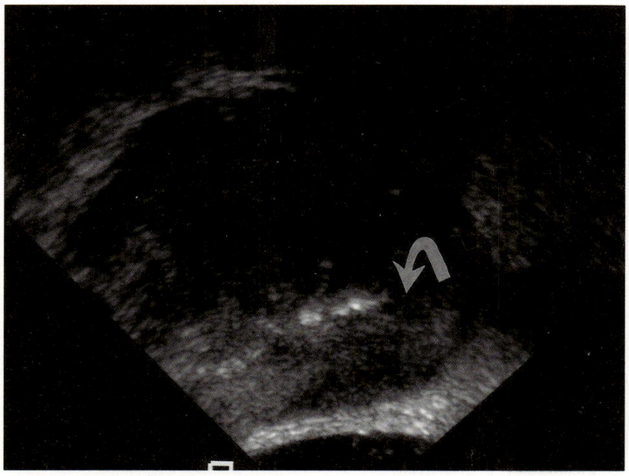

Figure 2.10 *(a) Diagram showing the technique of rectal guided biopsy. The probe within the rectum visualizes the lesion under suspicion whilst the biopsy needle within its triggering device (arrow) is passed down a guide, through the rectal wall; the biopsy is then taken. P, prostate. (b) Transverse axial section of the prostate in which there is a poorly demarcated echo-poor lesion in the left peripheral zone (arrow). (c) The lesion is imaged using an end-fire probe for rectal biopsy and the biopsy line is directed through the lesion. (d) The biopsy needle is pushed through the rectal wall (arrow) before the biopsy is taken. (e) The triggering device is fired and the needle can be seen to pass through the echo-poor lesion.*

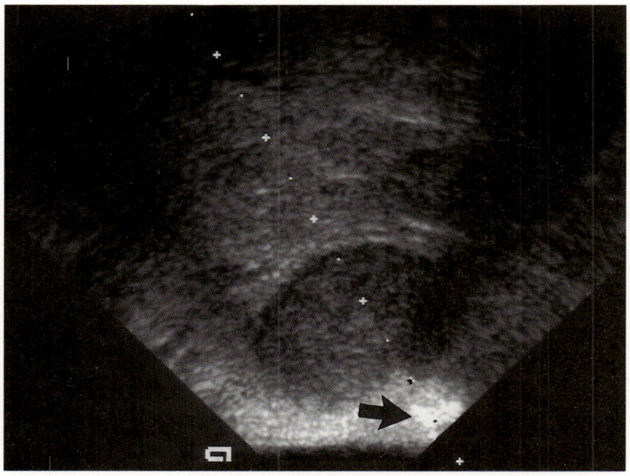

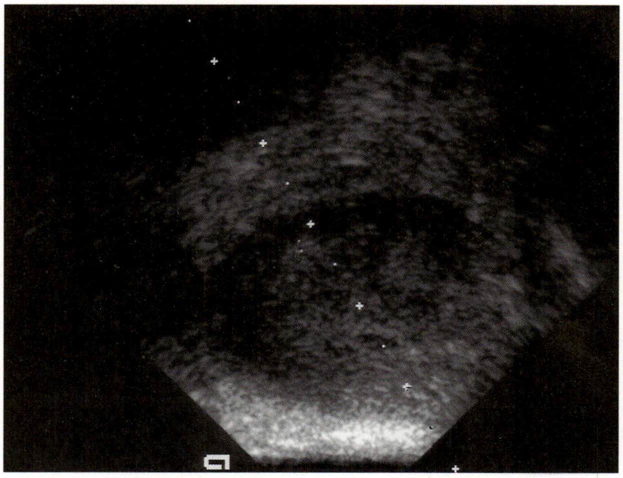

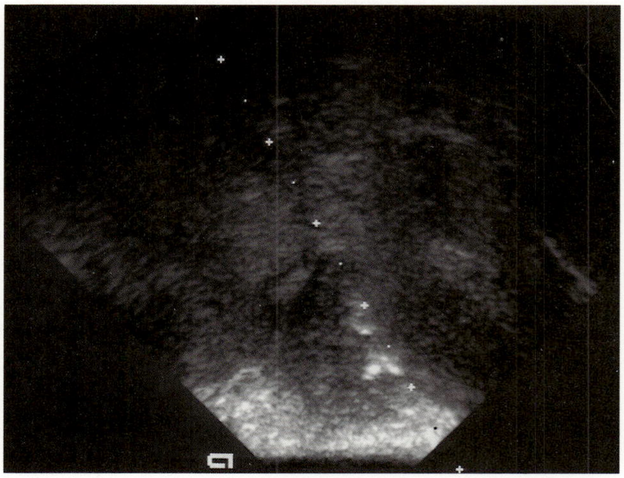

b

d

c

e

through the suspicious lesion. In many circumstances, in order to avoid taking a biopsy of the rectal wall, a 2-cm throw will enter the bladder. This will increase the chances of post-procedure haematuria. The patient needs to be warned that there will be some pain when the needle is about to enter the rectal wall and just before the biopsy is taken.

5. Once all the required biopsies have been taken, the probe is removed and a 500 mg Flagyl suppository inserted with a request to the patient to try and retain it for at least 1 h. Broad-spectrum antibiotics should be prescribed for 3 days following biopsy and the patient requested to drink plenty of fluids.

COMPLICATIONS OF PROSTATE BIOPSY

Post-biopsy sepsis is the most important potential complication following biopsy and one death has been reported.[11] Other complications are not serious (Table 2.3), but the patient needs to be warned.[12,13,14]

Table 2.3 Complications of TRUS guided prostate biopsy.

Complication	Transrectal (%)	Perineal (%)
Haematuria	58	2
Haemospermia	28	5
Rectal bleeding	37	1
Pyrexia	3	0.2
Pain/discomfort	20	10
Alteration in urine flow	7	3

It is prudent to supply the patient with a post-biopsy information sheet which advises of potential complications, stressing the potential implications of developing a temperature or dysuria. Rectal guided biopsy is associated with considerably more complications than perineal biopsy.

COMPARISON BETWEEN TRANSRECTAL AND PERINEAL BIOPSY TECHNIQUES (TABLE 2.4)

Both techniques are equally accurate in providing localization, but the transrectal route is associated

Table 2.4 Comparison between the transrectal and perineal approach for prostate biopsy.

Transrectal	Perineal
No anaesthesia	Local anaesthesia
Antibiotics	No antibiotics
Accurate biopsy	Accurate biopsy
Complications common	Complications uncommon
Should not be used for benign disease	Indicated in benign disease
Very short needle path	Long needle path

with more complications. The time taken to perform biopsies by either route is about the same and, as long as adequate anaesthesia has been given, the degree of discomfort experienced by the patient is about the same.

The incidence of complications will increase with the number of biopsies taken. If six or more are taken, 90 per cent of patients can expect minor rectal and urethral bleeding which will be persistent in up to 12 per cent.[15]

MEASUREMENT OF PROSTATE VOLUME

Labour-intensive planimetry is no more accurate than the more expedient elliptical methods. However, a simple variation of this, reflecting the non-elliptical shape of the prostate, the prolate-spheroid formula, is even more accurate over a wide volume range.[16,17,18]

Four basic methods are available. The step planimetry method calculates the volume of the gland by taking sequential transverse axial scans from the base of the prostate to the apex at specific intervals and summating these areas.[19] This is the most accurate method, but is time-consuming.[17,18] The prolate ellipsoid method uses the formula for the volume of an ellipsoid, and the last method is the machine-calculated volume derived from the maximum horizontal area of the gland outline planimetrically. All commercially available machines that can scan in two planes at right angles to each other have volume measurement packages already installed.

BENIGN PROSTATIC HYPERPLASIA

EPIDEMIOLOGY

BPH is the commonest pathological condition to affect elderly males and, after cataract extraction, prostatectomy is the second most frequent operation performed world-wide on males over the age of 60 years. Autopsy studies have shown that BPH begins to develop in males at about 40 years of age, commencing as small foci within the central zone, and is found with increasing frequency in older men to such an extent that BPH exists in the prostate in all men over the age of 90 years. The development of histological BPH does not necessarily imply that it is a clinically significant problem. It is well known that the size of the prostate does not correlate with the degree of obstruction that it might cause to the prostatic urethra. A minority of men consult their general practitioners about symptoms due to BPH, and many consider such symptoms to be a normal part of the ageing process.

The majority of the epidemiological studies of BPH have been performed within developed countries. It is difficult to estimate the prevalence of BPH in developing countries, since the life expectancy is short and large-scale investigation is not usually feasible in elderly males. It is now accepted that BPH is most common in black men and least common in men originating from south-east Asia, particularly Japan and China. Such data suggest that there might be a genetic predisposition to the development of BPH, but it is of note that Japanese men migrating to California acquire a higher rate of BPH than their counterparts remaining in Japan, which suggests an environmental factor. BPH does not develop in males castrated before puberty which implies that testicular androgens are a dominant factor in the pathogenesis of BPH, but no direct correlation has yet been proved. BPH is a gradually progressive disease that initially presents with mild symptoms of bladder outflow obstruction, and following gradual enlargement of the prostate leads to an incremental increase in both symptoms and objective measurements of outflow obstruction. BPH develops within the transition zone, and the relative increase in stroma and epithelial elements may vary between individuals. In some cases the hyperplasia may be predominantly stromal in nature to produce a more fibromuscular gland, whilst in others there may be a predominantly glandular/epithelial proliferation.

There are a number of similarities between BPH and prostate cancer. They display a parallel increase in prevalence with age, although prostate cancer lags behind BPH by 15–20 years. Both conditions are androgen-dependent, and about 83 per cent of prostate cancers develop in men with BPH. Unlike BPH, which usually arises in the transition zone, most prostate cancers arise from the peripheral zone.

SYMPTOMS

The symptoms of BPH can be divided into irritative and obstructive (Table 2.5). The onset of symptoms is gradual and the condition affects the older population, many of whom are poor historians. Objective assessment of outflow obstruction must always be performed, but scoring systems are now popular and attempt to provide an unbiased and reproducible evaluation of each patient's symptomatology. The American Urology Association has produced such a

Table 2.5 Symptoms due to benign prostatic hyperplasia.

Obstructive symptoms	Irritative symptoms
Poor urinary stream	Urgency
Long voiding time	Nocturia
Frequency	Urge incontinence
Hesitancy	
Retention of urine	
Post-micturition dribble	
Abdominal straining	

Table 2.6 Complications of benign prostatic hypertrophy.

Functional complications	Anatomical complications
Urinary tract infections	Bladder wall hypertrophy
Detrusor instability	Hydronephrosis
Detrusor failure	Haematuria
Urinary stasis	Bladder diverticula
Detrusor decompensation	

presence of bladder neck obstruction where the prostate becomes trapped.

TRUS APPEARANCES OF THE PROSTATE FOLLOWING SURGERY

The traditional surgical treatment by TURP for BPH is being challenged by less invasive treatments and ones that preserve the bladder neck and sexual function, as follows:

- Temporary prostate stents.
- Permanent prostate stents.
- Hyperthermia.
- Cryotherapy.
- Laser prostatectomy.
- Drug treatment.
- Balloon dilatation.

TRUS Appearances Following TURP

At TURP, the bladder neck and varying amounts of the central and transitional zones of the prostate are removed down towards the apex of the prostate gland, but not involving the distal sphincter mechanism. TRUS following TURP will show the cavity produced by surgery, but failure to see a cavity does not necessarily imply the absence of one (Fig. 2.15). To accurately assess the size of the cavity, the patient should have a full bladder and be asked to pass urine or strain in the attempt to do so whilst the prostate is continuously scanned. The full extent of the cavity will then be seen. Recurrent or persistent obstructive symptoms following TURP may have many causes (Table 2.7).

Postoperative strictures of the bladder neck will appear as a mid-prostatic cavity and a closed bladder neck (Fig. 2.16). Recurrent adenomas encroaching upon the operative cavity have similar appearances to preoperative benign tumours, and for a carcinoma to obstruct a cavity, it would have to be very extensive and would be obvious clinically.

Obstruction to the ejaculatory ducts is commonly seen following TURP and can cause perineal pain due to seminal vesiculitis. Dilatation of the ducts will be seen on TRUS (Fig. 2.17). Postoperative haematuria is often caused by prominent vessels lining the TURP cavity. These will be identified on CDI (Fig. 2.18).

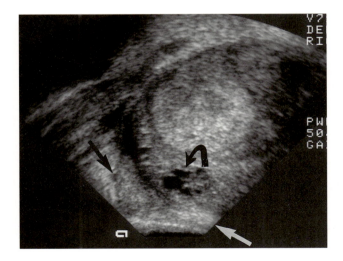

Figure 2.13 *Transverse axial section of the right lateral aspect of a large BPH. The peripheral zone (arrow) is compressed by adenomas of mixed echogenicity in which some cystic degeneration is seen (curved arrow).*

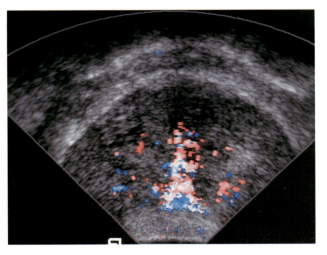

Figure 2.14 *Transverse axial colour Doppler scan of BPH. Considerably increased blood flow is seen with the central part of the gland, with no flow in the peripheral zones.*

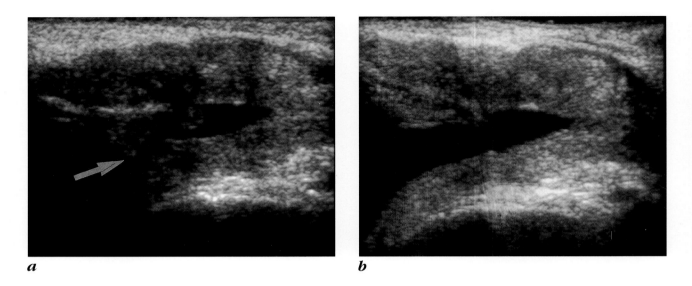

a   b

Figure 2.15 *(a) Following TURP of the prostate, the patient has symptoms of recurrent outflow obstruction. Sagittal TRUS suggests that there is recurrent growth obliterating the TURP cavity at the bladder neck (arrow). (b) The patient is asked to strain, and with the increase in total bladder pressure the bladder neck opens up normally to reveal a good TURP cavity.*

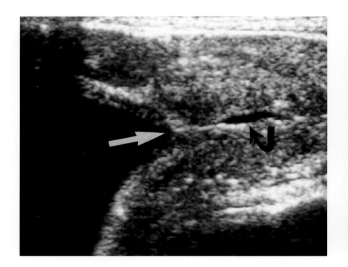

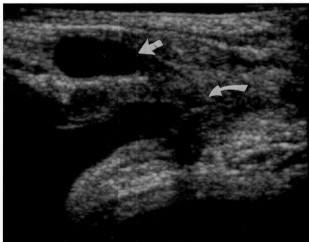

Figure 2.16 *Sagittal section of the prostate gland following TURP. There is a stricture at the bladder neck (arrow) and a residual mid-prostatic TURP cavity (curved arrow). This required further surgery.*

Figure 2.17 *Sagittal section of the prostate gland showing a good TURP cavity and obstruction to an ejaculatory duct (arrow) due to fibrosis at its opening (curved arrow) as a result of surgery.*

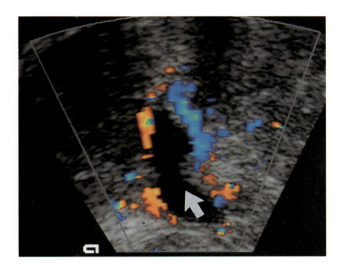

Figure 2.18 *Transverse axial colour Doppler TRUS in a patient with haematuria following TURP. The TURP cavity is well seen (arrow), as are very prominent blood vessels lining the TURP cavity which on cystoscopy were identified to be the cause of the haematuria.*

Table 2.7 Causes of persistent or recurrent obstructive symptoms following transurethral resection of the prostate gland.

Problem	TRUS appearances
Inadequate resection	Small or no TURP cavity
Recurrent hyperplasia	Adenoma attenuating a TURP cavity
Stricture of the bladder neck	Normal mid-prostatic TURP cavity
	Closed bladder neck
Bladder failure	Normal TURP cavity
Urethral or sphincter stricture	Normal TURP cavity
Development of prostate cancer	Echo-poor mass attenuating a TURP cavity

TRUS Appearances Following Stent Insertion

Temporary stents have a closely woven mesh that attenuates the ultrasound beam to such an extent that it is not possible to image the intrastent lumen or the relationship of the stent to the bladder neck; not that it is important to do so, as the stents extend into the bladder by design. This is best done by urethrography. The positions of permanent stents are clearly defined by TRUS. For accurate scanning, the bladder needs to be partially full. This will allow for very accurate depiction of the relationship of the stent to the bladder neck. The position of the distal end of the stent and its relationship to the distal sphincter and apical prostatic tissue are then assessed. Postoperative incontinence may be due to pre-existing instability, as a result of instrumentation or compromise of distal sphincter function because the stent is partly or wholly covering it. TRUS will help to differentiate between poor positioning and a functional abnormality.[22,23]

In the first few months following insertion, permanent stents invoke a hyperplastic reaction, but this settles within 6 months to leave a smooth urothelial covering of the stent (Fig. 2.19). The extent and uniformity of urothelium can be assessed by TRUS. Usually, the stent is covered by a uniform thickness of urothelium 1–2 mm in thickness, leaving an adequate intrastent lumen. Occasionally, focal areas of overgrowth are seen. CDI in the transverse axial or forward-looking sagittal planes allows for definition of the vascularity of the neurothelium (Fig. 2.20).[24]

Misplacement of the stent at the bladder neck with free wires which are not in contact with urothelium results in the wires becoming encrusted. TRUS will demonstrate such free wires and show if small stones are forming on them. Perineal pain following stent insertion may be due to the development of prostatic inflammatory disease, prostate abscess or blockage to the prostatic and ejaculatory ducts. TRUS will differentiate between these entities and point the clinician to the appropriate therapeutic course. Prolonged haematuria following stent insertion may be caused by prominent vessels supplying the urothelial covering. TRUS combined with CDI will demonstrate such vessels.

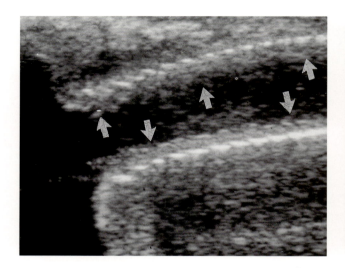

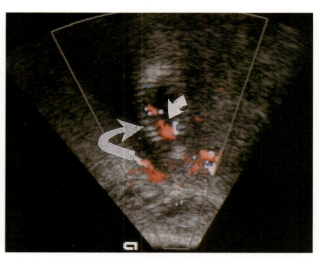

Figure 2.19 *Sagittal section of the prostate following the insertion of a permanent metal stent (Wallstent) into the posterior urethra for the relief of outflow obstruction due to BPH. The stent is perfectly situated at the bladder neck and there is a uniform amount of epithelium covering the stent (arrows).*

Figure 2.20 *End-fire sagittal colour Doppler section of the prostate in a patient with a Wallstent and heavy haematuria. CDI shows prominent vessels lying within the stent (arrows).*

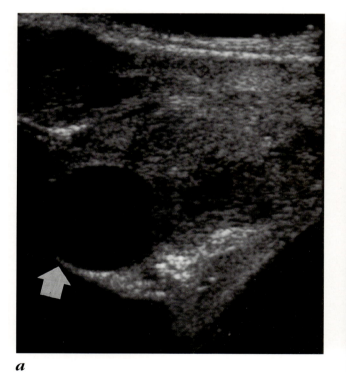

a

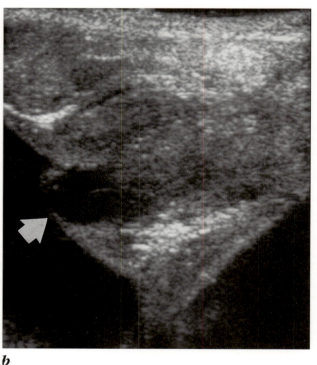

b

Figure 2.21 *(a) Sagittal TRUS in a patient with signs and symptoms of severe outflow obstruction and maximum urinary flow rates of 7 ml/s. There is a large cystic lesion lying just anterior to the bladder neck (arrow). (b) The cyst was aspirated under TRUS control with a 22 gauge needle using the perineal approach. The cyst has been almost aspirated to completion (arrow). Immediate post-aspiration urinary flow rates were 29 ml/s. The cyst required surgical removal at cystoscopy.*

OTHER CAUSES OF BLADDER OUTFLOW OBSTRUCTION WITH SPECIFIC ULTRASOUND APPEARANCES

Prostate Cysts

Cysts at the bladder neck can obstruct the outflow tract and can herniate down the posterior urethra during micturition. They appear as thin-walled transonic lesions in the midline of varying sizes (Fig. 2.21). These lesions can be multiple. To prove they are the cause of micturition difficulties, the cysts should be punctured under TRUS control using the perineal route and repeat uroflowmetry performed. Such cysts are likely to recur and require operative ablation.

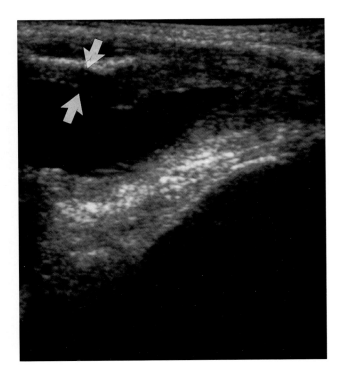

Figure 2.22 *Sagittal TRUS in a patient with detrusor sphincter dyssynergia. The prostate is small, but the bladder neck is wide open. Note the hypertrophied bladder wall (arrows).*

Detrusor Sphincter Dyssynergia

Detrusor sphincter dyssynergia has many neurological causes, e.g. multiple sclerosis and neuropathic bladder, and causes the bladder neck to become incompetent due to permanently high pressures within the bladder. The TRUS appearances are characteristic, with a wide-open bladder neck and dilatation of the posterior urethra down to the distal sphincter mechanism in a prostate that appears otherwise normal (Fig. 2.22).

Prostate Cancer

Prostate carcinoma can originate in the periurethral tissue of the prostate, but is usually associated with BPH and rarely causes obstruction on its own.

Bladder Neck Obstruction

Bladder neck obstruction is a common cause of outflow obstruction in young men, many of whom do not seek medical help because they either are not aware they have a problem or have historically been referred to as having a 'weak bladder'. Many of these men only come to medical attention when the underlying bladder neck obstruction is augmented by increasing benign hyperplasia, which has an accelerating effect upon the degree of obstruction. The definitive diagnosis depends upon the demonstration of trapping of contrast between the bladder neck and distal sphincter on interruption of micturition. This occurs because the little residual urine left in the posterior urethra when micturition is interrupted by closure of the distal sphincter mechanism cannot get back into the bladder past the obstructing bladder neck. The resultant rise in pressure within the posterior urethra can give rise to intraprostatic reflux and a chemical prostatitis.

TRUS in these patients characteristically shows a large echo-poor lesion around the proximal posterior urethra, this echo-poor area often extending down through the prostate (Fig. 2.23a). The prostate is usually of normal size, unless there is coexistent BPH. Intraprostatic reflux appears as subcapsular or intraprostatic echo-free lesions, often linear in nature and complicated by small periurethral ductal calculi, which are a feature of intraprostatic reflux (Fig. 2.23b).

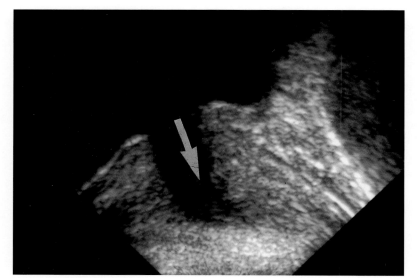

a

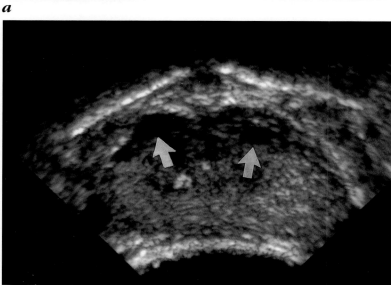

b

Figure 2.23 *(a) End-fire sagittal section of the prostate gland in a patient with bladder neck obstruction. There is an echo-poor area that is surrounding the urethral complex (arrow) and extending well down into the prostate itself. These are classic appearances. (b) Transverse axial section of the prostate in a patient with bladder neck obstruction and intraprostatic reflux. There are transonic subcapsular collections (arrows) seen.*

PROSTATE CANCER

EPIDEMIOLOGY

Prostate cancer now exceeds lung cancer as the most commonly diagnosed cancer in American men after skin cancer, and is the second major cause of cancer death in this group.[25] There has been a 17 per cent increase in deaths from this disease in the last 4 years alone (1988–1992).

Approximately 1 in every 11 men will have prostate cancer, and a 5-year survival of 88 per cent can be expected if malignancy is confined to the gland, reducing to 29 per cent if distal metastases are present at the time of diagnosis.[26] It is estimated that during the years 1985–2000 there will be a 37 per cent increase in prostate cancer deaths per year and a 90 per cent increase in prostate cancer diagnosed.[27] The impact and progress of the disease is similar to that of breast cancer, which has the profile of a more significant disease. The fourfold difference in research funding and research publications testifies to this lower status. However, the incidence rates, mortality and 5-year survival patterns for both diseases are comparable. As breast cancer is seen to be a potentially curable disease, the perception of prostate cancer is shifting from it being a disease only amenable to palliation to one that can potentially be cured.[28]

Whatever doubts there are about the current vogue for radical surgery,[29] there is no doubt that TRUS can identify early disease, allowing improved palliation over treatment whose commencement is delayed.[30] However, set against this is the spectre of large-scale unnecessary treatment, with all its adverse effects for a disease whose natural history in the vast majority of cases may very well be completely indolent.[31] This section will concentrate on the important role TRUS currently plays in the diagnosis and management of symptomatic prostate cancer and in the elucidation of positive DRE and PSA results found on screening, the practice of which, whatever one's point of view, is now a fact of life.[32]

THE NATURAL HISTORY OF PROSTATE CANCER

Ten to twenty per cent of cancers originate in the transitional zone, 5–10 per cent in the central zone and 70 per cent in the periphery.[33,34] TRUS examination concentrates on the peripheral zone, partly on account of the high incidence of the disease here, but more importantly on account of its relative inaccessibility to the urethral resectoscope, as its lies beyond the so-called surgical capsule of the gland.

Serial sections of prostate glands at autopsy from men over 50 have revealed an unexpectedly high prevalence of microfoci of well-differentiated adenocarcinoma. Every decade of ageing nearly doubles the incidence, from 10 per cent in men in their 50s to 70 per cent in men in their 80s.[35] The current estimate of the probability of having prostate cancer in a lifetime is now 11 per cent,[36] but this only represents the tip of the iceberg, as 90 per cent of prostate cancers remain latent and clinically unimportant for decades.[37] This prevalence of 'latent' or 'incidental' tumour is possibly unique to prostate cancer, and poses major management implications for its unheralded detection by modalities such as TRUS and

increasing biopsy rates on account of TRUS and PSA levels.

The largest natural history study is based on 223 consecutively diagnosed patients.[38] All had confined tumour and a mean age of 72 years, and most had grade 1 or 2 disease; only nine had grade 3. There was a 10-year observation period in which 34 per cent experienced progression and 11.6 per cent had metastases but only 8.5 per cent died as a direct result of prostate cancer. These patients who were given no initial treatment had survival rates which, in the opinion of the authors, are comparable to those in uncontrolled trials of radical treatment for localized prostate cancer. Tumour grade at the time of diagnosis was the most important prognostic factor. In 148 patients with well-differentiated tumours, progression occurred in 19 per cent and death in 2.5 per cent. In nine with higher grade poorly differentiated tumours, progression occurred in 67 per cent and death in 56 per cent. Other smaller studies support the major contention of this study that the vast majority of patients with untreated prostate cancer will die from other causes.[8] In a further study of 94 patients with confined disease T1 (cancer occupying less than 5 per cent of the tissue resected and not poorly differentiated), 27 per cent died from other causes within 4 years and an 8-year follow-up of the remainder showed that only 9 per cent died from prostate cancer.[39]

The major predictors of the malignant potential of prostate cancer are histological grade, stage of disease (Table 2.8) and tumour volume. As lesions greater than 1.5 cm in diameter are more liable to metastasise, size is an important determinant in predicting the natural history of the disease and is an indirect indicator of capsular infiltration, differentiation and metastatic spread.[40,41] Histological grading, requiring core biopsy specimens, is the definitive indicator of malignancy, and the system of Gleason[42] has been incorporated rapidly into clinical practice and appears to correlate well other known prognostic indicators, especially tumour size,[43] metastasis to pelvic lymph nodes[44] and even the level of PSA.[2]

Tumours that attain clinical importance arise principally in the peripheral zone of the gland. They grow peripherally through the capsule of the gland,[45,46] and favour passage through the perineural spaces that perforate the capsule only at the upper outer corner and apex of the gland.[47] They frequently invade the seminal vesicles and the neck of the bladder. They rarely cross the fascial space into the rectal wall. Metastatic spread is both lymphatic and

Table 2.8 TNM staging of prostate cancer.

T0   No evidence of primary tumour.

T1   Incidental histological finding.
    1a   Three or fewer microfoci carcinoma.
    1b   More than three microfoci.

T2   Tumour present clinically or grossly, limited to the gland.
    2a. Tumour 1.5 cm or less in greatest dimension, with normal tissue on at least three sides.
    2b. Tumour more than 1.5 cm in greatest dimension or in more than one lobe.

T3   Tumour invades into the prostatic apex or into or beyond the prostatic capsule or bladder neck or seminal vesicle, but is not fixed.

T4. Tumour is fixed or invades into adjacent structures other than those listed in T3.

haematogenous. The former is usually orderly, affecting the obturator and iliac nodes first.[48]

THE APPEARANCES OF CARCINOMA ON TRUS AND PATHOLOGIES WHICH GIVE SIMILAR APPEARANCES

The original TRUS description of prostate cancer was of an echogenic lesion often indistinguishable from calcification.[49,50] These original descriptions were almost certainly of large infiltrating tumours extending into areas of benign disease associated with calcification which are usually in the central and transitional zones of the gland. The typical appearance of prostate cancer on TRUS is an area of low echogenicity in the peripheral zone[51] (Fig. 2.24). Because of the resolution of early technology and the subtle lower echogenicity of early peripheral lesions, the appearance was probably not well depicted and not easily appreciated. Also, it is very seldom that carcinoma occurs in isolation in a model-type gland; it usually coexists with varying amounts and patterns of BPH, corpora amylacea and adenoma formation which distort the expected architecture of the gland, and the adjacent peripheral zone can be thinned and splayed around a burgeoning central zone. Appreciation of this background variability is essential in assessing the peripheral zone, and the spectrum of elderly prostate appearances may have deflected attention from subtler coexisting changes in the periphery, resulting in the misleading early descriptions. Large imaging–pathological correlation studies have defined the appearance of carcinoma as seen on TRUS and clarified the earlier ambiguities.[52,53] Although the above is the typical appearance, not all carcinoma is evident on TRUS and up to 25 per cent of tumours are isoechoic with normal prostate tissue.[54] A series of radical prostatectomy specimens with serial section histopathology generated 125 cases with proven T0/T1 tumours, all of which had preoperative TRUS. Seventy-six per cent were correctly identified on account of their low echogenic nature, but the isoechoic 24 per cent were missed.[55] It is generally accepted that 25 per cent or possibly more tumours defy depiction or are missed at TRUS. The reasons for this extend well beyond the usual explanations for differences in ultrasound performance, such as variability in operator skill and experience. Leaving these aside, the biophysical characteristics that determine grey scale conspicuity are complex and are not a simple function of spatial resolution. The echogenic lesion has been attributed to tumour infiltrating pre-existing corpora amylacea, high grade comedonecrosis and the fine stippled calcification associated with central necrosis[56] (Fig. 2.25). Although these are almost certainly contributory, the explanation probably goes deeper. Tumour size, equipment sophistication and calcification affect tumour depiction but the relationship is not

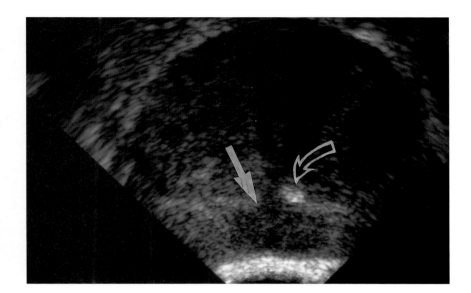

Figure 2.24 *Transverse axial section of the prostate. There is a peripherally situated echo-poor lesion (arrow) due to carcinoma. There is also BPH and a little corpora amylacea (open arrow).*

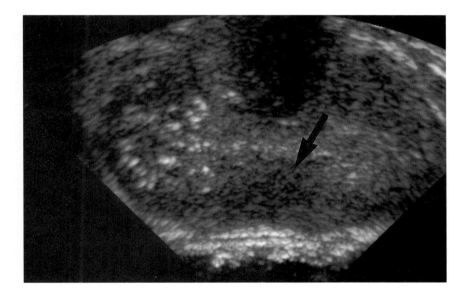

Figure 2.25 *There is an echo-poor lesion in the midline within the peripheral zone of the prostate (arrow), and the right peripheral zone is predominantly echogenic. Biopsy from both sites revealed carcinoma.*

straightforward. Several investigators using TRUS and MRI have noted a lack of correlation between tumour depiction at imaging and actual size when measured at pathological examination, suggesting that factors other than size determine detection.[57,58,59] Tumour morphology has been correlated with degree of echogenicity.[8] The relationship between tumour morphology and echogenicity appears to be directly proportional to the amount of intervening normal prostate tissue; the less normal tissue, the greater the density of malignant tissue and the lower the echogenicity. Larger infiltrative tumours are associated with stromal fibrosis, which normalizes echogenicity, reducing their representation at TRUS.

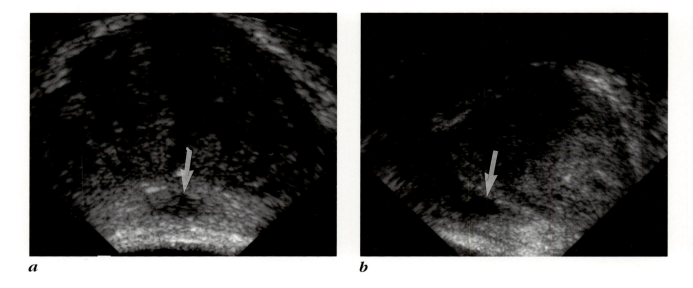

a *b*

Figure 2.26 *(a) Transverse axial TRUS. There is an echo-poor lesion in the midline within the peripheral zone of the prostate in a patient with coexistent BPH highly suggestive of malignancy (arrow). (b) Sagittal section of the prostate with an end-fire probe. The lesion is seen to be focal dilatation of an ejaculatory duct (arrow), not requiring biopsy.*

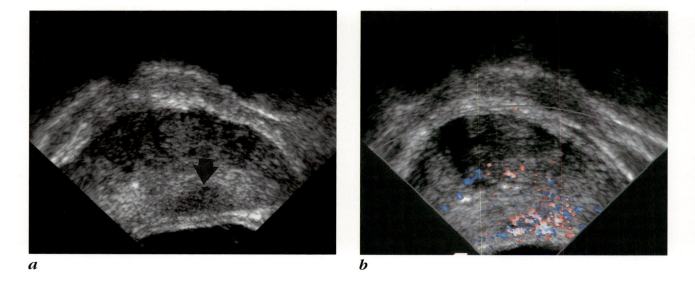

a *b*

Figure 2.27 *(a) Transverse axial section of the prostate showing a 1 cm peripherally situated echo-poor lesion (arrow). (b) CDI shows intense increased blood flow within the echo-poor lesion. Biopsy showed carcinoma.*

These observations may in part explain why up to 30 per cent of palpable nodules go undetected.

The peripheral zone sonographic hypoechoic nodule typical of malignant disease turns out to be a common and nonspecific finding, which is a second major difficulty with TRUS imaging.[60] Only 20 per cent of such lesions represent malignancy, which means a positive finding has an extremely low positive predictive value of 18–60 per cent, depending on who you read.[33,34,61] This low predictive value means high biopsy rates and tissue diagnosis for clarification, even if additional information known to improve the predictive value, such as DRE, PSA and colour Doppler, is available because missing a proportion of true positives is an acceptable and calculated part of screening practice but is wholly unacceptable in clinical practice.

A large range of anatomical variants and benign pathologies may masquerade as malignancy:

- Nodules of BPH.
- Prostate cysts.
- Granulomata.
- Granulomatous prostatitis.
- Haematoma.
- Muscle surrounding ejaculatory ducts.
- Dilated ejaculatory ducts.
- Malakoplakia.
- Prostate infarcts.

Nodules of benign glandular hyperplasia may extend into the peripheral zone or atypical conglomerations may occur there. Benign hyperplasia in the peripheral zone is more common than once thought and may cause focal bulging of the prostate capsule.[62] Other benign conditions simulate the appearances of prostate cancer. These include small benign prostate cysts, the normal ejaculatory ducts which with partial volume look like echo-poor lesions (Fig. 2.26), granulomatous prostatitis, cystic atrophy, prominent blood vessels, muscular tissue and malakoplakia. Granulomatous prostatitis, infarcts, cystic atrophy, blood vessels, haematomata, muscular tissue and malakoplakia all have a confounding similar appearance.[63] Rarer anomalies such as duct dilatation and muscle surrounding ejaculatory ducts may be mistaken for malignancy.[64]

COLOUR DOPPLER AND TRUS

The low predictive value of TRUS in diagnosing malignancy effectively necessitates biopsy of all peripheral zone lesions with an attendant high cost and a morbidity of questionable acceptability.[65,66] Accordingly, improving the predictive value of TRUS has important implications. It might enable a more selective biopsy policy or, if sufficiently good, obviate the need for biopsy altogether. It is already known that the size, site of lesion, DRE and PSA improve the positive predictive value of TRUS.[67] CDI is a convenient and integral adjunct to grey scale ultrasound, and emerging reports suggest a consistently increased colour flow signal in prostate malignancy (Fig. 2.27).

In a series of 158 biopsy-proven cases, colour Doppler did improve the positive predictive value of TRUS from 53 per cent to 77 per cent, but the authors concluded that the reduction in sensitivity was unacceptably large, and that colour Doppler alone only identified one additional case of malignancy independent of TRUS (1/75 cancers) and appeared to have little additional value over careful TRUS grey scale examination. Its routine application should therefore not alter established biopsy policy.[67] This study also showed that increased colour flow was not a universal accompaniment to malignancy, and 10 of 75 cancers were apparently avascular; this did not appear to relate to the size or staging of the tumour. The only other investigation into the possible role of colour Doppler is more enthusiastic but fails to define a clear benefit or role for this technology. Nine cancers (six patients) out of 132 were identified which had no demonstrable abnormality on grey scale ultrasound but had identifiable flow on colour Doppler (121 patients all had abnormal DRE or PSA), and conclusions drawn are that colour flow may assist biopsy guidance and improve conspicuity of subtle grey scale lesions for inexperienced operators.[66]

It was hoped that increased colour flow might consistently identify the difficult isoechoic lesion, but it is probable that an isoechoic lesion represents a larger tumour than the hypoechoic lesion, and larger tumours do not necessarily have relatively increased vascularity; indeed, the opposite may be the case. Tumour models demonstrate a relationship between vascularity and tumour size, being avascular less than 2 mm in diameter, uniformly vascular up to 1 cm^3 and developing central necrosis beyond this size with resultant loss in vascularity.[68] Unfortunately, the size of expected maximal tumour vascularity is also the same as maximal conspicuity on grey scale ultrasound, and intratumour blood flow also appears to show a wide heterogeneity in pattern of distribution. So there is no clear rationale for even an adjuvant

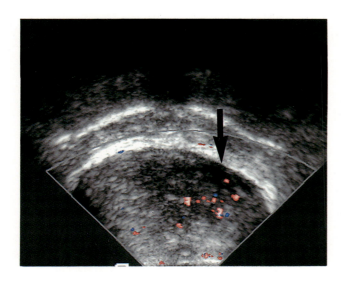

Figure 2.28 *Transverse axial colour Doppler image of the prostate. There is an echo-poor area in the left central zone associated with increased blood flow (arrow). Biopsy showed a carcinoma with no evidence of malignancy from the rest of the gland.*

role for colour Doppler. Colour Doppler can be useful in detecting tumours arising in the central zone of the prostate. They can appear as echo-poor, but indistinguishable from benign hyperplasia. Asymmetrically increased flow on colour Doppler suggests malignancy (Fig. 2.28).

The volume relationship between expected vascularity and tumour size suggests that poor conspicuity on grey scale imaging may also be accompanied by reduced vascularity on colour Doppler, so reliance on colour Doppler may be misleading and a case for careful grey scale scanning only could be made. Before any further clinical work on colour Doppler in prostate disease is embarked upon, more basic work on correlating colour Doppler and grey scale changes in malignancy with size and histological composition on fully mapped resection specimens is essential.

The overall benefit of colour Doppler is certainly not clear-cut, and its major contribution may be in consolidating the opinion of inexperienced scanners when presented with subtle grey scale lesions and possibly improving conspicuity in targeting biopsies.

THE ROLE OF TRUS IN PROSTATE CANCER

As well as its important and varied role in diagnosis, TRUS also influences the therapeutic management of prostate cancer and subsequent course. It contributes to the interpretation of equivocal clinical and biochemical findings, the diagnosis and staging of malignancy (Fig. 2.29), biopsy guidance and the follow-up of treated malignancy and assessment for local recurrence.

Assessment of prostate volume and diagnosis of other prostate afflictions may be extremely valuable in discriminating benign from malignant elevations in PSA. This assay is being increasingly used as a screening tool and many patients are now being referred for TRUS to clarify marginally high results. The difficulty starts with establishing an upper limit of normal for PSA; this remains controversial.[69, 70] It is now known that volume-adjusted PSA is a more accurate means of assessing normality.[17,18] Patients with a PSA value above the volume-adjusted 95th percentile have an estimated risk for prostate cancer up to nine times that of the normal population. Excluding possible malignancy and establishing alternative diagnoses such as acute prostatitis, which has a characteristic colour Doppler appearance,[71] or BPH and volume estimation for PSA adjustment may obviate the need for biopsy in these patients.

TRUS has a positive role to play in establishing the diagnosis of cancer when clinically suspected. TRUS is a sensitive technique and can easily detect impalpable malignancies.[58,59] Although the typical lesion has a nonspecific appearance with a low positive predictive value ranging from 18 to 60 per cent, assessment of additional parameters may improve this. In a series of 256 patients the positive predictive value of a hypoechoic lesion was 41 per cent, but this increased to 52 per cent if PSA was positive, 61 per cent if DRE was positive and 72 per cent if both were positive. Colour Doppler may improve the positive predictive value even more. Even when the PSA is normal, TRUS and biopsy may diagnose malignancy in a significant number of cases. In a series of 91 TRUS lesions in 83 men where the PSA was normal, biopsy revealed malignancy or premalignancy in 20 (21.5 per cent). In this scenario, if the TRUS lesion corresponds to the DRE there is a high likelihood of malignancy.[72] In patients where the nodule is confined to the gland and a T2 lesion is suspected, biopsy is usually mandatory for confirmation. The main role for TRUS is to guide biopsies to obtain cores for histological diagnoses. Several cores are necessary to enable accurate prediction of histological grade, which assists

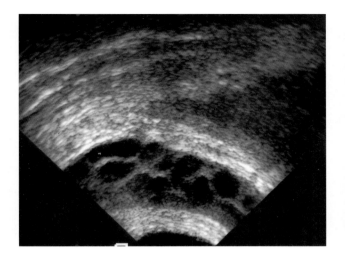

Figure 2.33 *Transverse axial section of a moderately dilated seminal vesicle.*

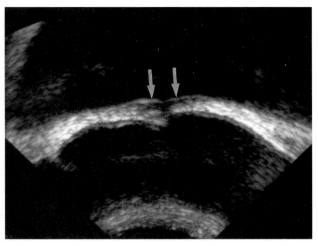

Figure 2.34 *Midline transverse axial TRUS showing gross dilatation of both seminal vesicles. The medial aspects of the vas deferens can be seen (arrows).*

value, and the ejaculatory ducts could only be visualized by operative vasography or seminal vesiculography.

ANATOMY OF THE GENITAL TRACT

The seminal vesicles are paired structures lying above the prostate and posterior to the bladder, measuring 5 cm in length and 1.5 cm in width; however, there is a great variation, depending upon age and the interval between ejaculation and scanning.[79] At their medial aspects, the seminal vesicles merge with the ipsilateral vas deferens to form the ejaculatory duct, which passes through the central part of the prostate to emerge in the urethra at the verumontanum. The normal duct narrows slightly in its distal half and is surrounded by smooth muscle. The whole of the urethra forms the rest of the genital tract. The ejaculate, which comprises predominantly secretions from the prostate itself, the contribution from the seminal vesicles and the testes accounting for 20 per cent of its volume, which is normally between 2 and 5 ml, enters the urethra at the verumontanum and is forced through the distal sphincter by contraction of the smooth muscle within the prostate. Retrograde flow of the ejaculate is prevented by an intact bladder neck mechanism.

INDICATIONS FOR TRUS OF THE GENITAL TRACT

These are as follows:

- Infertility.
- Haemospermia.
- Pyospermia.
- Low-volume ejaculate.
- Perineal pain.
- Pain on ejaculation.

Infertility

Infertility is usually caused by untreatable testicular abnormalities or congenital aplasia of the vas deferens or seminal vesicles, which may be partial or complete.[80] Where demonstrable obstruction to the genital tract exists, there is the potential of cure for infertility or at least improvement in the sperm count. As with other structures in the body, dilatation does not necessarily mean obstruction, but strongly suggests it.

The normal seminal vesicles have a variable appearance, but dilatation of them can be graded as moderate (Fig. 2.33) or severe. When it is severe, the seminal vesicles appear as paired cystic structures with thin walls (Fig. 2.34). To prove that obstruction exists, the seminal vesicle should be punctured with a 22 gauge

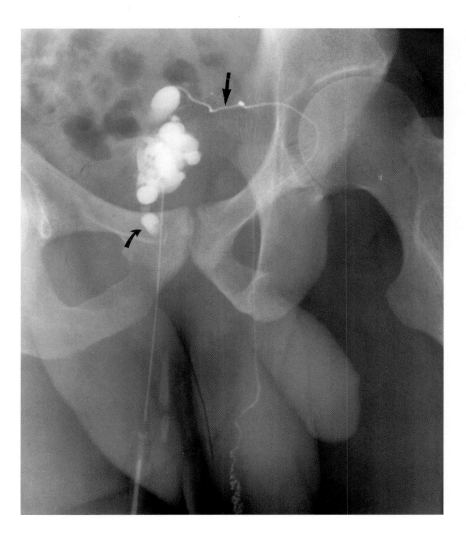

Figure 2.35 *Spot film taken during TRUS guided vasography. The dilated seminal vesicle was punctured via the perineal route and contrast injected. The dilated seminal vesicle is clearly identified and reflux down the ipsilateral vas is seen (arrow). The dilated ejaculatory duct is outlined (curved arrow) and there is no flow of contrast into the urethra. The obstruction was due to a distal ejaculatory duct stricture excised at urethroscopy.*

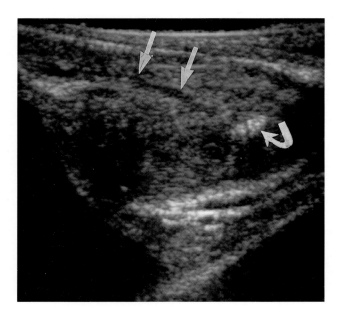

Figure 2.36 *Sagittal TRUS. There is mild dilatation of the ejaculatory duct (arrows) due to a collection of stones (curved arrow).*

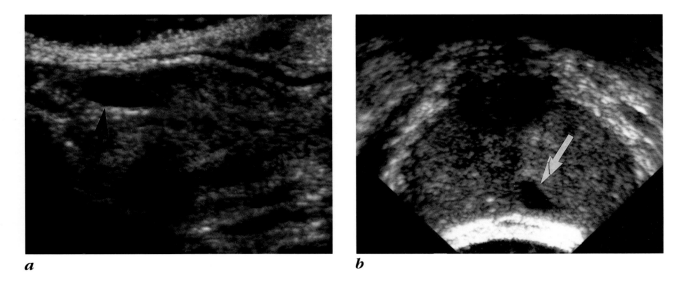

a   b

Figure 2.37 *(a) Sagittal section of the prostate showing localized dilatation of the ejaculatory duct (arrow). (b) Transverse axial image showing the ejaculatory duct to be to the left of the midline (arrow).*

needle using the perineal route under TRUS control. A small amount of seminal fluid is aspirated and under fluoroscopic control, contrast is injected. This will outline the distended vesicle and if no contrast enters the ejaculatory duct or urethra, but contrast passes retrogradely down the vas deferens, distal obstruction can be assumed and the level of obstruction will be identified (Fig. 2.35). This has considerable importance when the surgeon is planning to relieve the obstruction, the problem being that any surgery to the orifices of the ejaculatory ducts is close to the bladder neck mechanism, which if damaged may lead to retrograde ejaculation. Once the anatomy has been defined, patent blue dye is injected into the vesicle and the patient taken to theatre for immediate urethroscopy and resection of the ejaculatory ducts until a free flow of blue dye is seen. This will ensure that no more than is absolutely necessary is done.

Dilatation of the ejaculatory ducts is either focal or generalized.[81] The ducts are seen as distended echo-free structures passing through the prostate down to the obstructing lesion, which is commonly either a single stone (Fig. 2.36), a series of stones or a stricture at the distal end of the ejaculatory duct. On transverse axial imaging, the ejaculatory ducts are either side of the midline (Fig. 2.37) and should not be confused with Mullerian duct remnants, which are midline structures (Fig. 2.38).

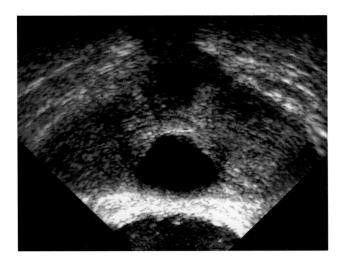

Figure 2.38 *Transverse axial TRUS showing a cystic midline lesion characteristic of a Mullerian duct remnant.*

Again, in an attempt to substantiate whether or not obstruction exists, the duct is punctured under TRUS control and saline injected into it whilst continually scanning. To make interfaces within the saline, it is vigorously shaken before injection. The saline will be seen to distend the duct, and obstruction is unlikely if the saline is seen entering the bladder through the bladder neck, which proves that the duct is patent. Contrast can then be instilled under fluoroscopic control and spot films taken. The lack of reflux down the ipsilateral vas deferens is a further indication that obstruction is not present.

Haemospermia

Blood in the sperm causes the patient a great deal of alarm, mainly because of the fear that cancer is the underlying cause,[82] but is rarely of clinical significance. It is a symptom that is becoming more commonly reported, presumably because of the increasing use of condoms as a protection against the acquired immune deficiency syndrome (AIDS). Haemospermia has a number of causes that can be identified by TRUS (Table 2.9).[83] In one series, TRUS was abnormal in 83 per cent of patients with haemospermia,[84] mainly because of calculi within the prostate or seminal vesicle (Fig. 2.39), but in most cases it is impossible to be certain that abnormalities seen on TRUS are responsible for the haemospermia, for calculi in prostatic ducts will be seen in hundreds of patients who do not have this symptom.

In the absence of any other genital symptoms, e.g. infertility, the indications for TRUS in men under 50

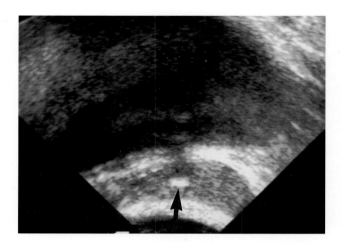

Figure 2.39 *Transverse axial TRUS of the left seminal vesicle in which a stone can be seen (arrow). The patient complained of haemospermia.*

years is to reassure them that no sinister pathology exists, as in most cases no treatment is needed. In those over 50, TRUS is essential to exclude malignancy.

Pyospermia

Pus in the semen is due to infective or inflammatory disorder of the prostate and seminal vesicles. It is usually associated with perineal pain and pyrexia. TRUS will identify such conditions and can guide aspiration of any abscess seen.

Low-volume Ejaculate

This condition is due either to pathology leading to diminished production of the various components that make up the normal male ejaculate, obstruction to the flow or the retrograde flow of ejaculate, and only becomes clinically significant if infertility coexists. TRUS will identify whether there is a significant lesion or not. Total ejaculatory failure in the absence of surgery to the bladder neck is usually due to congenital incompetence of the bladder neck, which is seen to be widely open on TRUS (Fig. 2.40). Such a finding is clinically important as it will direct treatment towards enhanced sperm retrieval,

Table 2.9 Classification and causes of haemospermia.

Classification	Causes
Haemospermia due to pathological conditions	Prostate cancer
	Ejaculatory duct stones
	Prostatic calculi
	Prostatitis
	Seminal vesiculitis
	Seminal vesicle tumours
Functional haemospermia	Excessive sexual indulgence
	Prolonged sexual abstinence
	Interrupted coitus
	Unbridled licence
Essential or idiopathic haemospermia	Bleeding from sudden emptying of distended seminal vesicles

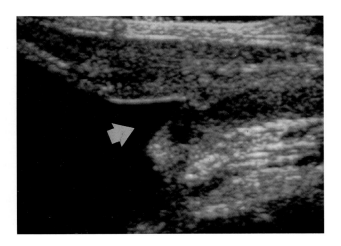

Figure 2.40 *Sagittal TRUS in a patient with total ejaculatory failure. The bladder neck (arrow) is wide open at rest.*

pharmacotherapy for the bladder neck or surgical reduction sphincteroplasty of the bladder neck. Unfortunately, there is a wide spectrum of the normal appearances of the bladder neck. Seemingly incompetent ones can be associated with normal antegrade ejaculation, but in the clinical context of infertility and no other demonstrable abnormality, an open bladder neck at rest on TRUS is likely to be clinically important.

Pain on Ejaculation

Pain on ejaculation has many causes:

- Seminal vesicle cystic disease.
- Stones in the genital tract.
- Prostatic inflammatory disease.
- Seminal vesiculitis.
- Urethritis.
- Urethral stones.

It is of great concern to the patient and TRUS should be the first line of investigation to identify a possible cause. Unilateral cystic disease or hypoplasia of the seminal vesicle is associated with other disorders of the development of the mesonephric duct,[85] usually ipsilateral renal dysgenesis in 80 per cent, or ectopic insertion of the ipsilateral ureter into a derivative of the mesonephric duct, either posterior urethra, ejaculatory duct or seminal vesicle, in 8 per cent of cases.[86] The finding on TRUS of a grossly distended, thin-walled seminal vesicle must encourage a search for other abnormalities. The pain is likely to be due to the mass effect of the dilated vesicle or haemorrhage within it and is always relieved by surgical removal. Infertility is not usually present because of the intact normal contralateral vesicle. Inflammation of the seminal vesicles is usually bilateral and appears on TRUS as thin-walled and slightly distended structures around which increased flow can be seen on colour Doppler imaging. Stones within the genital tract can cause pain as well as infertility and prostatic inflammatory disease usually causes a dull and persistent perineal pain exacerbated by ejaculation.

PROSTATIC INFLAMMATORY DISEASE AND PROSTATE ABSCESS

Inflammation of the prostate gland rarely occurs in prepubertal boys, but is common in men, accounting for 25 per cent of genitourinary complaints.[87] There are recognized types of prostatitis (Table 2.10). In a study involving 600 men attending a genitourinary clinic, bacterial prostatitis accounted for 5 per cent of cases, nonbacterial prostatitis for 64 per cent and prostatodynia for 31 per cent.[88] The pathogenesis of bacterial prostatitis is multifactorial, but includes ascending urethral infection and intraprostatic reflux into the ejaculatory ducts and the prostatic ducts themselves. When a carbon-particle solution was instilled into the bladders of men with nonbacterial prostatitis, macrophages impregnated with intracellular carbon particles were found in their expressed prostatic secretions 3 days later, thus proving intraprostatic reflux.[89] The reflux of infected urine will lead to bacterial prostatitis, whilst that of uninfected urine will result in a 'chemical' nonbacterial prostatitis and prostatodynia. In a study of 60 men with a clinical diagnosis of chronic prostatitis, TRUS guided biopsy showed chronic inflammatory infiltrate of low grade in 88 per cent of cases, whereas organisms were isolated from only 9 per cent and these were considered to be contaminants from perineal skin.[90]

Acute bacterial prostatitis presents as a severe febrile illness that is easily diagnosed clinically. Chronic prostatitis, whether nonbacterial or bacterial, is difficult to diagnose and is often a diagnosis made

Table 2.10 Classification of prostatitis.

Acute bacterial prostatitis	Associated with urinary tract infections
Chronic bacterial prostatitis	Associated with relapsing urinary tract infections
Nonbacterial prostatitis	No urinary tract infection, but inflammatory cells in prostatic secretions
Prostatodynia	No urinary tract infection and no inflammatory cells in prostatic secretions

by exclusion on no firm clinical, pathological or radiological grounds. Patients complain of perineal discomfort, irritative voiding symptoms (frequency and urgency), low back pain and pain radiating to the inner thighs and scrotum, ejaculatory pain and occasionally haemospermia. DRE is usually unremarkable and low-grade pathogens are cultured from the urine of men with chronic bacterial prostatitis.

Patients with prostatodynia have symptoms of prostatitis, but no pathogen can be cultured from urine and they have no history of urinary tract infection. Patients tend to be middle-aged and present with perineal pain and irritative voiding patterns.[91] Specific urodynamic features have been reported in these patients.[92] These include low urinary flow rates despite normal voiding detrusor pressures due to obstruction at the bladder neck and poor relaxation of the distal sphincter. Such urodynamic abnormalities are likely to result in increased pressures within the prostatic urethra and therefore intraprostatic reflux.

TRANSRECTAL ULTRASOUND

Many ultrasound abnormalities in prostatitis have been reported, as follows:

- Areas of focal increased echoes in the peripheral zone.
- Areas of decreased echoes in the peripheral zone.
- Prostatic calculi.
- Prominence of the periprostatic venous plexus.
- Oedema of the capsule of the prostate.
- Cavitatory changes.
- Prostatic abscess.
- Increased blood flow on colour Doppler in the central zone.

- Increased blood flow on colour Doppler in the peripheral zone.

The role of TRUS is to confirm the difficult clinical diagnosis of prostatic inflammatory disease, to assess the efficacy of treatment, to look for possible underlying aetiological factors and to search for complications.

Irrespective of the type of prostatitis or its severity, TRUS may be normal on both grey scale and colour Doppler studies. As prostatic inflammatory disease is predominantly a condition of the younger male, in whom the peripheral zones account for most of the prostate, it is not surprising that the commonest abnormality seen is altered echogenicity within the peripheral zone. Well-defined, unilateral echogenic foci not associated with acoustic shadowing are a feature (Fig. 2.41). Increased blood flow throughout the entire peripheral zone with or without underlying grey scale abnormalities occurs (Fig. 2.42), as well as localized increased blood flow associated with a grey scale abnormality. In the normal prostate, virtually no flow is seen in the periprostatic venous plexus except where the neurovascular bundles enter the prostate posterolaterally. In prostatitis, prominence of the venous plexus and increased flow within it is often seen (Fig. 2.43).

Potential underlying conditions that can be seen on TRUS are detrusor sphincter dyssynergia and bladder neck obstruction, both of which precipitate intraprostatic reflux; on TRUS the results of this appear as echo-free, linear structures or subcapsular collections (Fig. 2.44). TRUS should ideally be combined with an ultrasound cystodynamogram, which may go a long way in confirming a voiding dysfunction.

Medical treatment of prostatitis is directed towards the underlying voiding abnormality and long-term antibiotics. The grey scale abnormalities do not alter despite therapy, but the intensity and distribution of

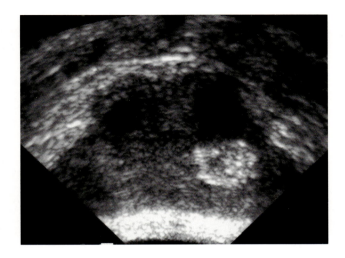

Figure 2.41 *Transverse axial TRUS in a patient of 23 years with chronic nonbacterial prostatitis showing an echogenic focus in the left peripheral zone.*

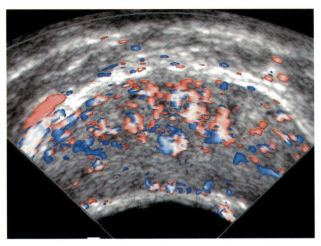

Figure 2.42 *Transverse axial colour Doppler TRUS in a patient with acute prostatitis. The underlying grey scale pattern is normal, but there is markedly increased blood flow throughout most of the peripheral zone.*

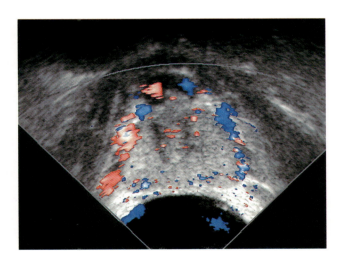

Figure 2.43 *Transverse axial TRUS showing increased flow in the periprostatic venous plexus in a patient with prostatitis.*

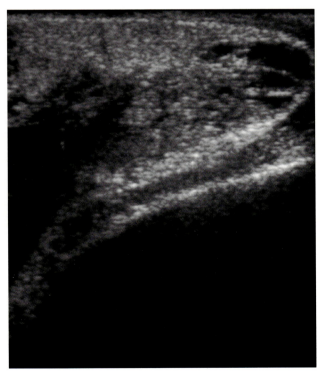

Figure 2.44 *Sagittal TRUS showing subcapsular collections due to intraprostatic reflux.*

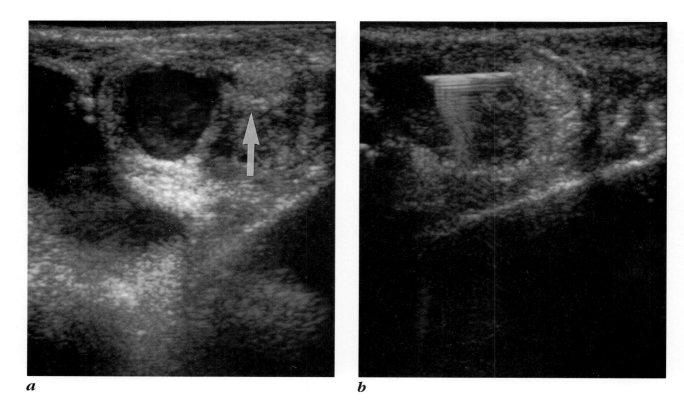

Figure 2.45 (a) Sagittal TRUS showing a thick-walled lesion with many internal echoes due to a prostatic abscess. Note the echogenic focus due to chronic bacterial prostatitis (arrow). (b) The lesion was needled via the perineal route to obtain a sample for microscopy.

abnormal blood flow does change and should revert to normal. Surgical treatment includes bladder neck incision, transurethral resection of the prostate and transurethral excision of prostatic calculi. Rarely, prostatitis can be complicated by the formation of a prostatic abscess, especially in immunocompromised patients.

PROSTATE ABSCESS

Abscesses within the prostate are becoming more common due to AIDS and prostate biopsy via the rectal route. Clinically, they present with perineal pain, pyrexia and a urethral discharge. TRUS will confirm the clinical diagnosis, assess the extent of the disease and monitor the effect of therapy, whether that be medical or decompression of the abscess by transurethral incision of it. TRUS guided perineal aspiration of a bacteriological sample is useful in the absence of a urethral discharge. TRUS guided perineal catheter drainage can be done.

On TRUS, abscesses appear as thick-walled, predominantly echo-poor lesions with numerous internal echoes (Fig. 2.45) and occasionally a fluid level.

REFERENCES

1. Lowsley OS, The development of the human prostate gland with reference to the development of other structures of the neck of the urinary bladder, *Am J Anat* (1912) **13**:299–349.

2. McNeal JE, Regional morphology and pathology of the human prostate, *Am J Clin Pathol* (1986) **49**:347–57.

3. Papsidero LD, Wang MC, Valanzuela LA, A prostate antigen in sera of prostatic cancer patients, *Cancer* (1980) **40**:2432–8.

4. Catalona WJ, Smith DS, Ratliff TL, Measurement of prostate specific antigen in serum as a screening test for prostate cancer, *N Engl J Med* (1991) **324**:1156–61.

5. Oesterling JE, Prostate specific antigen:a critical assessment of the most useful tumour marker for adenocarcinoma of the prostate, *J Urol* (1991) **145**:907–23.

6. Benson MC, Whang IS, Olsson CA,The use of prostate specific antigen density to enhance the predictive value of intermediate levels of serum PSA, *J Urol* (1992) **147**:817–21.

7. Cooner WH, Mosely BR, Rutherford CL, Prostate cancer detection in a clinical urological practice by ultrasonography, digital rectal examination and prostate specific antigen, *J Urol* (1990) **143**:1146–54.

8. Whitmore WF, Warner JA, Thompson IM, Expectant management of localised prostatic cancer, *Cancer* (1991) **67**:1091–6.

9. Rifkin MD, Choi H, Implications of small, peripheral hypoechoic lesions in endorectal ultrasound of the prostate, *Radiology* (1988) **166**:619–22.

10. Rifkin MD, Alexander AA, Pisarchick J, Matteucci T, Palpable masses in the prostate: superior accuracy of US-guided biopsy compared with accuracy of digitally guided biopsy, *Radiology* (1991) **179**:41–2.

11. Stamey TA, Presented specific antigen in the diagnosis and treatment of adenocarcinoma of the prostate, *Urol Monogr* (1989) **10**:

12. Clements R, Aideyan OU, Griffiths GJ, Peeling WB, Side effects and patients acceptability of transrectal biopsy of the prostate, *Clin Radiol* (1993) **47**:125–26.

13. Aus G, Hermansson CG, Hogosson J, Pedersen KV, Transrectal ultrasound examination of the prostate: complications and acceptance by patients, *Br J Urol* (1993) **71**:457–9.

14. Collins GN, Lloyd SN, Hehir M, McKelvie GB, Multiple transrectal ultrasound-guided biopsy–true morbidity and patient acceptance, *Br J Urol* (1993) **71**:460–3.

15. Hodge KK, McNeal JE, Terris MK, Stamey TA, Random systematic versus directly guided transrectal core biopsies of the prostate, *J Urol* (1989) **142**:71–5.

16. Terris MK, Stamey TA, Determination of prostate volume with transrectal ultrasound, *J Urol* (1991) **145**:984–7.

17. Littrup PJ, Kane RA, Williams CR et al, Determination of prostate volume with transrectal ultrasound for cancer screening. Part 1 Comparison with prostate specific antigen assays, *Radiology* (1991) **178**:537–2.

18. Littrup PJ, Williams CR, Egglin TK, Kane RA, Determination of prostate volume with transrectal ultrasound for prostate screening. Part 2 Accuracy of in vitro and in vivo technique, *Radiology* (1991) **179**:49–53.

19. Hastak SM, Gammelgaard J, Holm HH, Transrectal ultrasound volume determination of the prostate–a pre- and post-operative study, *J Urol* (1982) **127**:1115–18.

20. Stamey TA, Prostate specific antigen in the diagnosis and treatment of adenocarcinoma of the prostate, *Urol Monogr* (1989) **10**:50–64.

21. Boothroyd AE, Dixon PJ, Christmas TJ et al, The ultrasound cystodynamogram–a new technique, *Br J Radiol* (1989) **63**:331–2.

22. Chapple CR, Milroy EM, Rickards D, Permanently implanted urethral stent for prostatic outflow obstruction in the unfit patient–preliminary report, *Br J Urol* (1990) **66**:58–65.

23. Milroy EM, Chapple CR, Cooper JE, A new treatment for urethral stricture, *Lancet* (1988) **1**:1424–7.

24. Rickards D, Advances in ultrasound. In: Kirby, RS, Hendry WF, eds, *Recent Advances in Urology* (Churchill Livingstone: London, 1993) 2–15.

25. Coffey DS, Prostate cancer: an overview of an increasing dilemma, *Cancer* (1993) **70**:880–6.

26. American Cancer Society, *Cancer Facts and Figures* (ACA: Atlanta GA, 1992).

27. Carter HB, Coffey DS, The prostate: an increasing medical problem, *Prostate* (1990) **16**:187–97.

28. Walsh PC, Radical retropubic prostatectomy with reduced morbidity: an anatomic approach. *NCI Monograph* No. 7. (NIH Publication no. 88–3005) (Government Printing Office: Washington DC, 1988) 133–7.

29. Carr TW, Natural history of prostate cancer, *Lancet* (1993) **1**:91.

30. Robey EL, Schellhammer PE, Local failure after definitive therapy for prostate cancer, *J Urol* (1987) **137**:613–19.

31. Chodak GW, Questioning the value of screening for prostate cancer in asymptomatic men, *Urology* (1993) **42**:116–18.

32. Pollack HM, Resnick MI, PSA and screening for prostate cancer: much ado about something, *Radiology* (1993) **189**:353–6.

33. Lee F, Torp-Pederson S, Siders DB et al, TRUS in the diagnosis and staging of prostate cancer, *Radiology* (1989) **170**:609–15.

34. Lee F, Torp-Pederson S, Littrup PJ. Hypoechoic lesions of the prostate: clinical relevance of tumour size, digital rectal examination and prostate-specific antigen, *Radiology* (1989) **170**:29–32.

35. Sheldon CA, Williams RD, Fraley EE, Incidental carcinoma of the prostate: a review of the literature and critical reappraisal of classification, *J Urol* (1980) **124**:626–31.

36. American Cancer Society, *Cancer Facts and Figures* (ACA: Atlanta GA, 1991).

37. Gittes RE, Carcinoma of the prostate, *New Engl J Med* (1991) **324**:236–45.

38. Johansson JE, Adami HO, Andersson SO et al, High 10 year survival rate in patients with early untreated prostate cancer, *JAMA* (1992) **267**:2191–6.

39. Epstein JC, Paull G, Eggleston JC, Walsh PC, Prognosis of untreated Stage A1 prostatic carcinoma: a study of 94 cases with extended follow up, *J Urol* (1986) **136**:837–9.

40. Stamey TA, McNeal JE, Freiha FS, Morphometric and clinical studies on 68 consecutive radical prostatectomies, *J Urol* (1988) **139**:1235–41.

41. Gleason DF, Histological grading and clinical staging of prostate carcinoma. In: Tannenbaum M, ed., *Urologic Pathology: the Prostate* (Lea and Febiger: Philadelphia, 1977) 171–98.

42. McNeal JE, Bostwick DG, Kindrachuk RA, Patterns of progression in prostate cancer, *Lancet* (1986) **1**:60–3.

43. McNeal JE, Redwine EA, Freiha FS, Stamey TA, Zonal distribution of prostate adenocarcinoma: correlation with histological pattern and direction of spread, *Am J Surg Pathol* (1988) **12**:897–906.

44. Osterling JE, Brendler CB, Epstein JI et al, Correlation of clinical stage, serum prostatic acid phosphatase and prooperative Gleason grade with final pathologic stage in 275 patients with clinically localised adenocarcinoma of the prostate, *J Urol* (1987) **138**: 92–8.

45. Byar DP, Mostofi FK, Carcinoma of the prostate: prognostic evaluation of certain pathologic features in 208 radical prostatectomies: examined by the step section technique, *Cancer* (1972) **30**:5–13.

46. Villiers A, McNeal JE, Redwine E et al, The role of perineural space invasion in the local spread of prostate carcinoma, *J Urol* (1989) **142**:763–8.

47. Fowler JE Jr, Whitmore WF Jr, The incidence and extent of pelvic lymph node metastases in apparently localised prostate cancer, *Cancer* (1981) **47**:2941–5.

48. Resnick MI, Willard JW, Boyce WH, Transrectal sonography in the evaluation of patients with prostatic carcinoma, *J Urol* (1980) **124**:482.

49. Brooman PJC, Griffiths CW, Roberts EE et al, Per rectal ultrasound in the investigation of prostatic disease, *Clin Radiol* (1981) **32**:669–76.

50. Dahnert WF, Hamper UM, Eggleston JC et al, Prostatic evaluation of TRUS with histological correlation: the echopeic appearance of early carcinoma, *Radiology* (1986) **158**:97–102.

51. Griffiths GJ, Clements R, Jones DR et al, The ultrasound appearance of prostatic cancer with histological correlation, *Clin Radiol* (1987) **38**:219–27.

52. Lee F, Gray JM, Mcleary RD et al, Transrectal ultrasound in the diagnosis of prostate cancer. Location, echogenicity, histopathology and staging, *Prostate* (1985) **7**:117–29.

53. Salo JO, Ranniko S, Makinen J, Lehtonen T, Echogenic structure of prostate cancer imaged on radical prostatectomy specimens, *Prostate* (1987) **10**:1–9.

54. Hamper UM, Sheth S, Walsh PC et al, Capsular transgression of prostatic carcinoma: evaluation with transrectal US with pathologic correlation, *Radiology* (1991) **178**:791–5.

55. Hamper UM, Sheth S, Walsh PC, Epstein JI, Bright echogenic foci in early prostatic carcinoma: sonographic and pathologic correlation, *Radiology* (1990) **176**:339–43.

56. Carter HB, Hamper VM, Sheth S et al, Evaluation of transrectal ultrasound in early detection of prostate cancer, *J Urol* (1989) **142**:1008–10.

57. Carrol CL, Sommer SG, McNeal JE, Stamey TA, The abnormal prostate: MR imaging at 1.5T with histopathologic correlation, *Radiology* (1987) **163**:521–5.

58. Lee F, Bronson JP, Lee F et al, Cancer of the prostate assessment with transrectal ultrasound, *Radiology* (1991) **178**:197–9.

59. Lee F, Siders DB, Soren T, Prostate cancer, transrectal ultrasound and pathology comparison, *Cancer* (1991) **67**:1132–42.

60. Mettlin C, Lee F, Drago J, Murphy GP, The American Cancer Society National Prostate Cancer Detection Group. Findings on the detection of early prostate cancer in 2425 men, *Cancer* (1991) **67**:2949–58.

61. Ragde H, Bageley CM, Aldape HC, Blasko JC, Prostate cancer screening with high resolution transrectal ultrasound, *J Endourol* (1989) **3**:115–23

62. Chantelois AE, Parker SH, Sims JE, Horne DW, Malakoplakia of the prostate sonographically mimicking carcinoma, *Radiology* (1990) **177**:193–5.

63. Baran GW, Golin AL, Bergsma CJ et al, Biologic aggressiveness of palpable and non-palpable prostate cancer: assessment with endosonography, *Radiology* (1991) **178**:201–6.

64. Hinman F, Screening for prostatic cancer, *J Urol* (1991) **145**:126–30.

65. Chang P, Friedland GW, The role of imaging in screening for prostate cancer. A decision analysis perspective, *Invest Radiol* (1990) **25**:591–5.

66. Rifkin MD, Sudakoff GS, Archibald AA, Prostate: techniques, results and potential application of color Doppler US scanning, *Radiology* (1993) **186**:509–13.

67. Kelly IMG, Lees WR, Rickards D, Prostate cancer and the role of color Doppler ultrasound, *Radiology* (1993) **189**:153–6.

68. Folkman J, Cotran R, Relation of vascular proliferation to tumour growth, *Int Rev Exp Pathol* (1976) **16**:207–48.

69. Hortin GL, Bahnson RR, Daft M et al, Differences in values obtained with 2 assays of prostate specific antigen, *J Urol* (1988) **139**:762–5.

70. Chan DW, Bruzek DJ, Oesterling JE et al, Prostate specific antigen as a marker for prostate cancer: a monoclonal and polyclonal immunoassay compared, *Clin Chem* (1987) **33**:1916–20.

71. Lees WR, Kelly IMG, Rickards D, The diagnosis of prostatitis by colour Doppler imaging, *Radiology* (1992) **185**:106.

72. Spencer JA, Alexander AA, Gomella L et al, Clinical and US findings in prostate cancer: patients with normal prostate specific antigen levels, *Radiology* (1993) **189**:389–93.

73. Walsh PC, Jewitt HJ, Radical surgery for prostate cancer, *Cancer* (1980) **45**:1906–11.

74. Rickards D, Gowland M, Brooman P et al, CT and TRUS in the diagnosis of prostatic disease. A comparative study, *Br J Urol* (1983) **55**:726–32.

75. Schnall MD, Imai Y, Tomaszewski J et al, Prostate cancer: local staging with endorectal surface coil MR imaging, *Radiology* (1991) **178**:797–802.

76. Egawa S, Carter SS, Wheeler TM, Scardino PT, Ultrasonographic changes in the normal and malignant prostate after definitive radiotherapy, *Urol Clin North Am* (1989) **16**:741–9.

77. Clements R, Griffiths GJ, Peeling WB, Edwards AM, Transrectal ultrasound in monitoring response to treatment of prostate disease, *Urol Clin North Am* (1989) **16**:735–40.

78. Salomom CG, Flisak ME, Olson MC et al, Radical prostatectomy: transrectal sonographic evaluation to assess for local recurrence, *Radiology* (1993) **189**:713–19.

79. Littrup PJ, Lee F, McCleary RD et al, Transrectal ultrasound of the seminal vesicles and ejaculatory ducts: clinical correlation, *Radiology* (1988) **168**:625–8.

80. Carter SC, Shinohara K, Lipshultz LI, Transrectal ultrasound in disorders of the seminal vesicles and ejaculatory ducts, *Urol Clin North Am* (1989) **16**:773–90.

81. Clements R, Griffiths GJ, Peeling WB, Conn IG, Transrectal ultrasound of the ejaculatory apparatus, *Clin Radiol* (1991) **44**:240–4.

82. Murphy NJ, Weiss BD, Hematospermia, *Am Fam Physician* (1985) **32**:167–71.

83. Ganabathi K, Chadwick D, Feneley RCL, Gingell JC, Haemospermia, *Br J Urol* (1992) **69**:225–30.

84. Etherington RJ, Clements R, Griffiths GJ, Transrectal ultrasound in the management of haemospermia, *Clin Radiol* (1990) **41**:171–5.

85. Kenny PJ, Leeson MD, Congenital anomalies of the seminal vesicle: spectrum of computed tomographic findings, *Radiology* (1983) **149**:247–51.

86. King BF, Hattery RR, Lieber MM et al, Congenital cystic disease of the seminal vesicle, *Radiology* (1991) **178**:207–11.

87. Lipsky BA, Urinary tract infections in men, *Ann Intern Med* (1989) **110**:138–40.

88. Brunner H, Weidner W, Schiefer H-G, Studies of the role of *Ureaplasma urealyticum* and *Mycoplasma Hominis* in prostatitis, *J Infect Dis* (1983) **147**:807.

89. Kirby RS, Lowe D, Bultitude MI, Intraprostatic reflux: an aetiological factor in abacterial prostatitis, *Br J Urol* (1982) **54**:729–33.

90. Doble A, Thomas BJ, Furr PM et al, A search for infectious agents in chronic abacterial prostatitis using ultrasound guided biopsy, *Br J Urol* (1989) **64**:297–301.

91. Meares EM, Barbalias GA, Prostatitis: bacterial, nonbacterial and prostatodynia, *Semin Urol* (1983) **1**:146–50.

92. Barbalias GA, Meares EM, Sant GR, Prostatodynia: clinical and urodynamic characteristics, *J Urol* (1983) **130**:514–18.

Chapter 3 Transrectal Scanning: The Rectum and its Surroundings

John Beynon
A Roger Morgan

INTRODUCTION

Clinical evaluation of the rectum has relied traditionally on subjective digital examination, proctoscopy and rigid sigmoidoscopy. Where more objective assessment is of importance, such as in the evaluation of degrees of local invasion in rectal cancer, imaging methods have been introduced. The most successful of these to date has been rectal endosonography (RES).

Although endosonography was used initially to image the prostate, it has found a role in the examination of the rectum. Numerous studies have now reported its effectiveness in staging primary rectal cancer, and comparisons have been made with both clinical examination (i.e. digital) and other radiological techniques such as computed tomography (CT). Endosonography has also been used to review patients who have undergone sphincter-saving rectal resection, in order to detect or evaluate the extent of local recurrence.

ENDORECTAL SONOGRAPHY

The assessment of extent of local invasion in rectal cancer and thus its resectability has until recently relied on digital assessment. However, even in experienced hands, the accuracy varies from 60–80 per cent.[1,2] Similarly, involvement or otherwise of pararectal lymph nodes is poorly assessed clinically. Digital examination is also limited in that only the lower third of the rectum is accessible to the examining digit.

Management decisions regarding surgical or adjuvant treatment would be assisted by more accurate information. The main areas where this sort of information would be of benefit are in:

- The accurate preoperative staging of both local invasion and pararectal lymph node involvement, thus guiding the choice of individual surgical procedures, whether radical surgery or peranal local excision, or whether patients should be included in trials of adjuvant therapy.
- Identifying patients who have advanced local disease and are not candidates for primary surgical treatment and should be considered, for instance for primary radiotherapy. Re-evaluation using RES following radiotherapy could show that some of these cases would then be possible surgical candidates.
- The detection and evaluation of local recurrence, particularly if that recurrence is arising outside the rectal lumen.

THE HISTORY AND DEVELOPMENT OF RES

RES was first introduced by co-workers Wild and Reid with their development of an 'echoendo probe' in 1952.[3–5] The first instrument produced, like those available today, was hand-held, but also had a flexible shaft. Its ellipsoidal soundhead contained the piezo-electric crystal, drive shaft and drive motor. A water-filled balloon covered the transducer, which produced a sound beam at right angles to its long axis. A second instrument with a rigid shaft soon followed which allowed introduction into the rectum through a sigmoidoscope. Images could be taken for each revolution of the soundhead within the bowel. The first layered image of the bowel wall was produced using this early equipment and subsequently the first crude images of a rectal cancer. Limitations in technology resulted in this form of imaging of the gastrointestinal tract only being introduced into clinical practice over 30 years later by

Dragsted and Gammelgaard.[6] Using a Bruel and Kjaer (now B & K Medical) ultrasound scanner Type 8901 and rigid probe equipped with a 4.5-MHz transducer initially designed for prostatic imaging, 13 primary rectal cancers were assessed and results compared with postoperative histopathology. Invasion was correctly predicted in 11 cases. Despite their success with this promising technique they did not define their reporting criteria. The only real limitation noted was that in two patients the tumour could not be imaged due to the presence of stricture. The potential benefits of this new modality were similarly predicted by other investigators though using, at that stage, low frequency transducers of 3.5 MHz.[7,8] Hildebrandt and Fiefel, for example, successfully staged 23 of 25 patients using the same equipment with a transducer of 4.0 MHz. They found that in 25 patients examined, 8 tumours could not be assessed digitally but 15 of the others were correctly assessed by the examining finger, with two patients being overstaged. Their suggestion that an ultrasonic variation of the UICC system for staging should be adopted for use in ultrasonic staging by the use of the prefix 'u', i.e. uT1–uT4, has found favour with endosonographers. Initial problems that were encountered in this report were the distinction between T1 and T2 tumours using the 4-MHz probe and the examination of stenotic tumours. As with the previous report by Dragsted and Gammelgaard, no reporting criteria were defined for determining the degree of invasion.

TECHNIQUE AND EQUIPMENT

Most ultrasound scanners on the market at present have various forms of endocavity probes which can be purchased for this type of work. The plane of scanning is either transverse or longitudinal and there are some probes which scan in both planes. In the assessment of local invasion we feel it is important to have a degree of stand-off from the rectal wall. This allows the particular area of interest to lie within the focal range of the transducer being used. Surgical images produced by a radial scanner are easier to interpret, as they can be directly related to the appearances at operation in the pelvis. These 360° images are produced by mechanically rotating probes, requiring the presence of a water-filled balloon to cover the transducer for acoustic contact. Another major advantage of the balloon is its distension of the rectum, preventing distortion by infolding.

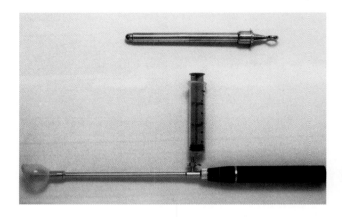

Figure 3.1 *The B & K Medical rectal endoprobe. A balloon covers the 7.0-MHz transducer for the purposes of examination. To place the probe at the level of the tumour, it may be introduced through a modified short rectoscope.*

Of the authors who have published data related to RES the majority have used equipment produced by B & K Medical (Denmark) (Probe type 1850) used in conjunction with a 5.5-MHz or 7.0-MHz transducer (Fig. 3.1) and more recently a 10.0-MHz transducer. In most series the 7.0-MHz transducer has been the one of choice, with a focal length of 2–5 cm. For the best imaging the rectum should be clear of faeces, and this can be accomplished using a disposable enema or suppositories. Examinations have traditionally been performed in the left lateral position, with the endoprobe either introduced blindly or through a rectoscope. This latter method is advantageous when examining higher or stenotic lesions. Following insertion, the balloon is inflated and the transducer switched on. The probe is then positioned to scan the area of interest. To obtain optimum images both the position of the probe and the volume of water in the balloon can be altered.

IMAGE INTERPRETATION

Correct identification of the image and its relationship to the histological structure of the rectal wall is

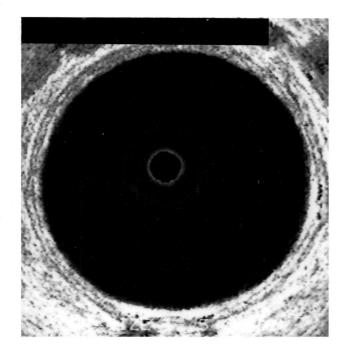

Figure 3.2 *An endosonogram demonstrating the five basic layers of the rectal wall. In rectal examinations anterior is always in the 12 o'clock position and the patient's left is to the right side of the scan.*

imperative for interpretation of endosonographic images of the rectum and particularly the extent of local invasion.

Five separate layers can be clearly identified in the rectal wall in most endosonographic scans. There are three hyperechoic layers separated by two hypoechoic.

The identification of the muscularis propria is crucial to accurate staging. There has been general agreement that the fourth hypoechoic layer represents the histologically discrete muscularis propria.

In the evolution of RES most controversy has surrounded the interpretation of the intermediate hyperechoic layer. It was originally reported by Hildebrandt et al that this intermediate layer represented a boundary echo between the hypoechoic mucosa/submucosa and the hypoechoic muscularis propria.[9] Thus:

- First hyperechoic layer — interface between water/balloon and mucosa.
- Second hypoechoic layer — mucosa and submucosa.

- Third hyperechoic layer — interface between mucosa/submucosa and muscularis propria.
- Fourth hypoechoic layer — muscularis propria.
- Fifth hyperechoic layer — interface between muscularis propria and perirectal fat.

However, Beynon et al, by performing anatomical studies, clearly showed that the five basic layers seen on RES of the rectal wall correspond directly to the anatomical layers present in the rectal wall.[10]

The five-layered system of interpretation is now recognized as the standard for routine clinical rectal sonography and is recognized now by most endosonographers (Fig. 3.2).

Hence:

- First hyperechoic layer — interface between the water/balloon and the mucosal surface.
- Second hypoechoic layer — combined image produced by the mucosa and muscularis mucosae.
- Third hyperechoic layer — submucosa.
- Fourth hypoechoic layer — muscularis propria.
- Fifth hyperechoic layer — interface between the muscularis propria and perirectal fat or serosa if present.

When an examination is being performed an additional hyperechoic layer will occasionally be seen within the fourth hypoechoic layer (the muscularis propria). Although not proven, it is thought this most probably represents an interface created by the two true muscle layers of the rectum (circular and longitudinal). Thus the true morphological layers of the rectum, with the exception of the muscularis mucosae, which gives a combined image with the mucosa, are represented by the five-layered image.

The perirectal fat has a mixed appearance on endosonographic examination. The mesorectum contains a variable number of lymph nodes which normally will not be imaged.

In the male the bladder, seminal vesicles, prostate, bulbar urethra and bulbo-urethral glands form the anterior relationships (Figs. 3.3a–c). The fascia of Denonvilliers separates the rectum and prostate in the male, while the rectovaginal septum separates the rectum and the vagina in the female. The uterus and ovaries can also be imaged in female patients.

The balloon covering the transducer during patient examinations produces a hyperechoic image of its own which merges with that of the mucosa–water interface. Imaging may be affected by the presence of artifacts, such as those produced by bubbles in the balloon or solid faeces in the rectum (Fig. 3.4).

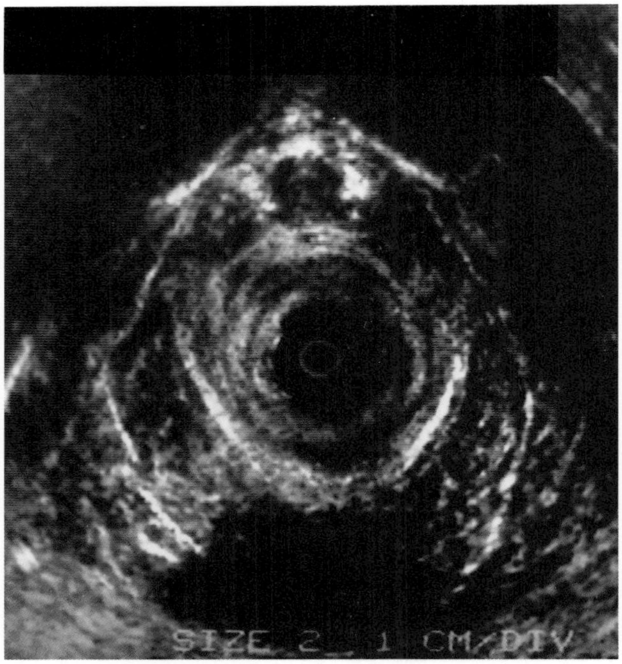

Figure 3.3 *The anterior relationships seen in the male during endosonographic examination. (a) The pelvic floor demonstrating the levator muscles, the inferior rami of the pubis, the upper part of the sphincter complex, bulbar urethra and bulbo-urethral glands. (b) The seminal vesicles in a patient treated for rectal cancer. (c) The prostate in a postoperative patient just at the level of the anastomosis.*

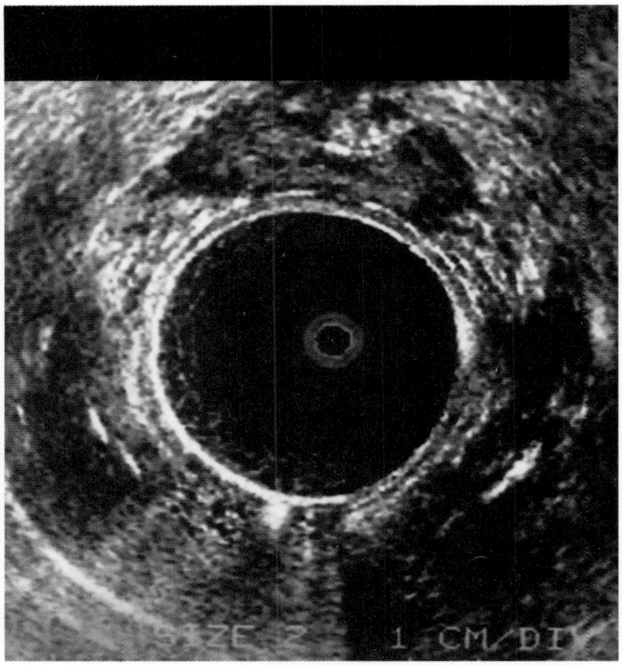

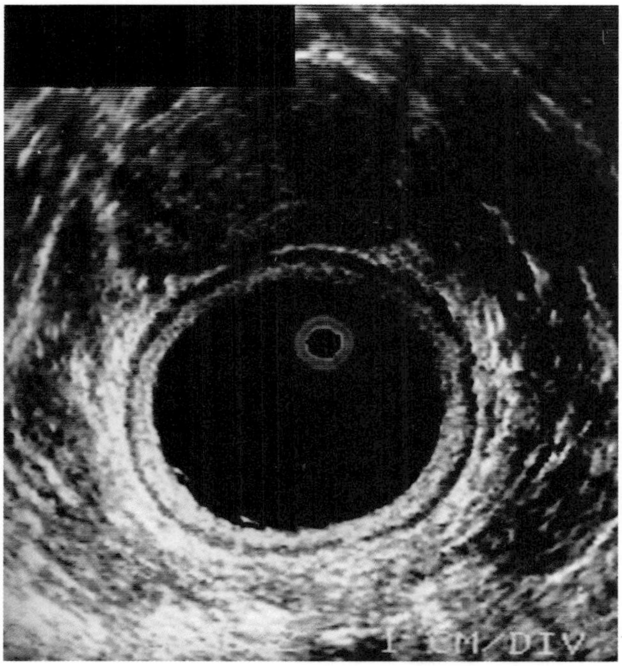

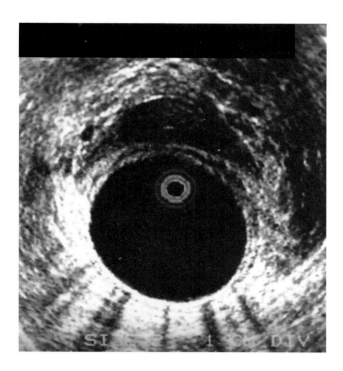

Figure 3.4 *Shadows due to the presence of faecal residue are seen in this female patient examined postoperatively at the 6 o'clock position. The uterus is clearly seen anteriorly.*

THE ASSESSMENT OF LOCAL INVASION IN RECTAL CANCER

On the whole, carcinomas of the rectum can be easily staged, as they appear ultrasonically to be uniformly hypoechoic and the degree of penetration is readily assessed. The TNM classification has been used to stage tumours, as all anatomical layers can be imaged. It has been suggested as a result that a prefix 'u' should be used to indicate an ultrasonic staging,[8] i.e.

- Benign adenoma — by definition an adenoma with severe dysplasia does not become a cancer until the submucosa is involved.
- uT1 — Tumour confined to the submucosa with an intact bright middle hyperechoic layer.
- uT2 — Tumour limited by the hypoechoic layer of the muscularis propria with no disruption of the bright interface between it and the surrounding fat.
- uT3 — Tumour penetrating the wall of the rectum to invade the adjacent fat. The tumour edge is usually irregular with sawtooth projections.
- uT4 — Tumour invading an adjacent structure.

Imaging is not difficult once the endosonographer/examiner has an understanding of the appearances of the normal rectum and also the method of staging. Examples of a uT2 tumour with an adjacent lymph node and two uT3 tumours are shown in Figs. 3.5, 3.6 and 3.7. The difference in the images is easily seen, with a hyperechoic interface between muscularis propria and fat in Fig. 3.5 which is disrupted with invasion into the surrounding fat in Figs. 3.6 and 3.7. A more obvious uT3 tumour with a typical irregular sawtoothed edge is seen in Figure 3.8. To tell the difference between a benign polyp and an early T1 tumour using endosonography is very difficult unless there is slight erosion of the submucosa on the scan. To make this sort of distinction, a high-quality scan with good resolution is necessary (Fig. 3.9). To demonstrate the extremes of invasion, an example of a uT4 tumour is shown in Fig. 3.10 with local invasion into the prostate.

Over the last 10 years various studies on the effectiveness of endosonography in staging rectal cancer have appeared in the literature.

Using various scanners, both radial (B & K Medical 1846 and/or 1849, or Aloka 520) and linear (Toshiba SAL50A, Aloka 280 SL, Kramed, GE RT3000), Rifkin and co-workers identified all 7 patients with extension of their tumours into the pararectal fat out of 26 patients with rectal cancers who were examined.[11,12] They later reported that tumour was identified in 79 of 85 patients, with two failures of examination. Patients were classified more crudely endosonographically into those confined or extending beyond the rectal wall. Invasion was identified in 25 patients through the muscularis propria but 8 were overstaged. Forty-three patients were correctly identified without invasion but five patients were understaged. Prediction of extension had a sensitivity of 83 per cent, specificity of 84 per cent, positive predictive value (PPV) of 76 per cent and negative predictive value (NPV) of 90 per cent.

An accuracy for sonographic staging of rectal cancer of 85.8 per cent was achieved by Fiefel et al with their first 60 patients, 42 of whom had been examined by endorectal sonography prospectively and subsequently subjected to surgery.[13] They later reported the results with a total of 129 cases, using in the more recent examinations a 7.0-MHz transducer.[9] Eighteen patients had no preoperative sonogram and 19 examinations were inadequate because of stenosis. Palliative treatment was offered in 15 cases. In the remaining 76 cases both endosonographic and histological assessments were available. In this later series one tumour was understaged and eight tumours were overstaged.

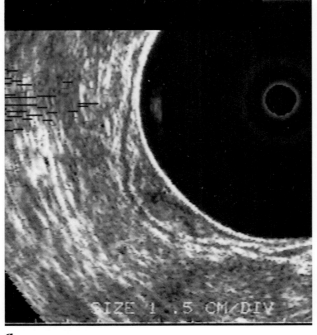

a

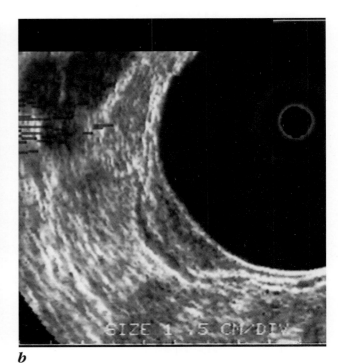

b

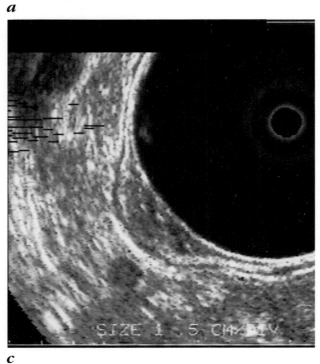

c

Figure 3.5 *(a) An adenocarcinoma of the rectum showing at this level the appearances of a uT1 tumour or a benign rectal polyp with an intact intermediate layer of submucosa. (b) The same tumour at a slightly different level demonstrating invasion of the submucosa. The interface between the muscularis propria and the surrounding fat is intact, thus making this a uT2 tumour. (c) The same tumour was thought to be node positive on the basis of this image demonstrating an adjacent hypoechoic node. This, histologically, was inflammatory.*

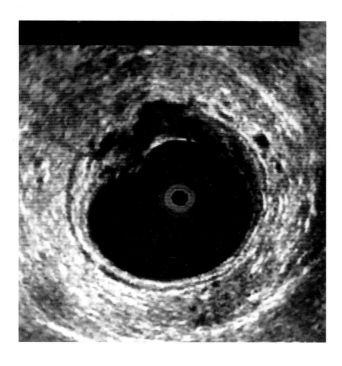

Figure 3.6 *An early uT3 tumour.*

Using an Olympus-Aloka ultrasonic endoscope (GF UM1, UM2, 7.5 MHz and Aloka probes of 7.5 MHz and 5 MHz), Saitoh et al defined three degrees of invasion, the first two broadly comparable to Dukes' histological staging:[14]

- Group 1 — tumour confined to the rectal wall.
- Group 2 — tumour invasion beyond the muscularis propria.
- Group 3 — tumour invasion into an adjacent organ.

Of their 99 patients, one could not be examined due to stenosis. Accuracy rates were 92.9 per cent in group 1, 91.9 per cent in group 2 and 75 per cent in group 3. Eight patients were overstaged and one understaged.

An early Italian study in which 23 patients with histologically proven rectal cancers were examined similarly gave good results using a CGR (SONEL 3000).[15] Using a 3.5-MHz transducer, radial scans were initially obtained but they used a 7.5-MHz

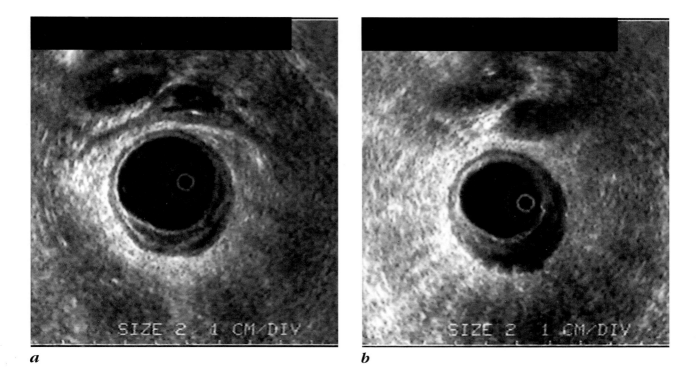

a   *b*

Figure 3.7 *(a) An endosonogram of a female patient demonstrating at this level the appearances of a uT2 tumour. The uterus and fallopian tubes are clearly seen anteriorly. (b) The same tumour at a higher level, now with clear invasion into the perirectal fat — a uT3 tumour.*

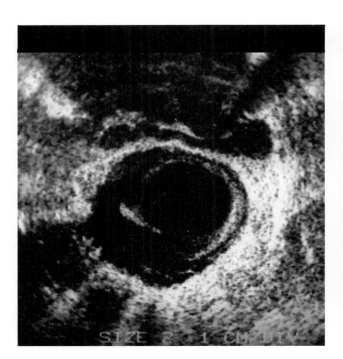

Figure 3.8 *A more advanced uT3 tumour showing the characteristic sawtooth projections into the adjacent tissue.*

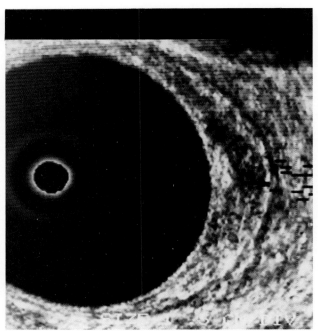

Figure 3.9 *A benign rectal adenoma.*

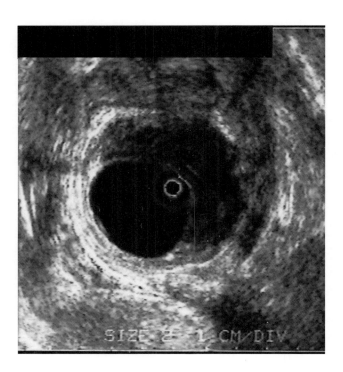

Figure 3.10 *A uT4 tumour with invasion into the prostate anteriorly and into the obturator internus on the left side of the patient.*

probe which provided 135° transverse sections of the rectal wall. Tumours were staged ultrasonically according to the UICC TNM system correctly in 20 cases. One tumour was overstaged as T2 and two tumours understaged as T2. Again, no attempt was made to define reporting criteria.

Glaser et al and Holdsworth et al, studying 86 and 36 patients, found that RES was accurate in 88 and 86 per cent of cases respectively.[16,17] Invasion through the rectal wall in the latter study was predicted with a sensitivity of 96 per cent and specificity of 50 per cent but was limited in that a transducer of 5.5 MHz was used.

A radial scanner (SSD-520, Aloka) and rigid endoprobe (ASU58, 7.5 MHz) were used in a large study from Japan on 122 patients.[18] An accuracy of 78 per cent was achieved. Endosonography overestimated the depth of cancer invasion in 21 patients. A suggested cause for the overestimation was inflammatory cell infiltration, while one possible cause of underestimation was microscopic invasion of cancer.

In order to define tumours suitable for peranal local excision, RES has been used to image small rectal tumours.[19] In discriminating between T1 and T2/3 tumours and between T1/2 and T3 tumours, the PPVs were 93 and 100 per cent respectively, while the NPVs were 94 and 93 per cent.

Table 3.1 Accuracy of digital, CT and RES for 42 palpable rectal adenocarcinomas.

	Accuracy	Sensitivity	Specificity	PPV	NPV
Digital	61.9	69.7	100	100	44.4
CT	71.4	76.5	62.5	89.7	38.5
RES	95.2	97.1	100	100	88.8

PPV = positive predictive value.
NPV = negative predictive value.

A large Italian series of 214 patients has been more recently reported. Tumours were located between 2 and 16 cm from the anal verge and RES achieved an accuracy of 94 per cent.[20]

Recently, flexible scanners have been used for the assessment of 120 rectal cancers. Similar degrees of accuracy have been reported to those with rigid probes, at 92 per cent.[21] The development of flexible echoendoprobes and their use in staging more proximal tumours is of little value, as little, if any, disagreement exists that surgery is the best form of treatment.

Beynon et al, in a prospective study of 100 patients, have also reported the accuracy of the technique. Accuracy has been compared with digital examination and CT in a combined study on 50 patients.[22–24] RES achieved in their hands an accuracy of 93 per cent in staging local invasion. It compared extremely favourably with the other modalities (Table 3.1). In 42 of the 50 patients who had palpable tumours, digital examination achieved an accuracy of 62 per cent, CT 71 per cent and RES 95 per cent.

Orrom et al have attempted to quantify the learning curve in RES by studying three groups of patients during consecutive periods of time.[25] The overall accuracy was 75 per cent; 60 per cent for the first 27 patients, 77 per cent for the next 30 patients and 95 per cent for the final 20 patients.

What are the effects of radiotherapy on the staging using RES? The accuracy of RES in predicting local invasion following radiotherapy fell from 86 per cent in those patients not given preoperative radiotherapy to 47 per cent in those given radiotherapy.[26] Poor resolution of the rectal wall and its post-radiotherapy thickening probably hamper interpretation of the extent of invasion (Fig. 3.11).

RES is therefore an accurate method of assessing local invasion in rectal cancer, as these studies from various authors and countries show. Further results are given in Table 3.2. Results in one study, however, appear poor, i.e. the report from Konishi et al from Japan.[27] The comparison and conclusion made in this study was not justified, as a hand-held linear scanner was compared with a fixed radial scanner (the 'Aloka chair'). This outdated instrument is of limited value in staging rectal cancer, as imaging is limited to the lower third of the rectum.

A high degree of correlation between RES predictions of local invasion and postoperative histopathology has been shown in the vast majority of studies quoted here. These predictions of the extent of local invasion compare very favourably with clinical assessment in the form of digital examination.

Table 3.2 Accuracy of endosonography in staging primary rectal cancer.

	No. patients	Accuracy (%)
Dragsted and Gammelgaard[6]	13	85
Hildebrandt and Fiefel[8]	25	92
Konishi et al[27]		
Linear scan	38	84
Radical scan	24	54
Romano et al[15]	23	91
Saitoh et al[14]	88	90
Hildebrandt et al[9]	76	88
Rifkin and Wechsler[12]	81	84
Accarpio et al[28]	54	94
Beynon[24]	100	93
Holdsworth et al[17]	36	86
Orrom et al[25]	77	75
Glaser et al[16]	86	88
Goldman et al[29]	32	81
Candio et al[30]	55	90
Yamashita et al[18]	122	78
Tarroni et al[20]	214	94
Katsura et al[21]	120	92

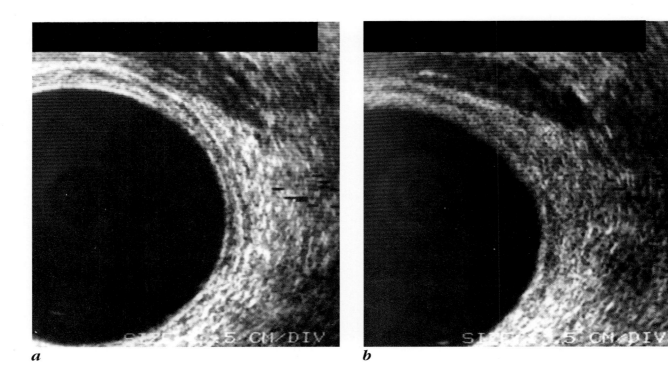

a   *b*

Figure 3.11 *(a,b) The rectal wall at two levels following radiotherapy. In (a) the layers can easily be identified while in (b) they are indistinct.*

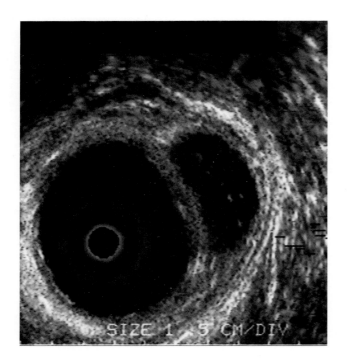

Figure 3.12 *A basiloid tumour of the anal canal imaged at the anorectal junction.*

In an attempt to see whether RES can differentiate between inflammatory and malignant infiltration, Beynon et al have prospectively measured the maximum depths of tumour infiltration both ultrasonically and histologically.[31] Depths of maximum tumour infiltration on RES were compared with those from the fixed specimen and histological slides. There was good correlation between the ultrasonic estimations of depth of penetration and the histological ones ($r = 0.36$, $P = 0.05$, CI = 95%; and $r = 0.46$, $P < 0.001$, CI = 99%). In 12 cases ultrasonic depths of tumour were measured in the laboratory on resected specimens and comparisons with pathological depths showed similar degrees of accuracy. RES may therefore help to distinguish between inflammatory and malignant infiltration, since it appears that both in vivo and in vitro what is seen ultrasonically reflects the true extent of the tumour.

RES has been used to assess extrarectal tumours such as leiomyosarcomas and rarer forms of rectal malignancy such as carcinoids, and assists with management decisions in these patients. In addition, with the advent of anal RES, tumours of the anal canal, such as squamous cell carcinomas and basiloid tumours, can also be imaged (Fig. 3.12).

LYMPH NODE ASSESSMENT

Of major independent prognostic significance for each patient is the involvement or not of perirectal lymph nodes by rectal adenocarcinoma. Involvement of lymph nodes is associated with decreasing survival rates and increasing local recurrence. In addition it has been observed from clinicopathological studies that the number of involved nodes is of importance, the presence of more than four nodes being associated with a poorer prognosis.

Patients such as these are those that would probably benefit from inclusion in trials of adjuvant therapy. The identification of these patients prior to surgical resection of the tumour has always been a problem. The success of RES in staging local invasion naturally led onto studies on the detection of lymph node metastases. There are now a few reports on the effectiveness of endosonography in the detection of mesorectal nodes.[9,12,14]

Hildebrandt et al, since using a 7-MHz transducer, reported the detection of lymph node metastases.[9] Metastatic involvement of pararectal lymph nodes was predicted in 12 of their 27 patients scanned preoperatively. However, these predictions were confirmed in only six cases, while the other six showed reactive changes. There was one false-negative case.

Ten of 13 patients with positive nodes were identified by Rifkin and Wechsler, with 6 false positives in the remaining 66 patients.[12] An overall sensitivity of 67 per cent was achieved, with a specificity of 91 per cent, PPV of 63 per cent and NPV of 92 per cent.

An accuracy of 73.2 per cent for the node-positive group using an ultrasonic endoscope has been achieved, and similarly 82.3 per cent for the node-negative group (19 false positives and 3 false negatives). Metastatic and non-metastatic nodes as small as 5 mm could be detected.[14]

Beynon et al have also reported their experience in detecting lymph node metastases (Table 3.3). Although there remains a problem with false positives, involved mesorectal nodes can undoubtedly be imaged.[32] Additionally, involved lymph nodes are of a significantly larger size than inflammatory nodes but the difference is not sufficient to make this of use clinically.

Despite this, when hypoechoic nodes are imaged and called positive the accuracies in the various series lie between 61 and 88 per cent. The lowest of these figures was in a study performed using a 5.5-MHz transducer.[17] It is probable that improved results

Table 3.3 The accuracy of endosonography in predicting N1 nodal involvement.

	No. patients	Accuracy (%)
Hildebrandt et al[9]	27	74
Rifkin and Wechsler[12]	81	88
Saitoh et al[14]	71	73
Beynon et al[32]	95	83
Holdsworth et al[17]	36	61
Tarroni et al[20]	214	84
Orrom et al[25]	77	82
Glaser et al[16]	73	79
Hildebrandt et al[33]	113	79

would have been obtained with the increased resolution afforded by a 7-MHz transducer.

Katsura et al, using a flexible instrument, have tried to differentiate inflammatory nodes from metastatic nodes based on the differing echo patterns.[21] Nodes were divided into two types based on sonographic appearances. 'A' nodes had an ill-defined border and an even and hyperechoic pattern. The incidence of metastases in these was 18.4 per cent. In type 'B' nodes with a well-defined border and an uneven and markedly hyperechoic intranodal pattern the incidence of metastases was 72 per cent. These observations do not reflect the experience of other endosonographers, who have observed that involved nodes tend to have a hypoechoic appearance (Fig. 3.13).

The learning curve in predicting lymph node involvement has been investigated in a study from Minnesota.[25] Twenty-one patients were assessed in the first year with a 71 per cent accuracy, while in the second year 40 patients were assessed with an accuracy of 88 per cent.

In an in vitro study, attenuation coefficients between nonspecific inflamed nodes and metastatic nodes have been compared and differences found.[33] Reactive nodes tended to have internal echoes and metastatic nodes none. Attempts to differentiate inflammatory nodes from tumour-involved nodes were subsequently made based on their appearance, i.e. hyperechoic or hypoechoic. Using these criteria, metastatic nodes were predicted with a sensitivity of 72 per cent, while inflammatory nodes were predicted with a specificity of 83 per cent and overall accuracy of 78 per cent. Micrometastases, mixed

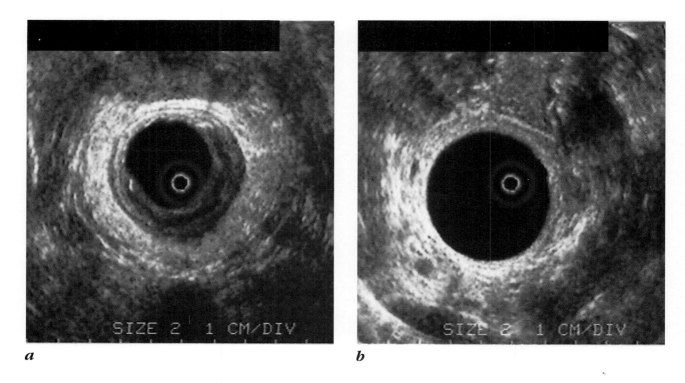

a   *b*

Figure 3.13 *(a) A uT3 tumour, with (b) involved lymph node above the level of the tumour.*

lymph nodes and changing echo patterns within inflammatory nodes were thought to explain the lack of improvement compared to other studies.

How does endosonography compare with other modalities in predicting nodal involvement? Beynon et al, in a comparative study, found CT to be inferior to RES in predicting the presence of lymph node metastases (Table 3.4).[32]

Milsom et al have approached the problem by performing ultrasonically guided biopsy of suspicious nodes to obtain a definitive staging.[34]

Lindmark et al have, in 53 patients, used Doppler ultrasound to help discriminate between lymph nodes and blood vessels.[35] The evaluation of nodal status was correct in 43 patients (accuracy 81 per cent). Nine of their patients had one or several metastases but RES did not identify all involved nodes in each case. Thirty-four patients had no involved nodes. There were two false positives and eight false negatives.

RES can therefore clearly identify extrarectal manifestations of malignancy as circumscribed echo-poor areas. Islands of tumour due to local invasion cannot be distinguished from involved nodes. The limitation of RES is that false-positive diagnoses occur which are not explained by the

Table 3.4 The accuracy of RES and CT in predicting nodal involvement, in a series of 46 patients with adenocarcinoma of the rectum.

	Accuracy	*Sensitivity*	*Specificity*	*PPV*	*NPV*
CT	56.5	25.0	90.9	75.0	52.6
RES	87.0	91.7	81.8	84.6	90.0

PPV = positive predictive value.
NPV = negative predictive value.

architecture of the nodes or their size. RES is more accurate than CT in the prediction of nodal involvement.

No direct comparison has been made with clinical assessment but it is hard to envisage that digital examination will achieve similar levels of accuracy as RES.

THE DETECTION OF LOCAL RECURRENCE

Despite apparently successful primary radical surgery, local recurrence occurs in 5–30 per cent of patients.[36]. Local recurrence is more common in tumours in the lower third of the rectum, which are large and locally invasive, and in those with lymphatic metastases.[37] Implantation of viable cells at surgery, giving true suture line recurrence readily detectable on sigmoidoscopy, is probably rare. The more usual so-called anastomotic recurrence results from local recurrence within the pelvis which presents at the anastomosis. This arises as a result of incomplete excision of the mesorectum.[38]

Is there any evidence that RES, which is so accurate in preoperative staging of rectal cancer, is of any use in the assessment and diagnosis of local recurrence? Since it is relatively inexpensive and portable, and the examination is brief, it can be included in a routine follow-up with clinical examination and sigmoidoscopy.

Female patients treated by restorative resection or abdominoperineal excision can also be scanned transvaginally.

Assessment of the neorectum is no different to preoperative examination in that five layers can be clearly identified. The appearance of an anastomosis may vary from normal to thickening of the rectal wall either completely circumferentially or locally (Figs. 3.14a,b). The localized thickening may be due to imaging of the teniae coli, which is the incomplete longitudinal muscle coat of the colon which forms the neorectum following surgery. The presence of staples does not affect the interpretation of the images as the staples are seen as small bright echoes and do not throw any significant shadow.

The ultrasonic anatomy of the pelvis may alter following surgery, and care is needed. Interpretation is aided by scanning approximately 3 months after treatment. Organs such as the uterus or segments of small bowel may prolapse alongside the neorectum and be mistaken for recurrent tumour.

Established locally recurrent cancer detectable by digital and sigmoidoscopic examination has endosonographic appearances identical to those of a primary rectal cancer, being echo-poor (Figs. 3.15 and 3.16). The extent of invasion can be assessed as with primary tumours, since there is again disruption of the ultrasonic layers.

Extrarectal locally recurrent tumour can be detected at an early stage. Tumour appears as a circumscribed echo-poor area in the para-anastomotic tissues. The presence of tumour cannot be diagnosed, however, just from the endosonogram. In these situations one of two policies can be adopted:

1. A repeat ultrasound scan can be performed after a suitable period of a month or 6 weeks. An increase in size will usually indicate recurrent malignancy.
2. A percutaneous transperineal biopsy can be performed using the endoprobe to guide the needle.

The effectiveness of RES in the follow-up of patients has been reported from a few centres.

Twenty-two recurrences were detected by Hildebrandt et al but only six of these were noted with ultrasound alone.[9] Three cases also had an elevated carcinoembryonic antigen (CEA), while ten cases had digital or endoscopic signs and an elevated CEA.

Eight local recurrences were detected by Romano et al[15] in their follow-up group of 42. Two ultrasonically false positives were detected but were subsequently shown to be due to fibrosis, diagnosis being confirmed by percutaneous biopsies.

Beynon et al imaged 22 recurrences in 85 patients, of which only 3 were detected solely by RES.[39] The others could be palpated digitally or were obvious on sigmoidoscopic examination.

In a study from Italy, 120 patients were followed up.[40] Seventeen recurrences were detected, six of which were asymptomatic. Twelve recurrences were detected by endorectal sonography, and five by endovaginal sonography. An accuracy of 97 per cent was reported, with a 94 per cent sensitivity and 98 per cent specificity. In six of their patients recurrences could be detected by either digital examination or endoscopy.

The Nottingham group made similar observations and they also noted that definition at the level of the anastomosis was lost because of loss of continuity of the layers.[41,42]

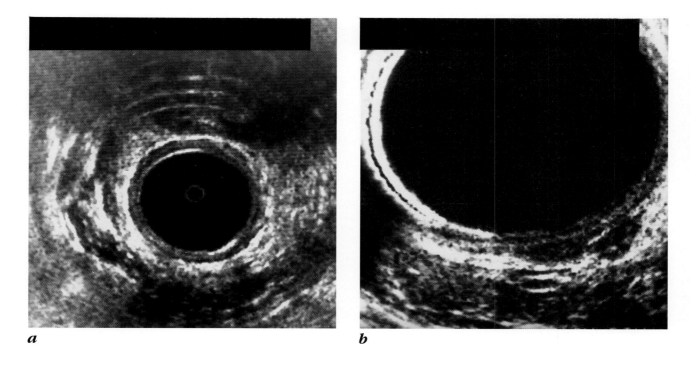

a b

Figure 3.14 *(a) Uniform thickness of the rectal wall at the level of an anastomosis following rectal surgery for carcinoma. (b) Localized thickening of the rectal wall at the site of an anastomosis.*

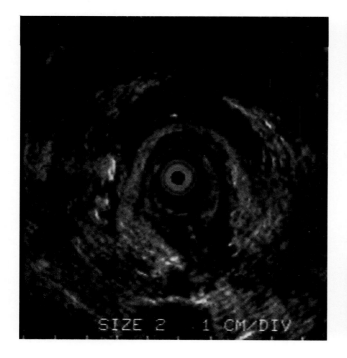

Figure 3.15 *A recurrent rectal carcinoma.*

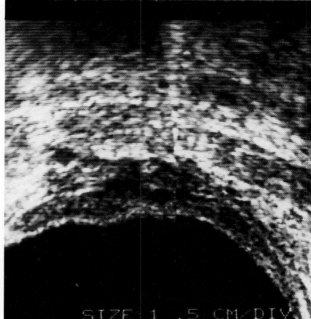

Figure 3.16 *A recurrent rectal carcinoma at the level of an anastomosis.*

Small extrarectal recurrences can therefore be detected before there is any evidence of luminal recurrence. Routine use of RES following the surgical treatment of rectal cancer allows a detailed examination of the pelvis, not previously possible without the use of more expensive techniques such as CT scan.

Used routinely from 3 months after surgery, RES would possibly allow the detection of early recurrence in a larger number of patients. Whether its use will allow second attempts at curative surgery remains to be seen.

PERIRECTAL AND RECTAL INFLAMMATORY DISEASE

The normal rectal wall thickness during examination varies depending on the distension of the balloon within the lumen. However, some reports have suggested that there is an increase in the overall thickness in active Crohn's disease and also in the absence of active proctitis in Crohn's.[43,44]

Perirectal abscesses are echo-poor with some reflective elements due probably to the presence of debris or air. Fistulae have been noted to be hypoechoic with occasional echogenicity due to the presence of air within the track. Cataldo et al[45] examined 24 patients with suspected perirectal sepsis and identified all 19 with pathology. They concluded that RES maybe an important addition to the clinical assessment of patients with complex perianal sepsis.

Various other perirectal lesions have been demonstrated using RES.[46] Carcinoid tumours, leiomyosarcomas (Fig. 3.17), melanomas and endometriosis tend to have a hypoechoic appearance. Similarly, rectal reduplication (Fig. 3.18), dermoids and retroperitoneal cystic hamartomas are hypoechoic. Lipomas tend to be hyperechoic, whereas chordomas have small internal bright areas due to calcification.

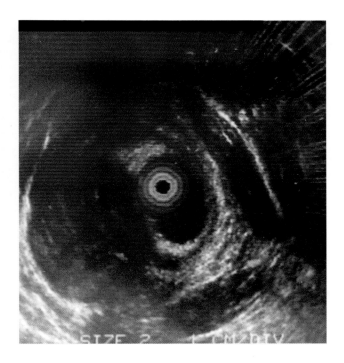

Figure 3.17 *A leiomyosarcoma of the rectum.*

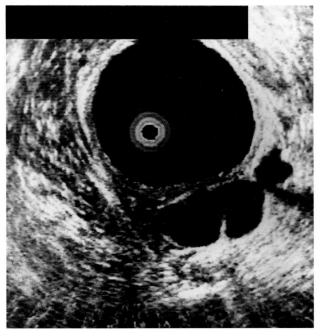

Figure 3.18 *Rectal reduplication seen as cystic areas posterior to the rectum.*

SUMMARY

What then is the future for RES? It has undoubtedly caught on more in the USA and Europe than in the UK. This may unfortunately be a reflection of the monetary constraints under which we practise.

It is likely that RES will have a role in deciding the treatment of benign rectal lesions, primary rectal cancer and recurrent rectal cancer, particularly in:

1. the identification of those lesions, benign and malignant, suitable for peranal local excision, and conversely those that are not;

2. the determination of whether locally advanced tumours are resectable or whether radiotherapy should be considered as a primary form of treatment before surgery;

3. the close follow-up of patients following treatment to detect local recurrence;

4. the investigation of pelvic abnormalities.

Undoubtedly, considering the accuracy of the technique, there should be a place for its use in the accurate allocation of patients with rectal malignancy into groups in trials of adjuvant therapy.

REFERENCES

1. Nicholls RJ, York Mason A, Morson BC et al, The clinical staging of rectal cancer, *Br J Surg* (1982) **69**:404–9.

2. Beynon J, Mortensen NJMcC, Foy DMA et al, Endorectal sonography: laboratory and clinical experience in Bristol, *Int J Colorect Dis* (1986) **1**:212–15.

3. Wild JJ, Reid JM, Diagnostic use of ultrasound, *Br J Phys Med* (1956) **19**:248–57.

4. Wild JJ, Foderick JW, The feasibility of echometric detection of cancer in the lower gastrointestinal tract I, *Am J Proctol Gastrol Colon Rectal Surg* (1978) Jan–Feb:16–25.

5. Wild JJ, Foderick JW, The feasibility of echometric detection of cancer of the lower gastrointestinal tract II, *Am J Proctol Gastrol Colon Rectal Surg* (1978) Mar–Apr:11–20.

6. Dragsted J, Gammelgaard J, Endoluminal ultrasonic scanning in the evaluation of rectal cancer, *Gastrointest Radiol* (1983) **8**:367–9.

7. Alzin HH, Kohlberger E, Schwaiger R, Alloussi S, Valeur de l'echographie endorectale dans la chirurgie du rectum, *Ann Radiol* (1983) **26**:334–6.

8. Hildebrandt U, Fiefel G, Pre-operative staging of rectal cancer by intrarectal ultrasound, *Dis Colon Rectum* (1985) **28**:42–6.

9. Hildebrandt U, Fiefel G, Schwarz HP, Scherr O, Endorectal ultrasound: instrumentation and clinical aspects, *Int J Colorectal Dis* (1986) **1**:203–7.

10. Beynon J, Foy DMA, Channer JL et al, The endosonic appearances of normal colon and rectum, *Dis Colon Rectum* (1986) **29**:810–13.

11. Rifkin MD, Marks GJ, Transrectal US as an adjunct in the diagnosis of rectal and extrarectal tumours, *Radiology* (1985) **157**:499–502.

12. Rifkin MD, Wechsler RJ, A comparison of computed tomography and endorectal ultrasound in staging rectal cancer, *Int J Colorectal Dis* (1986) **1**:219–23.

13. Fiefel G, Hildebrandt U, Dhom G, Die endorektale sonographie beim rektumcarcinom, *Chirurg* (1985) **56**:398–402.

14. Saitoh N, Okui K, Sarashina H et al, Evaluation of echographic diagnosis of rectal cancer using intrarectal ultrasonic examination, *Dis Colon Rectum* (1986) **29**:234–42.

15. Romano G, De Rosa P, Vallone G et al, Intrarectal ultrasound and computed tomography in the pre- and postoperative assessment of patients with rectal carcinoma, *Br J Surg* (1985) **72**:S117–19.

16. Glaser F, Schlag P, Herfarth Ch, Endorectal ultrasonography for the assessment of invasion of rectal tumours and lymph node involvement, *Br J Surg* (1990) **77**:883–7.

17. Holdsworth PJ, Johnston D, Chalmers AG et al, Endoluminal ultrasound and computed tomography in the staging of rectal cancer, *Br J Surg* (1988) **75**:1019–22.

18. Yamashita Y, Machi J, Shirouzu K et al, Evaluation of endorectal ultrasound for the assessment of wall invasion of rectal cancer, *Dis Colon Rectum* (1988) **31**:617–23.

19. Detry R, Kartheuser A, Endorectal ultrasonography in staging small rectal tumours, *Br J Surg* (1992) **79**:s30.

20. Tarroni D, Mascagni D, Urciuoli P et al, Endoluminal ultrasonographic accuracy in rectal cancer, *Br J Surg* (1992) **79**:s30.

21. Katsura Y, Yamada K, Ishizawa T et al, Endorectal ultrasonography for the assessment of wall invasion and lymph node metastasis in rectal cancer, *Dis Colon Rectum* (1992) **35**:362–8.

22. Beynon J, Foy DMA, Roe AM, et al, Endoluminal ultrasound in the assessment of local invasion in rectal cancer, *Br J Surg* (1986) **73**: 474–7.

23. Beynon J, Mortensen NJMcC, Foy DMA et al, Preoperative assessment of local invasion in rectal cancer: digital examination, endoluminal sonography or computed tomography? *Br J Surg* (1986) **73**:1015–17.

24. Beynon J, An evaluation of the role of rectal endosonography in rectal cancer, *Ann R Coll Surg Engl* (1989) **71**:131–9.

25. Orrom WJ, Wong WD, Rothenberger DA et al, Endorectal ultrasound in the preoperative staging of rectal tumours. A learning experience, *Dis Colon Rectum* (1990) **33**:654–9.

26. Napoleon B, Pujol B, Berger F et al, Accuracy of endosonography in the staging of rectal cancer treated by radiotherapy, *Br J Surg* (1991) **78**:785–8.

27. Konishi F, Muto T, Takahashi H et al, Transrectal ultrasonography for the assessment of invasion of rectal carcinoma, *Dis Colon Rectum* (1985) **28**:889–94.

28. Accarpio G, Scopinaro G, Claudiani F et al, Experience with local rectal cancer excision in light of two recent preoperative diagnostic methods, *Dis Colon Rectum* (1987) **30**:296–8.

29. Goldman S, Arvidsson H, Norming U et al, Transrectal ultrasound and computed tomography in preoperative staging of lower rectal adenocarcinoma, *Gastrointest Radiol* (1991) **16**:259–63.

30. Candio G, Mosca F, Campatelli A et al, Endosonographic staging of rectal carcinoma, *Gastrointest Radiol* (1987) **12**:289–95.

31. Beynon J, Mortensen NJMcC, Rigby H, Channer J, Rectal endosonography accurately predicts depth of penetration in rectal cancer, *Int J Colorectal Dis* (1992) **7**:4–7.

32. Beynon J, Mortensen NJMcC, Foy DMA et al, Pre-operative assessment of meso-rectal lymph node involvement in rectal cancer, *Br J Surg* (1989) **6**:276–9.

33. Hildebrandt U, Klein G, Schwarz HP et al, Endosonography of pararectal lymph nodes. In vitro and in vivo evaluation, *Dis Colon Rectum* (1990) **33**:863–8.

34. Milsom JW, Lavery IC, Stolfi VM et al, The expanding utility of endo-luminal ultrasonography in the management of rectal cancer, *Surgery* (1992) **112**:832–41.

35. Lindmark G, Elvin A, Pahlman L, Glimelius B, The value of endosonography in preoperative staging of rectal cancer, *Int J Colorectal Dis* (1992) **7**:162–6.

36. Phillips RKS, Hittinger R, Blesovsky L et al, Local recurrence following 'curative' surgery for large bowel cancer. II. The rectum and rectosigmoid, *Br J Surg* (1984) **71**:17–20.

37. Wood CB, Ratcliffe JG, Burt TW et al, Local tumour invasion as a prognostic factor in colorectal carcinoma, *Br J Surg* (1981) **68**:326–8.

38. Heald RJ, Ryall RDH, Recurrence and survival after total mesorectal excision for rectal cancer, *Lancet* (1986) **i**:1479–82.

39. Beynon J, Mortensen NJMcC, Foy DMA et al, The detection and evaluation of locally recurrent rectal cancer with rectal endosonography, *Dis Colon Rectum* (1989) **32**:509–17.

40. Mascagni D, Corellini L, Urciuoli P, Di Matteo G, Endoluminal ultrasound for early detection of local recurrence of rectal cancer, *Br J Surg* (1989) **76**:1176–80.

41. Charnley RM, Pye G, Amar SS, Hardcastle JH, The early detection of recurrent rectal carcinoma by rectal endosonography, *Br J Surg* (1988) **75**:1232.

42. Charnley RM, Heywood MF, Hardcastle JD, Rectal endosonography for the visualisation of the anastomosis after anterior resection and its relevance to local recurrence, *Int J Colorectal Dis* (1990) **5**:127–9.

43. Hulsmans F-jH, Bosma A, Mulder PJJ et al, Perirectal lymph nodes in rectal cancer: in vitro correlation of sonographic parameters and histopathologic findings, *Radiology* (1992) **184**:553–6.

44. Outreye van MJ, Pelckmans PA, Michielsen PP, Maercke van Y, Value of transrectal ultrasonography in Crohn's disease, *Gastroenterology* (1991) **101**:1171–7.

45. Cataldo PA, Senagore A, Luchtefield MA, Intrarectal ultrasound in the evaluation of perirectal abscess, *Dis Colon Rectum* (1993) **36**:554–8.

46. St Ville EW, Jafri SZH, Madrazo BL et al, Endorectal sonography in the evaluation of rectal and perirectal disease, *AJR* (1991) **157**:503–8.

Chapter 4 Anal Endosonography

Clive I Bartram

INTRODUCTION

Endosonography of the anal canal is a relatively new technique, of most value in assessing sphincter damage in faecal incontinence. The same apparatus may be used as for rectal endosonograpy,[1] although a hard cone[2] is preferable to a balloon system in the anal canal. Linear probes that were acceptable for endosonography in the rectum are not ideal in the canal. Sphincters, being circular structures, really require a radial image for assessment.

TECHNIQUE

The recommended modification is to use a hard plastic cone on the B & K Medical rectal endoprobe. The cone is made of a sonolucent TPX plastic, and is 1.7 cm in outer diameter (Fig. 4.1). A small hole at the top allows air to escape as the assembly is filled with degassed water.

No patient preparation is required. The probe may be coated with a little coupling gel and covered with a protective sheath, which is also lubricated before gently inserting into the anal canal. It is easiest to examine patients on their left side. It may be preferable to scan the patient in the same plane, to coordinate probe movements with the orientation of the pelvis. This means that on the screen the patient's left side is lowermost, with anterior on the right of the screen.

The probe should be cleaned with industrial spirit between cases, and if contaminated or after use, disassembled, washed and soaked in glutaraldehyde.

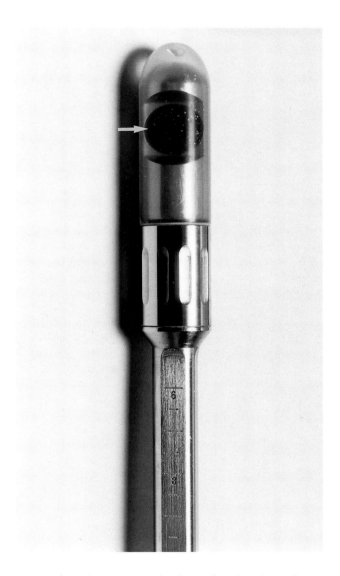

Figure 4.1 *The B & K Medical rectal endoprobe with water-filled hard cone. The 7-MHz transducer (arrow) is rotated mechanically to give a 360° image.*

NORMAL ANATOMY

The sonographic anatomy follows the pattern of the rectum, with the additional complexity of the striated

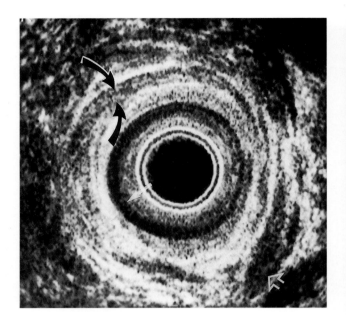

Figure 4.2 *Normal anatomy, mid-canal level in a male patient. The two bright reflections from the cone are innermost. Outside these is the hyperechoic subepithelial layer, surrounded by the hypoechoic internal sphincter (arrow). The longitudinal muscle is a broad hyperechoic band around this, with the external sphincter seen as a separate outer hypoechoic ring (curved arrows). All the images are orientated in the same plane as the patient was examined. The patient's anterior is on the right of the film, the posterior on the left, with the right side uppermost. The superficial transverse perineii are seen anteriorly (open arrow) meeting at the central point of the perineum.*

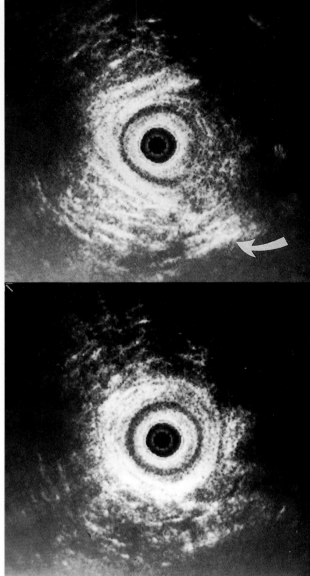

Figure 4.3 *Normal anatomy, with two views in a female patient. The upper image is at the deep level. The 'U' shape of the puborectalis and deep external sphincter extends anteriorly towards the pubic rami (curved arrow). Note the lack of any external sphincter anteriorly. The longitudinal muscle is poorly defined, probably due to a change in the orientation of the fibroelastic stroma so that it is less echogenic in this plane. In the lower image the intact ring of the external sphincter is now visible. The longitudinal muscle and external sphincter are of the same echogenicity, and so are indistinguishable – a typical finding in females.*

external sphincter muscle. The acoustic layers working from the inside outwards are as follows (Fig. 4.2):

- The cone causes two bright echoes.
- The mucosa is not defined.
- In the anal canal there is no muscularis mucosae to define a submucosa. Although this term is used, it is anatomically incorrect and 'subepithelial' is preferred. The subepithelial tissues are echogenic, in keeping with the submucosa of the rectum.
- The internal anal sphincter (IAS) surrounds the subepithelium. It is derived from the circular muscle of the rectum, and is a well-defined hypoechoic ring, ending at the level of the dentate line.

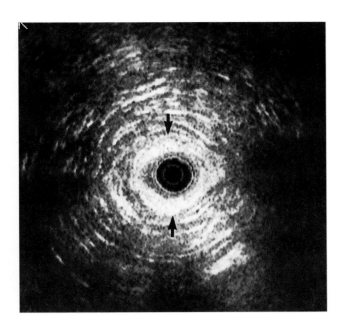

Figure 4.4 *The subcutaneous external sphincter is brightly echogenic (arrows). The internal sphincter is not visible, as the subcutaneous part of the sphincter is caudal to the termination of the internal sphincter.*

- Outside the IAS is the longitudinal muscle,[3] a complex structure, formed from the longitudinal muscle of the outer layer of the muscularis propria of the rectum. It is invested with a fibroelastic component from the fascia over the rectum and levator ani. It acts as an anchor, with its fibroelastic component permeating through the external anal sphincter (EAS), terminating in the perianal skin and perineal structures, so that the anal sphincter is held in place within the pelvis.

The EAS is striated muscle derived from the levator ani, and attached to the puborectalis. It forms a sling around the anorectum, and inserts anteriorly into the pubic rami. The EAS is divided into three layers: the deep, superficial and subcutaneous. In 60 per cent of females the EAS is similar in echogenicity to the longitudinal muscle,[4] and so is indistinguishable from it (Fig. 4.3). In the remaining 40 per cent of females and all males the EAS is mainly hypoechoic, and seen as a concentric ring around the longitudinal muscle. In both sexes the subcutaneous EAS is hyperechoic (Fig. 4.4). This part lies below the level of the IAS and tends to be conical, with the tail pointing posteriorly. The superficial part is elliptical, with muscle fibres inserting anteriorly into the perineal body and posteriorly into the anococcygeal ligament. The deep part is annular. There is an important difference in the configuration of the EAS between the sexes. In males it is more or less symmetrical, but in females it is shorter anteriorly, with the deep fibres running downwards and forwards into an anterior muscle bundle. When viewed in cross-section, this causes an apparent defect anteriorly high in the canal. Withdrawing the probe cuts through the sloping muscle bundles as they come around the sides, running anteriorly and inferiorly to fuse into the anterior muscle bundle at a lower level (Fig. 4.3).

The average thickness of the EAS is 8.6 ± 1 mm in males, and 7.7 ± 1.1 mm in females. The difference is related to the overall heavier weight of males. The longitudinal muscle is 2.5 ± 0.6 mm, and 2.9 ± 0.6 mm, and the IAS is 1.8 ± 0.5 mm, and 1.9 ± 0.6 mm respectively. An increase in the thickness of the IAS with age has been shown,[5] measuring 2.4–2.7 mm >55 years, and 2.8–3.5 mm >55 years. Other series have shown a 95 per cent confidence interval of 1–3.3 mm, also with a significant increase with age.[6] This relates to fibrous replacement of the smooth muscle of the internal sphincter, which makes the sphincter thicker as well as more echogenic.

SPHINCTER ABNORMALITIES

INTERNAL SPHINCTER

The IAS forms an intact ring. It should be of equal thickness all round at any given level, though it is often slightly thicker in the terminal portion. Any loss of continuity, or pronounced localized thinning, is abnormal.

Surgical division of the IAS, as at lateral internal sphincterotomy, produces a well-defined break in the IAS (Fig. 4.5). The ends are typically rounded and the

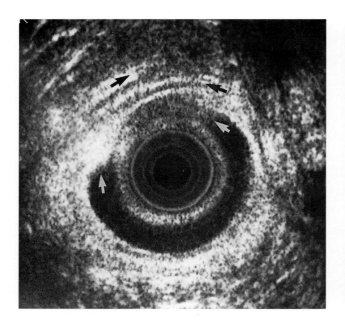

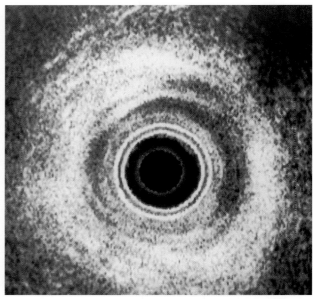

Figure 4.5 *Lateral internal anal sphincterotomy in a female patient for fissure. The rounded ends of the cut internal sphincter are clearly seen (white arrows). Unfortunately the external sphincter had also been incised (black arrows), rendering the patient faecally incontinent.*

Figure 4.6 *Fragmentation of the internal sphincter following a stretch procedure.*

remaining sphincter may bunch up a bit so that it seems thick. The surgical intention is to divide the lower third of the sphincter. Endosonography suggests that in men this is achieved,[7] but in women, who have shorter internal sphincters, sphincterotomy may inadvertently involve the entire length of the sphincter. This carries the risk of precipitating faecal incontinence.

Dilatation or stretch procedures are still common treatment for fissure or haemorrhoids. These may fragment the IAS (Fig. 4.6) and render the patient incontinent.[8] The endosonographic appearances are typical, with multiple defects and thin ragged remnants. The EAS may also be involved.

The IAS may be abnormally thick in some patients with obstructed defaecation.[9] Any sphincter >4 mm thick is abnormal. Very grossly thickened internal sphincters, up to 1 cm in thickness, have been associated with proctalgia fugax.[10]

EXTERNAL SPHINCTER

Abnormalities of the EAS are not so easy to recognize. Aberrant insertions of part of the EAS are relatively common, and it is important not to confuse normal variants with defects in the muscle.

Physical disruption of the EAS may be surgical, obstetric or traumatic in origin. Once the striated muscle ring is torn, the ends separate and heal by granulation tissue, leaving a fibrous scar. This creates an amorphous but relatively homogeneous segment, usually hypoechoic relative to the normal EAS and lacking its slightly striated texture (Figs. 4.7 and 4.8). Comparisons with surgery have shown[11] that endosonography was much more accurate in detecting sphincter defects than digital, manometric or concentric needle electromyography (EMG). Hitherto EMG has been the main method for clinically confirming EAS defects. It has been suggested that

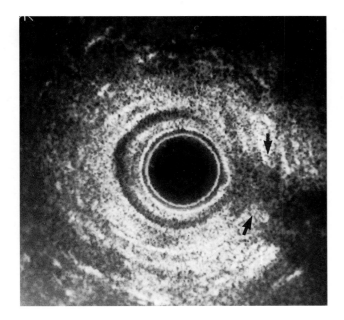

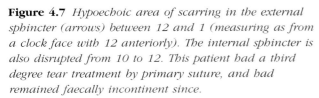

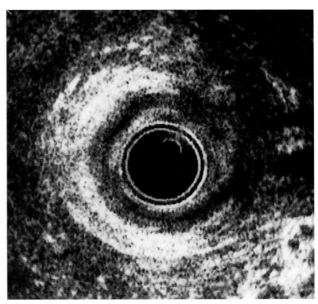

Figure 4.7 *Hypoechoic area of scarring in the external sphincter (arrows) between 12 and 1 (measuring as from a clock face with 12 anteriorly). The internal sphincter is also disrupted from 10 to 12. This patient had a third degree tear treatment by primary suture, and had remained faecally incontinent since.*

Figure 4.8 *Large obstetric injury with external and internal sphincter defects between 9 and 1, following a forceps delivery with rotation.*

anal endosonography (AES) is now the examination of choice[12] for this.

One of the commonest causes of sphincter damage is vaginal delivery. A tear in some part of the sphincter occurs during 35 per cent of first-time deliveries,[13] and is more common with forceps-assisted delivery. Clinically recognized third degree tears are much less common. It is usual to perform a primary repair for third degree tears. The results from this are less than perfect. Endosonography has shown that many still have residual sphincter defects[14,15] (Fig. 4.7). Childbirth injuries often have only transient symptoms of faecal incontinence. It is not until later in life, when the effects of ageing, the menopause and progressive neuropathy combine, that the pelvic floor becomes decompensated and overt symptoms develop. Two studies[16,17] suggest that sphincter defects will be found in 87–90 per cent of women presenting with faecal incontinence. AES is important in the investigation of faecal incontinence,[18–21] as sphincter damage may be missed on other tests, and the patient then denied their best opportunity of recovering continence, which is by surgical repair. Good functional results correlate with the restoration of an intact external ring.[22]

ANAL SEPSIS

Most fistulae *in ano* are straightforward, and it is really only complex fistulae that create difficulties. Extensive surgery may be needed to lay open all the tracks and drain abscesses. This will damage the sphincter so that there is a risk of the patient becoming incontinent. On the other hand, if any part of the fistula remains, by either being missed or not having

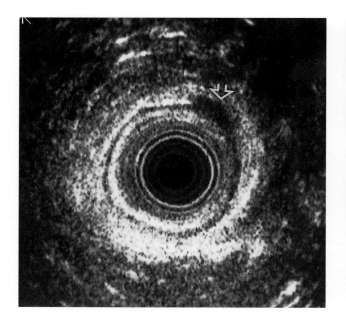

Figure 4.9 *Intersphincteric fistulous tract (arrow) adjacent to the internal sphincter at the site of an internal opening.*

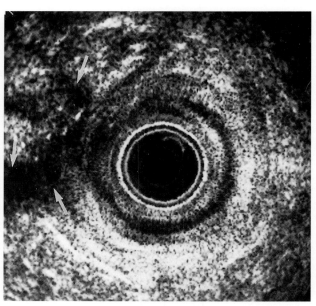

Figure 4.10 *Transphincteric extension of a fistula. Irregular hypoechoic tracking (arrows) through the external sphincter. Several bright foci are noted, which may be due to granulation tissue, foreign bodies or gas.*

been dealt with surgically, the fistula will recur. It would obviously be helpful to assess the fistula preoperatively, to be certain as to the full extent of the tracks and situation of abscesses. Fistulography has been used, but is not generally considered helpful.[23] Transrectal ultrasound has been found to be superior to computed tomography (CT) for detecting fistulae and abscesses.[24] The detection of internal openings and primary and secondary tracks by AES has been compared to clinical examination and operative findings.[25] Endosonography was found to be accurate in detecting tracks and openings within the anal ring, but failed to detect superficial or high tracks. Magnetic resonance imaging (MRI), with its capability for multiplanar imaging and detection of granulation tissue with fat suppression protocols, appears to be the examination of choice.[26]

Tracks appear as hypoechoic bands on endosonography. As the probe is moved within the canal, the course of the tracks can be traced. The clinical description of an intersphincteric track refers to a track between the external and internal sphincters which is running in the longitudinal muscle. Where the track merges into the internal sphincter, this is the site of an internal opening (Fig. 4.9). If the track extends through the EAS, transphincteric extension has occurred (Fig. 4.10). This is surgically important, as it then becomes more difficult to deal with the track, as the EAS cannot be incised at will, if incontinence is to be avoided. Abscesses are indicated by large irregular hypoechoic collections, and confirmed if these contain multiple bright echoes from gas bubbles (Fig. 4.11). Localized bright reflections may be due to granulation tissue or even foreign bodies.[27] After several operations, there is often considerable residual fibrosis and deformity (Fig. 4.12). Scarring is difficult to distinguish endosonographically from active low-grade inflammation, so that it is difficult to tell if there is sepsis present. At this stage it is important to assess how much normal sphincter remains, as this may affect surgical management.

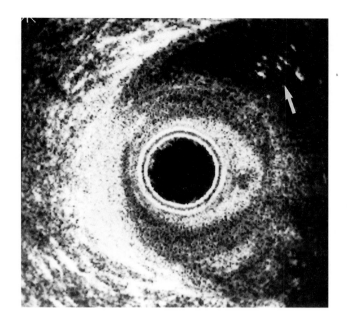

Figure 4.11 *A large anterior perisphincteric abscess in a patient with Crohn's disease. Gas bubbles are present within the abscess (arrow).*

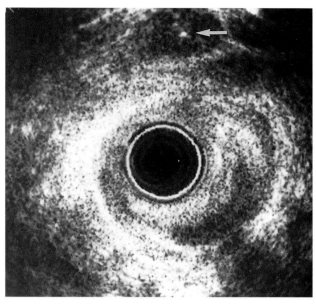

Figure 4.12 *Multiple operations for recurrent fistula-in-ano has left the sphincter extensively scarred in both the external and internal components. Inflammatory tissue around a Seton in an extrasphincteric track is seen.*

ANAL MALIGNANCY

Sphincter involvement by low rectal cancers may be demonstrated on AES (Fig. 4.13), but this has little practical value, as these patients require abdominoperineal excision irrespective of the degree of involvement. Treatment of anal cancer is not so clear-cut, and radiotherapy may be the preferred option. These tumours are currently staged by size (Table 4.1) and involvement of adjacent structures. Based on ultrasound findings, tumours may be classified more precisely (Table 4.2). In a review of 50 patients, Goldman et al[28] found that all tumours T1–2/uT1–2 had a complete response to radiotherapy, whereas those with a T1–2/uT3–4 had a 64 per cent response, and there was no response with T3–4/uT3–4. Recurrence will be indicated by a hypoechoic mass, so that AES is also useful in the follow-up of these patients.

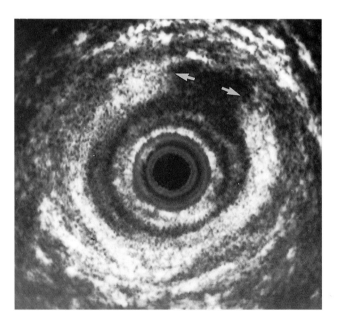

Figure 4.13 *This patient had a large low rectal carcinoma. The lower extent of this could be traced down into the sphincter, where the hypoechoic tumour mass is seen infiltrating the external sphincter (arrows).*

Table 4.1

T stage	Description of tumour
T1	<2 cm in greatest dimension
T2	2–5 cm
T3	>5 cm
T4	Involving adjacent organ

Table 4.2

uT stage	Description of tumour
uT1	Confined to subepithelium
uT2	Confined to sphincter
uT3	Penetrating outside sphincter
uT4	Involving adjacent organs

INDICATIONS – SUMMARY

- Faecal incontinence to assess internal/external sphincter damage.
- Anal pain (± constipation). Abnormally thick internal sphincter, suggesting a smooth muscle myopathy.
- Anal sepsis with a complex fistula. Transphincteric extension, or following multiple operations, state of residual sphincter.
- Anal malignancy to stage small tumours. Recurrent disease.

REFERENCES

1. Tjandra JJ, Milsom JW, Stolfi VM, Lavery I, Oakley J, Church J, Fazio V, Endoluminal ultrasound defines anatomy of the anal canal and pelvic floor, *Dis Colon Rectum* (1992) **35**:465–70.

2. Law PJ, Bartram CI, Anal endosonography: technique and normal anatomy, *Gastrointest Radiol* (1989) **14**:349–53.

3. Sultan AH, Nicholls RJ, Kamm MA, Hudson CN, Beynon J, Bartram CI, Anal endosonography and correlation with in vitro and in vivo anatomy, *Br J Surg* (1993) **80**:508–11.

4. Sultan AH, Kamm MA, Nicholls RJ, Bartram CI, Endosonography of the anal sphincters: normal anatomy and comparison with manometry, *Clin Radiol* (1994) **49**:368–74.

5. Burnett SJ, Bartram CI, Endosonographic variations in the normal internal anal sphincter, *Int J Colorect Dis* (1991) **6**:2–4.

6. Nielsen MB, Hause C, Rasmussen OØ, Sorensen M, Perdersen JF, Christiansen J, Anal sphincter size measured by endosonography in healthy volunteers, *Acta Radiol* (1992) **33**:453–6.

7. Sultan AH, Kamm MA, Nicholls RJ, Bartram CI, Internal anal sphincter division during lateral sphincterotomy, A prospective study, *Dis Colon Rectum* (accepted for publication).

8. Speakman CTM, Burnett SJD, Kamm MA, Bartram CI, Sphincter injury after anal dilatation demonstrated by anal endosonography, *Br J Surg* (1991) **78**:1429–30.

9. Nielsen MB, Rasmussen OØ, Pedersen JF, Christiansen J, Anal endosonography findings in patients with obstructed defecation, *Acta Radiol* (1993) **34**:35–8.

10. Kamm MA, Hoyle CHH, Burleigh DE et al, Hereditary internal sphincter myopathy causing proctalgia fugax and constipation, *Gastroenterology* (1991) **100**:805.

11. Sultan AH, Kamm MA, Talbot AC, Nicholls JR, Bartram CI, Anal endosonography for identifying external sphincter defects confirmed histologically, *Br J Surg* (1994) **81**:463–5.

12. Tjandra JJ, Milson JW, Schroeder T, Fazio VW, Endoluminal ultrasound is preferable to electromyography in mapping anal sphincter defects, *Dis Colon Rectum* (1993) **36**:689–92.

13. Sultan AH, Kamm MA, Hudson CN, Thomas JM, Bartram CI, Anal sphincter disruption during vaginal delivery, *New Eng J Med* (1993) **329**:1905–11.

14. Sultan AH, Kamm MA, Hudson CN, Bartram CI, Third degree obstetric anal sphincter tears: risk factors and outcome of primary repair, *Br Med J* (1994) **308**:887–91.

15. Nielsen MB, Rasmussen OØ, Pedersen JF, Christiansen J, Risk of sphincter damage and anal incontinence after anal dilatation for fissure-in-ano, *Dis Colon Rectum* (1993) **36**:677–80

16. Burnett SJD, Spence-Jones C, Speakman CTM, Kamm MA, Hudson CN, Bartram CI, Unsuspected sphincter damage following childbirth revealed by anal endosonography, *Br J Radiol* (1991) **64**:225–7.

17. Deen KI, Kumar D, Williams JG, Olliff J, Keighley MRB, The prevalence of anal sphincter defects in faecal incontinence: a prospective study, *Gut* (1993) **34**:685–8.

18. Law PJ, Kamm MA, Bartram CI, Anal endosonography in the investigation of faecal incontinence, *Br J Surg* (1991) **78**:312–14.

19. Cuesta MA, Meijer S, Derksen EJ, Boutkan H, Meuwissen SGM, Anal sphincter imaging in faecal incontinence using endosonography, *Dis Colon Rectum* (1992) **35**:59–63.

20. Nielsen MB, Hauge C, Pedersen JF, Christiansen J, Endosonographic evaluation of patients with anal incontinence, *AJR* (1993) **160**:771–5.

21. Felt-Bermsa RJ, Cuesta MA, Koorevaar M, Striyen RL, Menwissen SG, Dereksen EJ, Wesdrop RI, Anal endosonography: relationship with anal manometry and neurophysiologic tests, *Dis Colon Rectum* (1992) **35**:944–9.

22. Engel AF, Sultan AH, Kamm MA, Nicholls RJ, Bartram CI, Anterior anal sphincter repair in patients with obstetric trauma, *Br J Surg* (1994) **81**:1231–4.

23. Kuijpers HC, Schulpen T, Fistulography for fistula-in-ano. Is it useful? *Dis Colon Rectum* (1985) **28**:103–4.

24. Schratter-Sehn AU, Lochs H, Vogelsang H et al, Comparison of transrectal ultrasonography and computed tomography in the diagnosis of periano-rectal fistulas in patients with Crohn's disease, *Gastroenterology* (1992) **102**:A691.

25. Choen S, Burnett S, Bartram CI, Nicholls RJ, Comparison between anal endosonography and digital examination in the evaluation of anal fistulae, *Br J Surg* (1991) **78**:445–7.

26. Lunniss PJ, Armstrong P, Barker PG, Reznek RH, Phillips RK, Magnetic resonance imaging (MRI) of anal fistulae, *Lancet* (1992) **340**:394–6.

27. Law PJ, Talbot RW, Bartram CI, Northover JMA, Anal endosonography in the evaluation of perianal sepsis and fistulo in ano, *Br J Surg* (1989) **76**:752–5.

28. Goldman S, Norming U, Svensson C, Glimelius B, Transanorectal ultrasonography in the staging of anal epidermoid carcinoma, *Int J Colorect Dis* (1991) **6**:152–7.

Chapter 5 Transvaginal Ultrasound in Gynecology

Edward A Lyons
Clifford S Levi
Sidney M Dashefsky

INTRODUCTION

The assessment of the female pelvis has taken on a new dimension with the advent of endo- or transvaginal ultrasound (TVS). Due to the close proximity of the transducer to the pelvic organs, one now not only has detailed visualization of structures as small as 1 mm but also can use palpation to detect tenderness or the presence of adhesions. With the use of phased array transvaginal probes, Doppler ultrasound is used to study hemodynamics and further characterize normal and pathological processes.

TECHNIQUES AND INSTRUMENTATION

The patient lies on the examining table with knees bent and spread slightly apart. A sheet covers the lower abdomen and legs so as to maintain a degree of privacy. In some cases it is helpful to elevate the pelvis with several sheets rolled up or with a foam wedge. This allows better access for examining the fundus in the acutely anteverted uterus.

The patient usually arrives with a partially full urinary bladder. It is strongly recommended to do an initial assessment transabdominally to detect any masses which are either too attenuating, too large or out of the field of view of the transvaginal probe. Undegenerated fibroids are common and may be difficult to see due to their propensity for attenuation. Transvaginally, only a small portion of the mass may be seen adjacent to the probe, with the bulk of the mass being 'invisible'. Similarly, a solid, fat-filled dermoid teratoma may not be appreciated, as only the first few centimeters will be seen, due to the attenuation. Even a simple cyst, although easy to see sonographically, may be missed if it lies outside of the pelvis.

Higher frequency mechanical sector or phased array transducers (5.0–7.5 MHz) are commonly available. The high frequency and close proximity give better resolution. A disadvantage is the limited field of view, which may reach only 8 cm. Most transvaginal probes can image to a depth of approximately 8 cm, with a focal range from 2 cm to 6 cm. The image display angle is typically 90–100° but can be as wide as 270°.

The transducer should be cleaned thoroughly before and after use. In our laboratory it is stored in a bactericidal solution (Cidex) between examinations and overnight. We use the plastic storage tube of a 50-ml syringe which has been inserted into the end of a Rubbermaid trolley that sits adjacent to each scanner. It is used to hold towels, gel and the filming device. The probe is removed from the solution, dried and wiped. It is covered with a condom containing scanning gel. Sterile gel is then placed carefully on the outer surface of the condom as a lubricant for probe insertion. Care must be taken not to tear the condom while applying it to the probe or putting on the lubricant. In the infertile patient undergoing ovarian stimulation and follicle monitoring, lubricants with antispermicidal properties should be avoided and glycerin or warm water used instead.

CONSENT

It is very important to explain the procedure to the patient and obtain her verbal consent. The study is often likened to a conventional pelvic examination. A written consent is seldom necessary but this is a decision made by each individual facility. It is now common practice to have a female chaperon in the room during the procedure if it is done by a male sonographer.

PROBE INSERTION

The probe is inserted into the vagina either by the patient herself or by the sonographer or sonologist. It is inserted cautiously while observing the image on the screen. If it is inserted too far into the posterior fornix, orientation becomes difficult.

THE SCAN

The probe is placed in the coronal scan plane, and swept anteriorly to assess the position of the uterus; if this is anteverted, it is evaluated. Moving the probe in and out of the vagina optimizes visualization of the uterus from fundus to cervix. Having the patient tilt her pelvis up facilitates scanning of the uterine fundus.

Moving the probe from side to side gives the initial assessment of the adnexa and ovaries. It is sometimes helpful to apply gentle pressure on the anterior abdominal wall to move the ovaries closer to the transducer. The ovaries can be difficult to demonstrate in about 25 per cent of postmenopausal patients because of the absence of the characteristic cystic ovarian follicles. The internal iliac vessels also serve as an important landmark lying just posterior and lateral to the ovaries.

Transvaginal color Doppler is now being used to evaluate flow in the female pelvis. It is of particular value in analyzing small vessels that are difficult to identify by pulsed Doppler alone. Comparison of flow characteristics in pelvic masses may be significant in differentiating benign from malignant lesions.[1]

Trophoblastic flow can be detected with color and may be useful as an aid in diagnosing ectopic pregnancy. Color Doppler, which indicates direction, velocity and type of blood flow, combined with pulsed Doppler, which quantifies the flow, produces simultaneously a great deal of information regarding pelvic arterial and venous hemodynamics.

THE NORMAL PELVIS

UTERUS

The entire normal, non-gravid uterus may be easily examined with TVS. The usual scanning planes are sagittal and axial of the organ as opposed to the patient. The current standard for display of

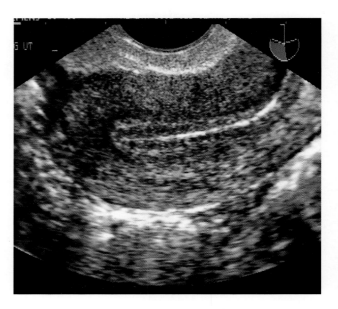

Figure 5.1 *Normal uterus—late proliferative phase. TVS shows the white echogenic central stripe of the endometrial canal. The echogenic secretory endometrium is surrounded by a thin hypoechoic inner layer of the myometrium.*

transvaginal images is with the fundus directed towards the left of the sector field of view in the anteverted uterus (Fig. 5.1). Alternatively, when the uterus is retroverted, the fundus will appear towards the right of the sector image. Some investigators may display the uterus in a reverse fashion. Uterine length, including the cervix, was a routine measurement with transabdominal sonography (TAS); however, due to a limited field of view it is usually not possible to make this measurement. In smaller, postmenopausal uteri, it may be possible to measure uterine length from external os to fundus.

For this chapter, examination of the uterus with TVS has been divided into five components: cervix, myometrium, size and contour, endometrium and endometrial cavity and common variants.

Cervix

The tip of the vaginal probe should be about 2–3 cm from the cervix in order to visualize it adequately. The cervix may be examined from side to side in the

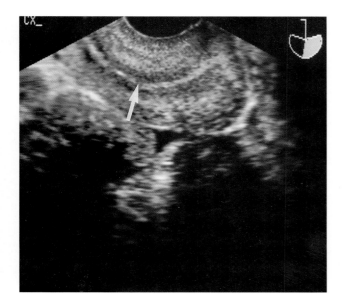

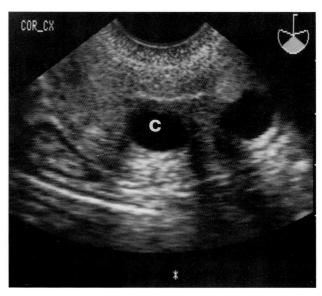

Figure 5.2 *Normal cervix. Sagittal TVS of the cervix (endocervical canal, arrow). Free fluid is present behind the cervix.*

Figure 5.3 *Nabothian cysts. Coronal TVS of cervix with two nabothian cysts (c).*

sagittal plane, and from external os to the level of the internal os in the semi-axial plane. The cervix may be examined as the initial structure in the scanning sequence, or it may be examined after scanning of the body and fundus is complete. For the latter case, this may be done by withdrawing the probe slowly until the cervix is recognized on the viewing screen.

The endocervical canal typically appears as a thin, central echogenic stripe similar to the endometrial cavity echo (Fig. 5.2). The endocervical canal may have a small amount of fluid during the periovulatory phase perhaps related to the higher fluid content of the mucus at this time.[2]

The echotexture of the cervix is similar to that of the outer two-thirds of the myometrium. There are no prominent vascular structures normally visible in the cervix; however, packets of paracervical vessels are typically seen just lateral to the cervix at the level of the internal os. These vessels appear as a complex of relatively convoluted, hypoechoic tubules. On occasion, flow echoes may be observed on real-time viewing as streaming low-amplitude echogenic particles in the vessels.

Small, simple cysts are frequently observed in the cervix adjacent to the endocervical canal (Nabothian cysts) and external os (endocervical cysts) (Fig. 5.3). The cysts may be singular or multiple and are usually less than 2 cm in diameter. They are typically echofree with prominent acoustic enhancement. The enhancement is increased on TVS, probably due to the use of a higher frequency transducer with the focal zone at the appropriate location in the imaging field.

Myometrium

The myometrium is divided sonographically into three zones, the internal, intermediate and external zones. The internal myometrium is relatively thin, the intermediate zone is the thickest portion, and is surrounded by the external myometrium, which is intermediate in thickness. Muscle bundles course in different directions within the three zones. The internal myometrium has longitudinal and circular fibers, the intermediate zone has two bundles of spiral

SINGLETON HOSPITAL
STAFF LIBRARY

fibers and the external zone is exclusively longitudinal fibers. The external and intermediate zones have an echotexture which is relatively homogeneous and of moderate echogenicity. The myometrium appears to remain relatively constant in echogenicity from childhood to menopause. Focal or multifocal, discrete sonographic inhomogeneity of the myometrium is almost always due to fibroids while focal or diffuse and ill-defined inhomogeneity is due to adenomyosis or, less commonly, invasive endometrial carcinoma.

Relatively large myometrial veins are typically seen in the periphery of the uterus between the external and intermediate zones. These veins can also be observed with TAS but not as frequently or as clearly. They may be more common in multiparous women. With TVS, weakly echogenic blood may be observed while scanning in real time. Anatomically, these vessels correspond to the arcuate venous plexus. The vessels appear spherical on axial scans and tubular on sagittal scans.

The inner third of the myometrium typically appears as a hypoechoic halo adjacent to the relatively echogenic endometrium (see Fig. 5.1). This myometrial halo increases slightly in thickness and sonographic visibility in the secretory phase of the cycle. Until 1986, this halo was believed to be part of the endometrium.[3,4] In 1986, Fleisher et al[2] indicated that the echopoor halo appeared to correlate with the internal layer of the myometrium based on histological correlations that he performed. This is also borne out by uterine magnetic resonance imaging.

Size and Contour

Uterine length is relatively difficult to measure because of a limited field of view in most TVS sector images, although some give a 140° angle that generally encompasses the entire organ. The transverse and anteroposterior dimensions of the uterus could be measured in the non-gravid uterus; however, plane selection may be difficult.

The outer, serosal surface of the uterus should be smooth and regular. Surface irregularity is invariably due to subserous leiomyomatous disease. The anterior surface is directly apposed to the posterior and superior walls of the urinary bladder. The posterior surface is usually interfaced with the rectum and sigmoid colon; however, fluid in the posterior cul-de-sac may separate the uterus from adjacent bowel (Fig. 5.4). The lateral surfaces of the uterus are related to the adnexa, including the ovaries.

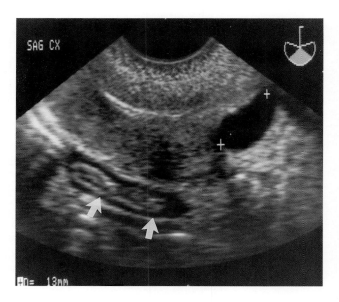

Figure 5.4 *Normal bowel. Sagittal TVS at the level of the cervix, showing a normal loop of bowel (arrows) in the posterior cul-de-sac (nabothian cyst, electronic calipers).*

Endometrium and Endometrial Cavity

The endometrial cavity is normally seen as a bright line or stripe in the center of the uterus. It is usually visible in all phases of the menstrual cycle as well as in the postmenopausal uterus. The line disappears when there is free fluid within the cavity.

The endometrium is divided into functional (zona compacta and zona spongiosa) and basal (zona basalis) zones. The functional zone consists of glands and stroma. The basal zone contains the closed or blind ends of the glands. Changes in the morphology of the functional zone of the endometrium account for the thickness and textural variation observed with transvesical and transvaginal sonography during the natural or stimulated menstrual cycle. The basal zone is relatively thin and does not change appreciably in thickness during the cycle.

It is recommended that the thickness of the endometrium be measured on a long-axis image of the uterus rather than on an axial scan because of more reliable and reproducible plane selection.[2] Total endometrial thickness measurements include the anterior and posterior wall layers of the endometrium. If fluid appears to separate the endometrial cavity, a single wall-thickness measurement should be made.

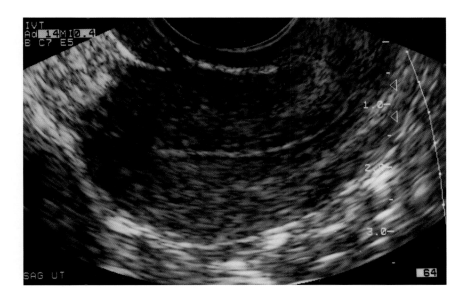

Figure 5.5 *Early proliferative phase of endometrial cycle. Thin endometrium at day 7 of the menstrual cycle.*

The thickness and echotexture of the endometrium varies with the phase of the menstrual cycle as well as the level of ovarian endocrinological activity.[2,4,5] During the menstrual phase, the endometrium appears as a relatively thin, interrupted interface of 1–4 mm in total thickness. During the early proliferative phase (days 5–9), the endometrium thickens to between 4 mm and 8 mm and has an echotexture which is isoechoic or slightly more echoic than the outer portion of the myometrium (Fig. 5.5). In the late proliferative (days 10–14) or preovulatory phase, a multilayered or triple-line endometrium may be seen. This pattern is related to a moderately echoic uterine cavity interface and spongiosa zone surrounding the inner hypoechoic compact zone. In the secretory phase (days 15–28), the endometrium achieves maximum thickness of between 8 mm and 16 mm and appears as a uniformly echogenic central band significantly greater in echo-brightness than the outer myometrium (Fig. 5.6). The normal decidualization of the endometrium associated with intrauterine and ectopic pregnancy cannot be reliably differentiated with TVS from the normal secretory endometrium of nonconception cycles. The hypoechoic halo representing the inner third of the myometrium may be seen in all phases of the menstrual cycle but is most prominent during the secretory phase.

Total endometrial thickness measurements greater than 14–16 mm in patients of childbearing age should raise suspicion of endometrial disease. In postmenopausal patients, the uterus is small and the normal unstimulated endometrium should be quite thin, measuring less than 8 mm[6,7] (Fig. 5.7). The endometrium may be 2–3 mm thicker in postmenopausal patients on estrogen replacement therapy.

An endometrium of normal thickness may appear falsely thickened (pseudo-thickening) if oblique slices are taken through the uterus or if there is a mass in the endometrial cavity which is isoechoic to the endometrium.

Common Variants

Uterine duplication of various types is a common finding on TVS. Depending on uterine position, it may not be possible to determine with certainty the exact type of developmental uterine anomaly present. In our experience, the septated and bicornuate uteri are the most frequent Mullerian abnormalities detected. These two types can usually be distinguished by a semi-axial section at the fundal level (Fig. 5.8). The bicornuate uterus will show a parting of the uterine

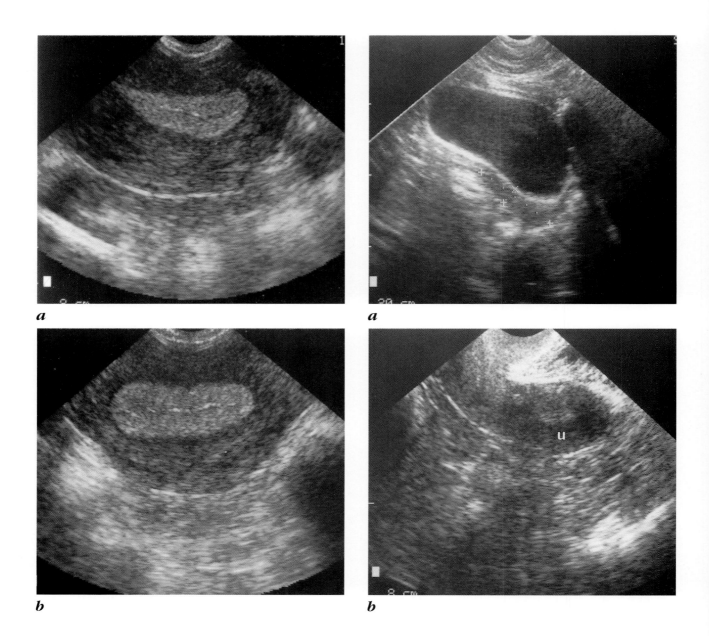

Figure 5.6 *Secretory phase of endometrial cycle. (a) Sagittal scan in a retroverted uterus. (b) Axial scan of the uterine body. The endometrium is uniformly echogenic and thickened.*

Figure 5.7 *Postmenopausal uterus. (a) Transvesical sonogram showing small uterus (electronic calipers) posterior to the echofree bladder. (b) TVS showing greater detail of the atrophic uterus (u) with the thin endometrium.*

fundi by a triangular area of echogenic fat. This feature is not evident with a complete or incomplete septated uterus. With both duplication anomalies, high semi-axial sections will show the endometrial echo complex separated by a band of myometrium. As scanning is directed towards the cervix, the bipoled endometrium may be seen to remain separated (uterus septus or uterus bicornis bicollis, or

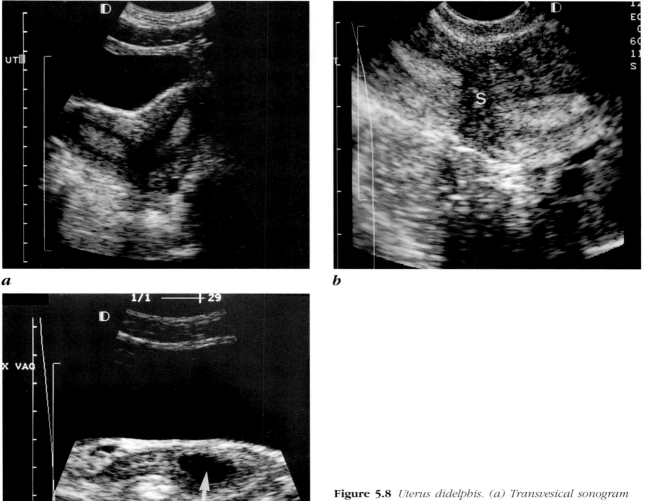

a

b

c

Figure 5.8 *Uterus didelphis. (a) Transvesical sonogram of bicornuate uterus. (b) TVS showing two endometrial canals separated by a midline septum (S). (c) Transverse sonogram through the upper vagina showing normal right vagina and hydrocolpos of the left vagina (arrow).*

uterus didelphis) or may be seen to join centrally (uterus subseptus or uterus subseptus). Indentation of the fundal portion of the endometrium may be seen on the semi-coronal scan in cases of uterus subseptus or uterus bicornis unicollis.

Uterine Vascular Anatomy

The common iliac arteries bifurcate just below the pelvic brim to form the internal and external iliac arteries. The internal iliac arteries supply the pelvic viscera, pelvic walls, perineum and gluteal regions. The external iliac arteries supply the lower limbs and exit the pelvis through the femoral canal after coursing through the false pelvis along its lateral walls. The internal iliac artery (hypogastric) is an important landmark, lying posterior to the uterus, ovaries and fimbriated ends of the fallopian tubes. It divides into anterior and posterior divisions retroperitoneally. The internal iliac veins are posterior to the arteries.

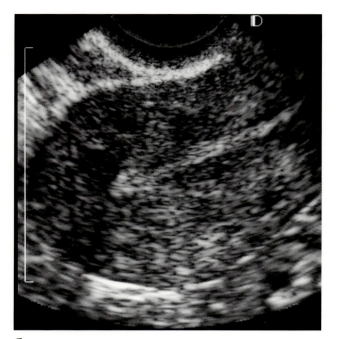

a

b

Figure 5.9 *Uterine blood flow. (a) Sagittal TVS of the uterus with (b) blood flow demonstrated by color flow Doppler.*

The uterine artery arises from the anterior trunk of the internal iliac artery and runs medially along the levator ani to the cervix. From the cervix it ascends lateral to the uterus in the broad ligament (parametrium) to the fallopian tube and ovary and ends with a branch that joins the ovarian artery. Anterior and posterior arcuate arteries anastomose with the uterine arteries and run within the broad ligament before entering the myometrium. High-resistance, high-velocity flow is characteristic of uterine arteries. The arcuate arteries and accompanying venous plexus lie between the intermediate and external layers of the myometrium. The radial branches of the arcuate extend into the intermediate layer of myometrium and end in the tortuous spiral arteries that penetrate the endometrium (Fig. 5.9).

VAGINA

The vagina is not usually the focus of attention when imaging the pelvis with TVS; however, it may be seen in sagittal and coronal planes when the tip of the probe is placed at the introitus. It appears as a hypoechoic tubular structure with an echogenic lumen that curves inferiorly over the muscular perineal body at the introitus. The bladder, trigone and urethra are anterior to the vagina, and the rectum is posterior. The distal ureters are lateral to the upper vagina and pass anteriorly to enter the bladder. The posterior fornix of the vagina is closely related to the rectouterine recess of the peritoneal cavity (posterior cul-de-sac) and is separated by the thickness of the vaginal wall and peritoneal membrane.

Potential applications of vaginal imaging with TVS include assessment of vaginal masses such as Gartner's duct cyst.

OVARIES

The normal ovary is best detected with the probe in the coronal plane and then by sliding it laterally from the uterine cornua and out to the lateral pelvic sidewall; sweep anterior and posterior along the sidewall to visualize the ovaries. The normal landmarks are the internal iliac artery and the ureter, which lie immediately posterior to or behind the ovary. At this level, the internal iliac artery branches into its anterior and posterior branches. Lateral to the ovary is the obturator internus muscle (OIM), seen as a striated band of tissue about 1 cm thick. Lateral to the OIM is a bright echogenic line which represents the medial wall of the bony ischium.

The ovaries are ellipsoid in shape and are located in the ovarian fossa of Waldeyer on either side of the uterus close to the pelvic sidewall. The ovarian fossa is bounded anteriorly by the obliterated umbilical artery, posteriorly by the ureter and internal iliac artery and superiorly by the external iliac vein. They are attached to the broad ligament and lie posterior and inferior to the fallopian tube. The ovaries have an echotexture similar to that of myometrium, frequently with small cystic follicles in varying stages of development. Ovarian location is variable, especially in women who have been pregnant. Rarely can they be found in the cul-de-sac or behind the fundus of the uterus. In less than 25 per cent of patients, the ovary is not found on the lateral pelvic sidewall but may be quite mobile, lying above the uterine fundus or in the posterior cul-de-sac. If it lies cephalad or anterior to its normal position the examiner may have to press down on the lower anterior abdominal wall to bring it into view.

In the premenopausal female the ovary itself is readily identifiable by the varying number and size of cystic Graafian follicles usually less than 2 cm in diameter (Fig. 5.10). In the postmenopausal patient no such follicles are present and the ovarian echogenicity is similar to that of the adjacent fibro-fatty tissue. It is most helpful to use the internal iliac artery as a landmark in these patients. In the postmenopausal patient, the ovaries are small and are visualized 65–70 per cent of the time, more if cysts are present within them. These can be present in 15 per cent of normal postmenopausal patients.

The suspensory ligament of the ovary, which arises from the pelvic sidewall, contains the ovarian vessels and nerves. The ovarian artery lies on the dorsal surface of the ovary and is seldom visualized due to its small diameter.

Ovarian size is variable, depending on menstrual status (premenarchal, menstruating or postmenopausal), age, height and weight, pregnancy history, and phase of menstrual cycle (follicular, preovulatory or luteal) (Fig. 5.11). Cohen et al[8] studied ovarian volumes in normal menstruating subjects and found that a range of 1.2–11.8 cm³ with a mean volume of 9.8 cm³ was typical. The mean volume for postmenopausal patients is approximately 3.7 cm³ and for premenarchal girls the

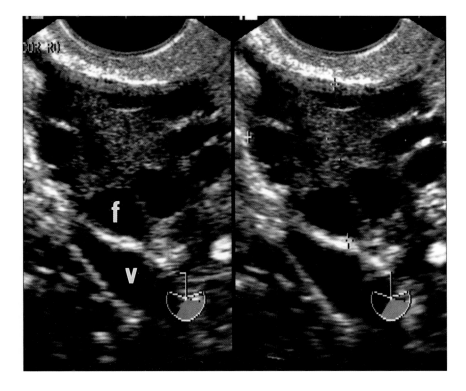

Figure 5.10 *Normal ovary. TVS coronal scan of the right ovary without calipers (left) and with electronic calipers (right). Multiple developing follicles (f) are present. v, iliac vein.*

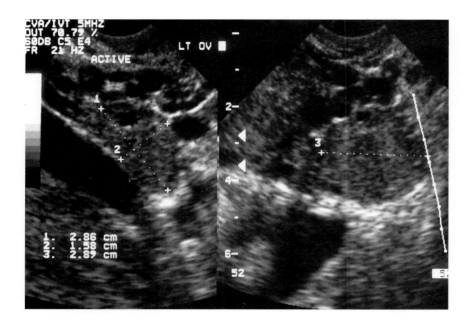

Figure 5.11 *Normal size of ovary. Sagittal (left) and axial (right) scans of the left ovary. Normal axial, coronal and longitudinal measurements (electronic calipers) using TVS.*

range is 0.75–2.32 cm³. Ovarian volume in Cohen's study was found to be highest in the preovulatory (days 11–16) phase and lowest in the luteal (days 17–35) phase. Factors affecting ovarian volumes in postmenopausal patients include years since the menopause, weight, parity, age at menopause, a history of hormone replacement therapy, and previously diagnosed breast cancer.[9]

Cyclical changes of the ovary are visualized with development of the dominant follicle at days 9–10 of a regular 28-day cycle. It is generally a thin–walled cyst measuring 8–10 mm in size[1] and enlarges daily until it ruptures at the time of ovulation. Occasionally the cumulus oophorus can be observed as a 'cyst within a cyst' in the dominant follicle and is a reliable sign of impending ovulation. Fluid from within the follicle is released at the time of ovulation, and this is followed by collapse of the follicle. Shortly thereafter the corpus hemorrhagicum, a cyst filled with echogenic blood, is formed and free fluid in the posterior cul-de-sac is frequently seen.

Transvaginal color Doppler can be used to follow the dominant follicle and corpus luteum. Differences in the resistance index of luteal flow have been observed in patients with early intrauterine pregnancy, in ectopic pregnancy and in non-pregnant patients. Studies have shown that 80–90

per cent of the blood flow to the ovary is supplied to the corpus luteum.[1]

Vascular impedance in ovarian vessels changes with fluctuations in estrogen levels due to its effects on arterial smooth muscle, causing vasodilatation in the early and late luteal phase. Differences in flow patterns in the postmenopausal ovary are being investigated for detection of ovarian neoplasms.[10,11]

In summary, one must note the following features of the ovary: its overall size and volume; its echogenicity; the size and number of follicles; the presence of any masses within or adjacent to the ovary; the presence of adjacent free fluid or any pain or tenderness elicited as the probe pushes against the ovary.

Ovarian Vasculature

The ovarian arteries arise directly from the abdominal aorta slightly inferior to the renal arteries. They enter the pelvis through the infundibulopelvic ligament on the lateral pelvic sidewall. They run along the dorsolateral aspects of the ovaries and divide into branches within the ovarian stroma. The parenchymal vessels are seen throughout (Fig. 5.12). Variations in vascular impedance in different phases of the menstrual cycle are observed, with highest systolic and diastolic flow just preceding ovulation and in the secretory phase. New vessel formation around a corpus luteum cyst of menstruation (normally seen in the luteal phase or second half of the menstrual cycle) gives rise to increased diastolic flow around the cyst.[1]

FALLOPIAN TUBES

The fallopian tube is approximately 10 cm in length and lies in the superior part of the broad ligament. The fimbriated end is open to the peritoneal cavity and has an ostium measuring approximately 3 mm in diameter. The medial third is referred to as the isthmus, and is round and cordlike. The intramural or interstitial portion of the tube is approximately 1 cm in length[12] and is well seen with transvaginal scanning.

Unfortunately, due to its small luminal dimension, its tortuous and variable course, and its lack of strong acoustic interfaces, the normal fallopian tube is usually not well visualized with TVS. This fact is particularly true for the distal end of the tube. However, a careful scan of the uterine fundus will often define the proximal portion of the tube and the broad ligament, which can be identified as a single moderately echogenic curvilinear structure arising laterally from the cornua. In fact, identification of the proximal tube, followed by a careful lateral sweep in the direction of the distal tube, will often help to direct the investigator to the location of the ovary. In addition, this technique is also very helpful when scanning the adnexa for the presence of an ectopic gestation.

As is true elsewhere in the body, pelvic fluid can be used as an acoustic window to better visualize anatomical structures. A significant quantity of free fluid of any etiology within the pelvis may help delineate the normal tube and may permit visualization of the infundibulum and fimbriae. Keeping the pelvis in a dependent position during the scan should help pool any free intraperitoneal fluid around the tube.

In contrast to the normal tube, the diseased tube is usually easily seen. It is frequently distended and fluid-filled and is usually initially identified as a large cystic adnexal mass. However, careful scanning in multiple planes of section will demonstrate the serpiginous and continuous nature of the tube, differentiating it from an ovarian cystic mass. Frequently, thickened mural involutions are seen to radiate from the wall into the distended lumen, giving the

diseased tube a characteristic 'cogwheel' appearance in cross-section.[13] In comparison to TAS, TVS provides improved visualization of the fallopian tubes, and by gentle maneuvering the probe can also be used to physically examine the tube for tenderness and for the existence of adhesions.

BOWEL

The examination of bowel has always been problematic for ultrasound, due to the presence of gas within the bowel lumen. Gas presents a highly reflective interface to the sound beam, causing very bright echoes to be displayed with insufficient variation in gray scale to permit distinction of detail. In addition, since the vast majority of the sound energy is reflected by the gas, the region deep to a gas interface is obscured in acoustic shadow. As a result, the typical pattern for normal gas-filled loops of bowel with the pelvis is an inhomogeneous display of regions of hyper- and hypoechogenicity surrounding the uterus and ovaries. Changes in the echogenicity and the appearance of this pattern, due to peristalsis, can usually be seen during the length of the scan. When bowel is filled with gas, distinction of the muscular bowel wall is usually difficult. If the TVS is being performed for investigation of a palpable pelvic mass, care should be taken to closely examine a region of non-peristalsing bowel. Ovarian dermoid cysts can produce a very similar appearance to gas-filled bowel. However, careful scanning in multiple planes should identify the fusiform nature of bowel and some characteristic peristalsis. If peristalsis is not seen, the examination should be repeated to identify any changes in the echo pattern. No change over time should arouse the suspicion of a dermoid cyst.

As was the case with the fallopian tubes, the existence of intra- and/or extraluminal fluid substantially improves the detail that is displayed. Fortunately, small bowel frequently contains fluid-filled loops, particularly if the TVS scan is being done following a TAS for which the patient had been hydrated.

In this situation, the hypoechoic muscular wall of normal loops of small bowel can often be seen surrounding the fluid-filled lumen. When the bowel contains fluid from chyme and the digestive products, low-level echoes are usually seen to swirl within the fluid and the lumen is seen to vary in shape and dimension as the bowel peristalses. Small bowel can usually be seen to peristalse frequently and to

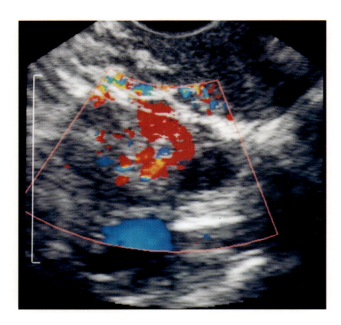

Figure 5.12 *Normal ovary in the periovulatory period—color flow Doppler demonstrates the ovarian vessels.*

contain numerous echogenic mural folds corresponding to the plicae circulares. In contrast, large bowel will peristalse less frequently and can usually be identified by its larger luminal diameter and the less numerous haustral folds. However, fluid-filled large bowel is an unusual finding and should alert the investigator to the possibility of pathology.

BLADDER, URETERS AND URETHRA

In contrast to TAS, TVS should be performed after the urinary bladder has been emptied. Due to the proximity of the TVS probe to the structures of interest and due to the improved spatial resolution, a fluid-filled urinary bladder is not required for TVS. In fact, a distended bladder will hinder the examination by displacing the uterus out of the focal zone of the transducer. However, a small amount of fluid in the bladder may help to position a severely anteverted uterus, and is also useful for examination of the bladder wall, ureters and urethra. In most cases, even immediately post-void, a small residual volume of urine will remain within the bladder.

As the probe is inserted, the bladder is the most easily recognizable structure that is initially seen and because of its constant position should be used by the investigator to orient the plane of section. Upon insertion, the posterior angle of the bladder can be identified by its moderately echogenic thick muscular wall surrounding the small anechoic volume of urine. Occasionally the bladder is completely empty with the superior and inferior walls apposed, making identification more difficult. The normal bladder wall should be of uniform thickness and display moderate echogenicity. The mucosal surface is smooth and echogenic. Due to the limited field of view of the TVS probe, the entire bladder can rarely be examined. However, the superior resolution of TVS provides an excellent method for evaluation of the bladder wall at its posteroinferior margin, the trigone, and the urethra.

The normal ureters are usually not identified on TVS. However, the ureterovesical junctions (UVJ) may be identified as small bilateral prominences in the posterior bladder wall. On occasion, a blush of echoes within the bladder from a urine jet will lead the investigator to the ureterovesical junction. The superior resolution of TVS facilitates the examination of this area for small calculi, masses or ureteroceles. A dilated distal ureter will be seen as a tubular anechoic structure angling obliquely from the UVJ and coursing laterally and superiorly from the level of the cervix. A negative Doppler sample will quickly distinguish a widely distended ureter from a pelvic blood vessel.

The short female urethra can commonly be seen extending inferiorly from the bladder and running just anteriorly to the vagina. The best view of the urethra is obtained with the probe at the introitus or only partially inserted into the distal third of the vagina. With a sagittal orientation the apposed mucosal surfaces of the urethra are seen as an echogenic line surrounded by the much more hypoechoic muscularis. But, on occasion, an anechoic sliver of urine can be seen distending the urethra. Much less commonly, an intraurethral mass may be defined.

LIGAMENTS AND MUSCLES

The pelvic ligaments and musculature are infrequently seen in the normal female pelvis on TVS. Both are usually obscured by bowel.

Free pelvic fluid may delineate the broad and round ligaments as they extend laterally from the uterus. Both appear as echogenic cord-like structures which may be separated from the adjacent fallopian tube. However, a large volume of pelvic fluid such as ascites is needed to well visualize the ligaments.

The majority of the pelvic musculature lies outside the focal zone of the high-frequency TVS probe, and, in addition, is usually obscured by bowel gas. Occasionally, the obturator internis muscle can be seen in the lateral pelvic wall deep to the uterus.

In coronal section, the muscle is displayed as a solid fusiform non-mobile mass extending obliquely to the lateral pelvic sidewall. It is more hypoechoic than the myometrium and contains linear echogenicities characteristic of striated muscle.

THE ABNORMAL PELVIS

THE UTERUS

Endometrium

TVS is an excellent modality for the assessment of the endometrial thickness and echogenicity, but even more important is its ability to identify even the earliest gestational sac at 36–40 days menstrual age. This confirms the diagnosis of an intrauterine gestation, or, on the other hand, would suggest the presence of an ectopic pregnancy.

Infertility

In the assessment of the infertile patient and in the monitoring of the uterine response to stimulatory agents, it has become the standard practice to evaluate endometrial thickness as well as its echogenicity during the menstrual cycle. The latter has been found useful as an indicator of ovulation and the time when the endometrium is most receptive. This pattern shows an echogenic peripheral zone with a central echopoor zone.

Endometritis

On TVS this appears as thickened endometrium with increased echogenicity (Fig. 5.13). Free endometrial fluid which may be clear or echogenic (pyometra) may be present. Hydrometra or hematometra may occur secondary to cervical stenosis due to neoplasm or radiation fibrosis and may be indistinguishable from pyometra in the absence of other clinical or sonographic signs. Endometritis may be associated with hydro- or pyosalpinx or tubovarian abscess.

Endometrial Carcinoma

Adenocarcinoma of the endometrium is presently the most common gynecologic cancer in the United States. The incidence has been rising over the past 50 years. It is primarily seen in obese postmenopausal women and has been associated with diabetes and hypertension. It is more commonly seen in the presence of unopposed estrogen such as in postmenopause, estrogen replacement without progesterone, estrogen-producing tumors, and polycystic ovary disease of premenopausal women.

It is usually well differentiated and low grade, I or II. Higher grade lesions with myometrial invasion have a poorer prognosis.

Sonographically, the echogenicity varies depending on the grade. Highly differentiated mucin-producing tumors are often echogenic (Fig. 5.14). Low-grade tumors are often hypoechoic. Disruption of the inner muscular layer or subendometrial 'halo' suggests myometrial invasion. Recent studies suggest that TVS may be able to estimate the degree of myometrial invasion and the stage of disease.

Color or conventional Doppler may be helpful in identifying a low-impedance flow in the altered neovasculature of the lesion.

Endometrial Appearance of Tamoxifen

There has been great concern expressed about the appearance of the endometrium in postmenopausal women with breast carcinoma treated with tamoxifen.[14] Tamoxifen is primarily an anti-estrogen but has an estrogen agonist effect on the endometrium. While there is an association between tamoxifen and endometrial carcinoma, tamoxifen-induced endometrial appearance is often abnormal without the presence of carcinoma. Thickened hyperechoic endometrium with cystic spaces has been seen after just 3 months of therapy (Fig. 5.15). Thickness of both walls measured an average of 22 mm (8–38 mm) in most patients. On curettage the findings are often atrophic endometrium or an inadequate specimen. Endometrial biopsy may yield little more; however, Hulka and Hall found patients with polyps, hyperplasia, endometritis, proliferative endometrium and 1 of 11 cases with carcinoma. These were detected with biopsy and not on hysterectomy, which may give additional findings.

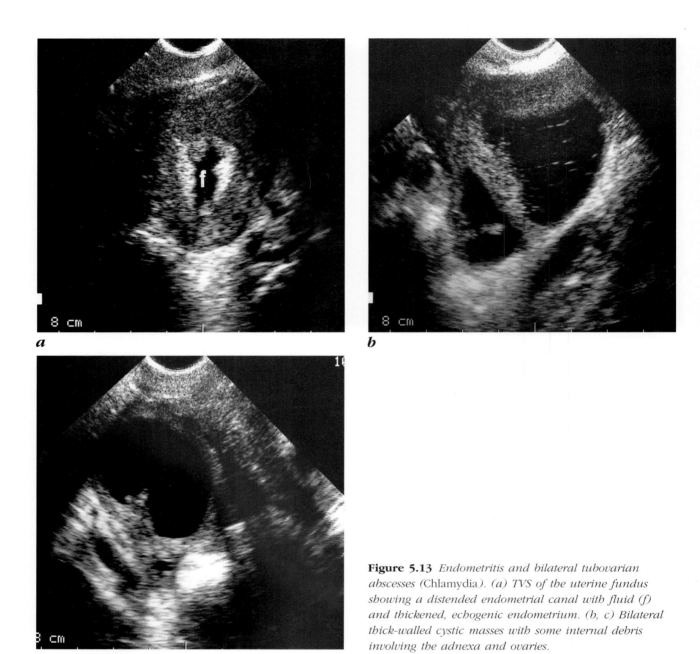

Figure 5.13 *Endometritis and bilateral tubovarian abscesses* (Chlamydia)*. (a) TVS of the uterine fundus showing a distended endometrial canal with fluid (f) and thickened, echogenic endometrium. (b, c) Bilateral thick-walled cystic masses with some internal debris involving the adnexa and ovaries.*

Postmenopausal Bleeding

The endometrium is usually the source of postmenopausal bleeding in cases of cystic proliferation, adenomatoid polyps, endometrial carcinoma, and degenerating or ulcerating fibroids. In all of the instances, the TVS evaluation may be very useful. In endometrial carcinoma one may see a mass of tissue with increased echogenicity. There have been reports that one can even assess the degree of extension of the neoplasm into the myometrium. Endometrial polyps and submucosal fibroids will be identified as intracavitary masses which may be echogenic or echopoor. The normal endometrium in the postmenopausal female is thin and echopoor. It measures 2 mm in thickness with a range of 1–12 mm. In women on

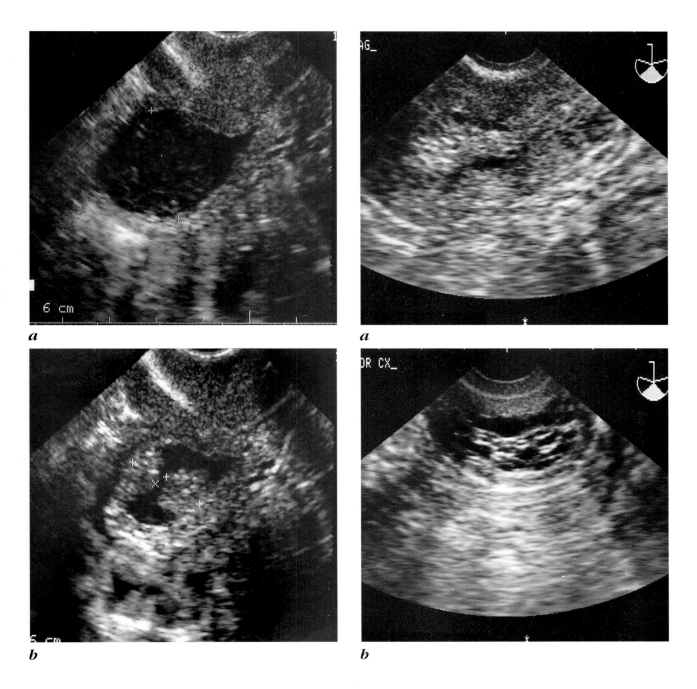

Figure 5.14 *Low-grade endometrial carcinoma. (a) Sagittal transvaginal scan of an anteverted postmenopausal uterus. There is debris and fluid within a distended endometrial canal. (b) Broad-based polypoid echogenic masses (electronic calipers) which do not extend into the myometrium.*

Figure 5.15 *Abnormal endometrium—tamoxifen. (a) Sagittal transvaginal scan of an anteverted uterus. Thickened echogenic endometrium with cystic areas in the region of the basal layer. (b) Coronal scan of the lower uterine segment, showing the prominent cystic changes.*

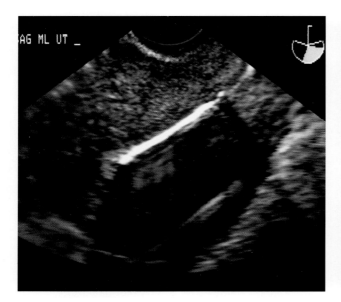

Figure 5.16 *IUCD. Longitudinal transvaginal sonogram showing the IUCD as a bright echo with shadow within the endometrial canal of the body and fundus of the uterus.*

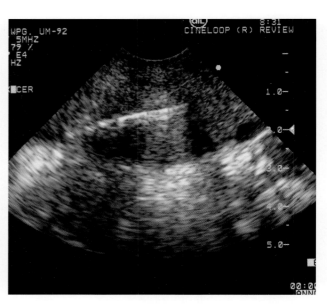

Figure 5.17 *Intramural IUCD. Axial transvaginal sonogram showing an 'off-axis' IUCD extending into the right side of the myometrium.*

estrogen therapy the endometrium will be thicker and more echogenic than in those without therapy.

Granberg et al[15] found that 87.3 per cent of patients with postmenopausal bleeding and an endometrial thickness of greater than 5 mm had some degree of endometrial pathology. Endometrial carcinoma was seen only in patients with an endometrial thickness of greater than 9 mm.

ENDOMETRIAL CANAL

Intra-Uterine Contraceptive Device (IUCD)

The best way to assess the presence and position of an IUCD is with ultrasound (Fig. 5.16). TVS has some advantages over the transvesical method. Both can identify the position of the IUCD within the canal but TVS should be able to identify invasion of the IUCD into the myometrium (Fig. 5.17). If the device lies outside of the uterus, neither technique is of value and an abdominal radiogram is needed. One can also determine which type of device is in place by their rather characteristic appearance.

Fluid

There is not normally any fluid within the endometrial canal except at mid-cycle when there is increased secretion or during menstruation (Fig. 5.18). At these times there may be only a small amount extending less than 1 cm within the canal. Fluid may be present in association with a decidual cast of ectopic pregnancy, with cervical stenosis secondary to cervical carcinoma or following cryosurgery.

Masses (Polyps, Fibroids)

Endometrial polyps may be seen within the canal as oblong or rounded, typically echogenic masses 1–3 cm in diameter. Most are less than 2 cm in size (Figs. 5.19 and 5.20). They may have small cysts within the mass, and with color Doppler vascularity can be appreciated. They are commonly made up of endometrial tissue and if uniformly hyperechoic they are as a rule benign. They commonly present with menometrorrhagia and have been reported in up to

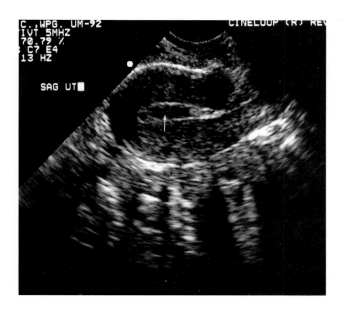

Figure 5.18 *Blood in the endometrial canal. Fluid (arrow) within the endometrial canal during menstruation.*

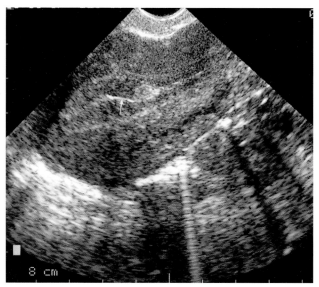

a

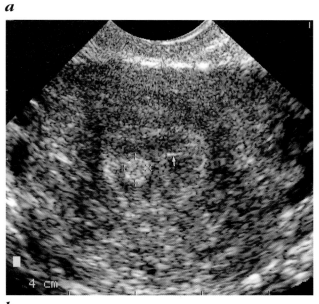

b

Figure 5.19 *Endometrial polyp. Transvaginal scans, sagittal (a) and coronal (b), of the uterus, showing an echogenic 3.8-mm endometrial polyp (electronic calipers, b) adjacent to the endometrial canal (arrow).*

24 per cent of symptomatic women.[16] They are most common in the fifth decade, with 20 per cent presenting after menopause.

The larger polyps of greater than 3 cm are usually heterogeneous in echogenicity and often abnormal. They may be infarcted, hemorrhagic, cystic or have metaplasia or carcinoma.

In premenopausal patients they have little or no malignant potential but in postmenopausal patients 10–15 per cent are associated with malignancy.

Submucous fibroids may protrude into and distort the canal or may actually prolapse out through the cervical os. They are generally small and uniformly hypoechoic. Saline installation into the endometrial canal makes identification of polyps or submucous fibroids much easier (Fig. 5.21).

MYOMETRIUM

Fibroids

Non-degenerated fibroids can be detected more frequently by TVS than by transvesical sonography

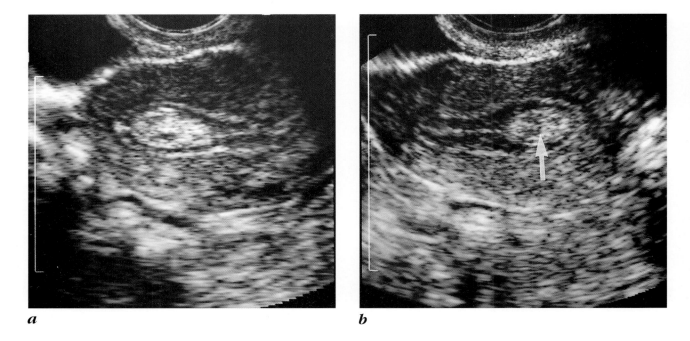

a   *b*

Figure 5.20 *Endometrial polyp. Transvaginal scans, sagittal (a) and coronal (b), of the uterus, showing an echogenic endometrial polyp (arrow, b) expanding the left side of the endometrial canal in the fundus.*

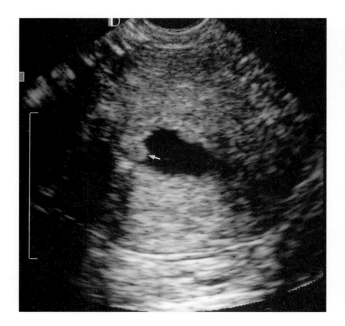

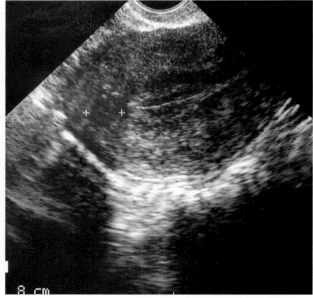

Figure 5.21 *Endometrial polyp—intrauterine saline infusion. An axial scan after 10 ml of intrauterine saline injection demonstrates a small echogenic mass (arrow) protruding into the fluid-filled endometrial canal.*

Figure 5.22 *Intramural uterine fibroid. Small hypoechoic fundal fibroid (electronic calipers).*

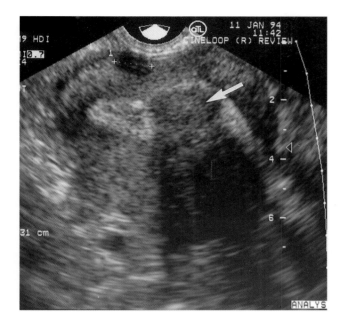

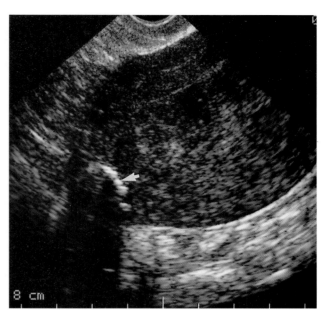

Figure 5.23 *Submucosal and subserosal uterine fibroids. Coronal TVS showing attenuating left-sided endometrial mass, a submucosal fibroid (arrow) and smaller subserosal fibroid (electronic calipers).*

Figure 5.24 *Calcified uterine fibroid. Calcified fibroid (arrow) casting a distal shadow within the peripheral myometrium.*

if one looks for variations in echogenicity within the myometrium. A non-degenerated fibroid may be as small as 5 mm in diameter and will only show a slight decrease in echogenicity. There may be increased attenuation of sound with some distal shadowing. These findings may be subtle. Larger ones are usually discrete, hypoechoic, rounded masses with distal 'shadowing' (Fig. 5.22). The distal shadowing is best appreciated with the higher frequency crystal of the transvaginal probe.

Fibroids may occur at all ages but are more commonly seen after 30 years of age. They are estrogen-dependent and usually regress after menopause. They may arise anywhere in the uterus from the fundus to the cervix and from a submucosal location out to a subserosal or pedunculated location (Fig. 5.23). Once a fibroid outstrips its vascular supply it undergoes central degeneration but this is not commonly seen. With degeneration there may also be dystrophic calcification, which may lie peripherally like a ring (Fig. 5.24) or more centrally like an amorphous mass. Malignant degeneration to a leiomyosarcoma is rare, occurring in 0.2 per cent of fibroids.

The very large fibroid masses may be difficult to fully appreciate on the transvaginal scan due to the limited field of view as well as the attenuation of the sound beam. In these situations transvesical sonography has the advantage of better orientation.

Location of fibroid

Submucosal masses are best seen by their distortion of the endometrial canal. The exact significance of the degree of cavity distortion versus the incidence of infertility or recurrent abortion is not yet known.

Intramural fibroids are more commonly seen and are usually multiple. They appear as discrete hypoechoic masses.

Subserosal fibroids distort the outer surface of the uterus, giving the typical lobulated appearance of the 'enlarged fibroid uterus'. Pedunculated subserous fibroids may appear as an extrauterine mass. The diagnosis may be made by demonstrating a whorled appearance or by applying gentle pressure with the transducer that will cause the mass to move with (as opposed to separate from) the uterus if the two are connected.

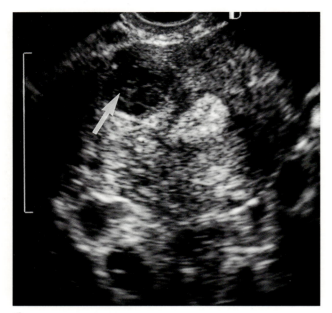

a

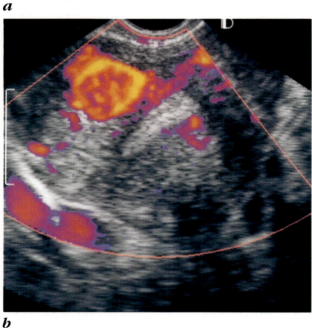

b

Figure 5.25 *Uterine fibroid—blood flow. (a) Transvaginal sonogram of subserosal uterine fibroid (arrow) with (b) blood flow within and around the fibroid demonstrated by power color Doppler (yellow ring).*

Size differences

The small ones are often multiple and may be very hard to see. If they lie in a submucosal location or are definitely hypoechoic, they can be visualized. On occasion they appear simply as areas of 'inhomogeneity'. The medium and large ones are most readily appreciated by their hypoechoic appearance with the distal shadowing.

Character

Non-degenerated ones may be isoechoic with myometrium, moderately echogenic or hypoechoic and highly attenuating. Whorled internal architecture may be present and correspond to concentric bundles of smooth muscle and connective tissue. Degenerated ones have areas of increased echogenicity or a cystic center. Up to 25 per cent have calcified areas within a fibroid as a result of dystrophic calcification. Calcification may be seen either centrally or peripherally.

The fibroid may cause distortion of the gestational sac but should not be confused with the 'mass-like' myometrial contraction.

The vascularity of fibroids has not been extensively studied. There have been recent advances in color flow Doppler using power mode. This has given rise to some initial images which show, in some fibroids, peripheral vascularity (Fig. 5.25). The significance of these findings is not yet clear.

Adenomyosis

Adenomyosis is benign invasion of endometrium into myometrium with associated diffuse overgrowth of muscle. The endometrial glands are of the basalis type and typically resistant to hormonal stimulation. Conservative drug therapy may be beneficial,[17] as opposed to the conventional management of hysterectomy.

This is a common diagnosis in some select series in France and South America with a sensitivity of 80 per cent and specificity of 74 per cent for diffuse disease and 87 per cent and 98 per cent for focal disease.[18,19] It does not appear to be a commonly made diagnosis in North America. The frequency has been reported in the literature to vary between 5 per cent and 70 per cent.[20]

On TVS the criteria used are: (1) thickening and asymmetry of the anterior and posterior myometrial walls; (2) increased myometrial echotexture; and (3) heterogeneous, indistinctly marginated areas. The findings are apparently more appreciable on MRI, with

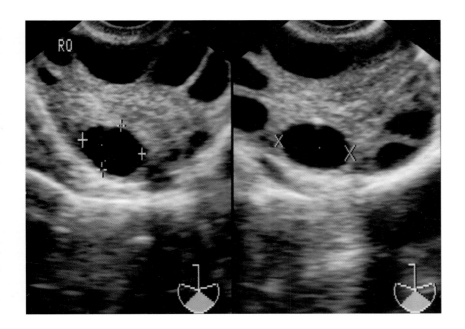

Figure 5.26 *Follicle monitoring. Measurement of follicle size on day 12 menstrual age in right ovary (electronic calipers).*

a myometrial mass with indistinct margins of primarily low signal intensity, or focal or diffuse widening (>0.5 cm) of the inner myometrial layer or junctional zone on T2 images.[21] These studies were performed in the luteal phase (days 20–26) of the cycle in patients suspected of adenomyosis with pain or menorrhagia and pathological confirmation. There may also be general myometrial thickening in the diffuse form.

THE OVARY

Follicle Monitoring

Induced ovulation is commonly used in the management of infertility in association with assisted fertilization or in vitro fertilization. It increases the number of available follicles and therefore oocytes. The two medications commonly used are clomiphene citrate (CC) and human menopausal gonadotrophin (HMG). CC is an estrogen antagonist which binds estrogen receptor sites in the pituitary and hypothalamus, leading to the release of more follicle-stimulating hormone (FSH). HMG contains both FSH and luteinizing hormone (LH). It recruits follicles directly. In patients with no exogenous estrogen or estrogenic activity it leads to the development of a small number of large follicles. The growth rate and the estrogen levels correlate well. In patients with estrogenic activity there is rapid recruitment of many follicles, which grow at different rates. There is poor correlation with serum estrogen and the risk of hyperstimulation is increased.[22]

Daily measurement of serum estradiol levels was the standard to assess follicular development prior to assisted fertilization in patients with infertility on an ovarian stimulation cycle. TVS has now become the standard mode of ovarian follicle assessment and development.[23] It was this use that accounted for the rapid development of the technology shortly after its introduction in the early 1980s. The number and size of follicles can best be seen transvaginally (Fig. 5.26). Once a follicle exceeds 15–18 mm, an injection of human chorionic gonadotrophin (HCG) is given to stimulate the release of LH and subsequent follicle rupture 48 h later. The monitoring is well tolerated and even preferred by these females who have to be scanned daily during ovulation induction. Mature oocytes can be retrieved from follicles of 10 mm to over 20 mm in average diameter. Within this range there is no significant difference in the percentage of mature oocytes retrieved or in the fertilization rates.

The cumulus oophorus in the mature Graafian follicle is more readily seen with TVS and indicates that ovulation will occur within 36 h. The cumulus is not currently used as a predictor of outcome, although it is said to be seen in 50–80 per cent of follicles greater than 18 mm in diameter.

The presence of low-level intrafollicular echoes may be a useful predictor of outcome. This finding may be due to released clumps of granulosa cells and has been associated with a higher pregnancy rate.[24]

Masses

Cyst

Cystic masses are readily seen, except those that are so large or are above the uterine fundus so as to be out of the field of view of the transvaginal probe. The character of the material within the cyst, the presence of septa, debris and solid components, can be more readily appreciated. Hemorrhagic cysts may present a very confusing pattern and should be followed closely.

Solid

The character of solid masses can be better seen transvaginally. The echogenic fat of the ovarian dermoid may show up more clearly; on the other hand, it may be very confusing, as the sound beam is totally attenuated. TVS may detect the presence of small masses which may be missed transvesically. The probe can also be used to 'palpate' the mass to assess tenderness and mobility, which will significantly assist in the differential diagnosis.

Non-neoplastic cystic masses

Polycystic ovary disease (PCOD)

This results from chronic anovulation with a 'steady state' of FSH and LH resulting in recruitment and early development of multiple follicles which do not mature appropriately and then become atretic. The sonographic appearance is variable but the 'classic' appearance is bilateral enlarged ovaries with multiple follicles measuring ≤8 mm situated peripherally (string of pearls) (Fig. 5.27). The tunica may be thickened and echogenic. Up to 30 per cent of patients have normal-sized ovaries with the rest exceeding 6 cm³ and usually twice normal size. The diagnosis depends, sonographically, on more than 11 follicles, generally small (<5 mm), no dominant follicle, enlarged ovarian volume (>6 cm³) and increased ovarian stromal echogenicity. The maximum number of follicles in normal controls was 11 in a recent transvaginal study.[25] Median values of the mean size

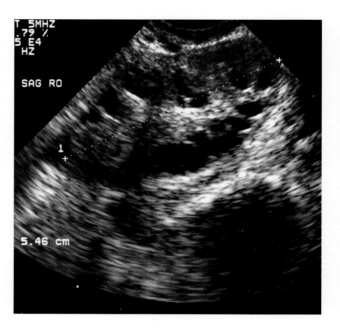

Figure 5.27 *Polycystic ovary. TVS shows an enlarged right ovary containing multiple small peripherally situated cysts.*

and number of follicles, ovarian volume, and percentage with moderate or markedly increased stromal echogenicity were, respectively, 5.1 mm, 5.0, 5.9 ml and 10 per cent in control subjects, and 3.8 mm, 9.8, 9.8 ml, and 94 per cent in patients with PCOD.[25]

Follicular cysts

These are cysts which arise from atretic follicles and are the most common form of ovarian cyst. They are usually 3–8 cm in diameter. Smaller follicular cysts cannot be differentiated from follicles on single examination. Most are unilocular and smoothly marginated while many have internal septations and debris which simulate a mural nodule. They regress spontaneously or with hormonal suppression on sonographic follow-up 4–6 weeks later.

Corpus luteum cysts

These result from failure of absorption or, commonly, excess bleeding into the cyst. Hemorrhagic corpora lutea are more commonly symptomatic than a follicular cyst, are evanescent and often regress in 4–6 weeks. They are unilocular and tend to be thin-walled (Figs. 5.28–5.30).

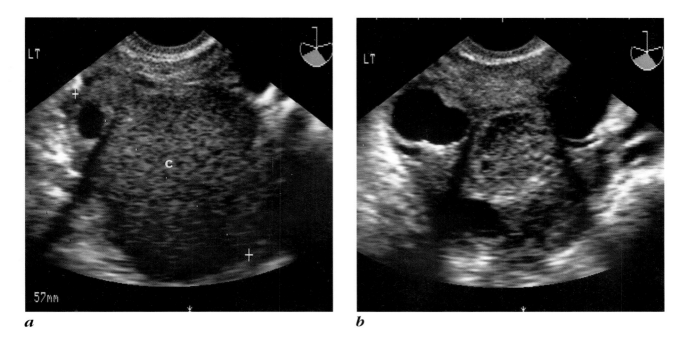

Figure 5.33 *Endometriosis. (a, b) Sagittal scans of a complex left adnexal mass with cystic components and a large cyst (c) containing diffuse low-level internal echoes.*

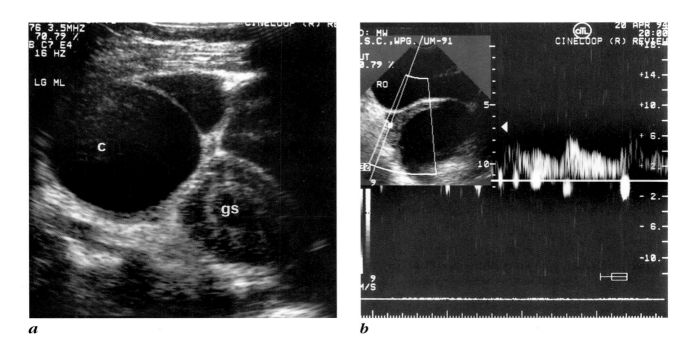

Figure 5.34 *Ovarian torsion in early pregnancy. (a) Transabdominal midline sonogram shows the uterus and gestational sac (gs). The right ovary, situated above and to the left of the uterus, was tender and contained large cysts (c). (b) Transvaginal pulsed Doppler of the right ovary demonstrated residual low-level arterial flow. The torsion was reduced laparoscopically.*

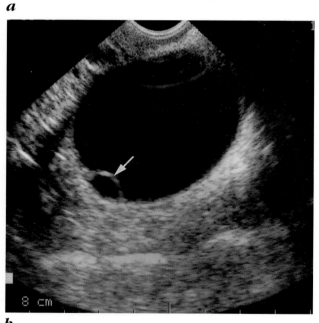

a

b

Figure 5.35 *Ovarian serous cystadenoma. TVS shows (a) a cystic left adnexal mass containing a mural nodule (electronic calipers) and (b) a single peripheral septation (arrow).*

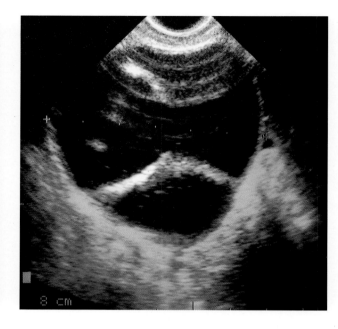

Figure 5.36 *Ovarian cystadenoma—thick septum. Thick septum in the lower half of the large cystic mass.*

postmenopausal age group, occurring in 14.8 per cent of patients.[26] The incidence of simple cysts is 200 times more common than that of ovarian cancer and these cysts should not be considered to be neoplastic. Regular sonographic follow-up may be indicated, as they will fluctuate in size and often disappear.

They should have a high resistance pattern on duplex ultrasound.

Ovarian neoplasia

Epithelial tumors

This group comprises 65–75 per cent of ovarian tumors and 90 per cent of ovarian malignancies. Tumor spread is primarily intraperitoneal but may also be by direct extension, lymphatics (paraortic) and, in late stages, hematogenous.

(1) Serous cystadenoma and cystadenocarcinoma – These are the most common accounting for 30 per cent of all ovarian neoplasms. Serous cystadenoma represents 20 per cent of all benign ovarian neoplasms, 20 per cent of which are bilateral. Cystadenocarcinoma accounts for 40 per cent of

ovarian malignancies, 50 per cent of which are bilateral. The larger the size of the lesion, the greater the likelihood of malignancy. The sonographic findings of serous cystadenoma usually include a large, thin-walled, unilocular cyst which may contain thin septations (Figs. 5.35 and 5.36). Occasional papillary projections are present. The cysts are detectable sonographically in 70 per cent of cases. Of interest in a recent series, all false-positive diagnoses of serous cystadenoma were benign tumors. Endometriomata and dermoid cysts may have similar sonographic features to those of serous cystadenoma. The sonographic findings of serous cystadenocarcinoma usually include a multilocular cystic mass with multiple papillary projections. There is often echogenic solid internal debris, thick septae and cyst walls. The mass may be fixed due to external papillary projections. Ascites is frequently present. Cysts with borderline malignancy may appear grossly at pathology as a multiloculated cystic lesion with internal papillary excrescences. Sonography has not been sensitive, suggesting malignancy in only 36 per cent of these tumors. Doppler detection of neovascularization may improve detection.

(2) Mucinous cystadenoma and cystadenocarcinoma – These account for 20 per cent of all ovarian neoplasms with cystadenoma, and 20 per cent of all benign ovarian neoplasms; 5 per cent are bilateral. Cystadenocarcinoma is bilateral in 25 per cent of cases and accounts for 6–10 per cent of all malignant ovarian neoplasms. Sonographically, mucinous cystadenomas are often huge, multiseptated masses with low-level internal echoes. Papillary projections are rare. Sonographically, the findings of mucinous cystadenocarcinomas are similar in appearance to those of serous cystadenocarcinoma, with multiple loculations, papillary projections and low-level echoes (Fig. 5.37). Differentiation from a benign mucinous tumor is notoriously difficult.

(3) Other epithelial tumors – There are three other kinds of epithelial tumor, endometrioid, clear cell and Brenner. Endometrioid tumors account for 20 per cent of ovarian malignancies, 30–50 per cent are bilateral. Sonographically, there is a cystic mass with papillary projections or occasionally a solid mass with internal hemorrhage or necrosis. Clear cell tumors are a variant of endometrioid tumors; 40 per cent are bilateral. They account for 5–10 per cent of primary ovarian carcinomas and have non-specific sonographic findings of a solid complex mass. Brenner tumors are rare, comprising 1–2 per cent of

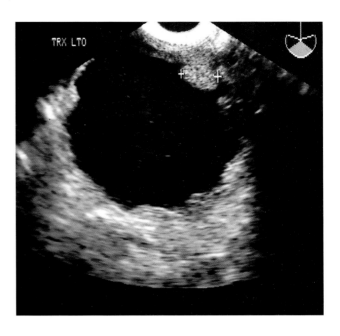

Figure 5.37 *Mucinous cystadenoma with borderline malignancy. Transverse sonogram of the left adnexa shows a cystic mass with a mural nodule (electronic calipers). Pathological examination revealed a mucinous neoplasm with borderline malignant potential.*

all ovarian tumors; <10 per cent are bilateral. They are almost always benign. Thirty per cent are associated with cystic neoplasms. Sonographically, there is a hypoechoic solid mass.

Germ cell tumors
(1) Dermoid cyst (benign cystic teratoma) – These comprise 10–15 per cent of ovarian neoplasms; 10–15 per cent are bilateral. They are most common at childbearing age and are invariably benign. Immature malignant teratomas represent <1 per cent of all teratomas, are usually seen in the first two decades of life and are generally solid with internal necrosis or hemorrhage. Sonographically, a benign dermoid cyst is predominantly cystic with a mural nodule which may contain hair, teeth or fat. This component usually casts an acoustic shadow (Figs. 5.38 and 5.39). Extensive sonic shadowing may be mistaken for bowel gas, and the full extent of the mass may not be appreciated. It may have fat–fluid or hair–fluid level with the echogenic fat or hair in a non-dependent position. In difficult cases the sonographer may need to confirm the presence of the mass palpated by the

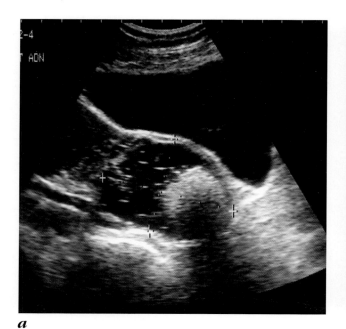

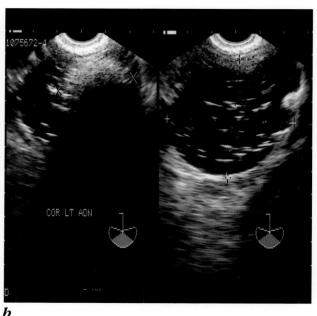

a   *b*

Figure 5.38 *Ovarian dermoid cyst with a fat–hair mass. (a) Transabdominal left parasagittal scan through a full bladder. The predominantly cystic mass is outlined by the electronic calipers. The echogenic solid mass is seen caudally. (b) Transvaginal sonograms using a split screen. On the right is the cystic component with patchy internal echoes from debris. On the left is the echogenic mass outlined by calipers measuring 32 mm. Only the proximal portion of the mass is seen, with marked attenuation distally.*

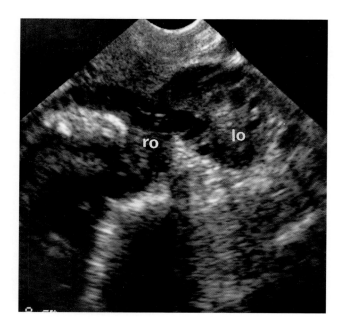

Figure 5.39 *Ovarian dermoid with a calcific mass. Coronal transvaginal sonogram shows a calcified mass in the right ovary (ro) adjacent to the normal left ovary (lo).*

clinician and with the patient's permission, may perform a combined examination with either a digital vaginal examination and transvesical sonography, or a transvaginal examination with palpation on the anterior abdominal wall. This may demonstrate a hard, palpable, echogenic, attenuating mass that may not have been 'visible' initially.

(2) Dysgerminoma – These account for 3–5 per cent of ovarian malignancies and form the most common type of malignant germ cell tumor. They are bilateral in 5–15 per cent of cases, and 80–90 per cent occur in women under 30 years of age. They are common in adolescence and are the second most common ovarian neoplasm in pregnancy. They are often associated with mixed germ cell tumors. Sonographically, they usually feature an echogenic solid mass which may have areas of necrosis or hemorrhage (Fig. 5.40).

(3) Endodermal sinus (yolk sac) tumor – These are the second most common malignant germ cell tumors; they have low-grade malignant potential but

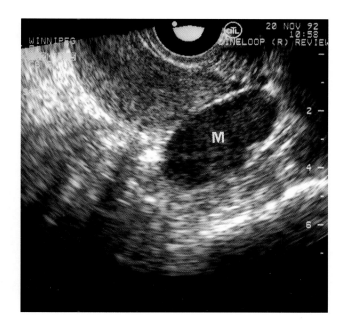

Figure 5.40 *Ovarian dysgerminoma. Solid oblong homogeneous mass (M) which replaces the right ovary.*

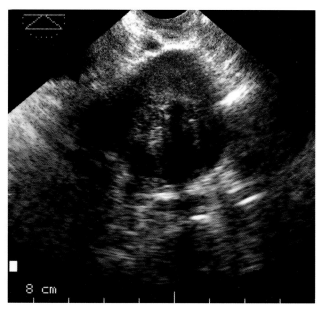

Figure 5.41 *Ovarian thecoma. Longitudinal sonogram of the right ovary with a 3 cm solid mass with some acoustic shadowing.*

are very fast growing and virulent. The patients have a median age of 19 years. Serum α–fetoprotein is positive. The sonographic appearance is similar to dysgerminoma.

(4) Other germ cell tumors (embryonal carcinoma, choriocarcinoma) – These are rare. They are solid with necrosis or hemorrhage. There are no specific sonographic findings.

(5) Mixed germ cell tumors – These comprise 8 per cent of all malignant germ cell tumors. There are no sonographic features to allow differentiation from other germ cell tumors.

Sex cord–stromal tumors of the ovary
(1) Granulosa–stromal cell tumors – Mixed granulosa–theca cell tumors are more common than either granulosa or theca cell tumors. There is a wide age range but they are most common in postmenopausal patients. They have low malignant potential; only 3 per cent are bilateral. An estrogen-producing tumor may present with uterine bleeding in older women

and precocious puberty in premenarchal females. There is a 10–15 per cent incidence of associated endometrial carcinoma. Sonographically, they are small masses, predominantly echogenic and solid. Larger masses may be multiloculated, simulating cystadenomas.

(2) Thecomas and fibromas – These are rare, commonly benign, and usually unilateral, with 70 per cent occurring in postmenopausal patients. Fibromas may be multiple (10 per cent). Estrogen production is frequent in thecomas and rare in fibromas. Both appear sonographically as solid and attenuating with an acoustic shadow corresponding to the entire extent of the tumor (Fig. 5.41). Fibromas may be associated with ascites and pleural effusions (Meig's syndrome). Association with ascites is not specific for fibromas.

(3) Sertoli–Leydig cell tumor – These are very rare, and comprise less than 0.4 per cent of ovarian tumors. The mean age is 24 years; 70 per cent are masculinizing and 20 per cent are malignant. The

sonographic appearance is similar to granulosa–theca cell tumors.

Metastatic carcinoma of the ovary

Metastatic involvement of the ovary accounts for up to 29 per cent of all malignant ovarian cancers. The commonest primary tumors are colon, breast and gastric carcinomas. The Krukenberg tumor is an infiltrative mucinous carcinoma of the signet ring cell type. It is usually metastatic, with 80 per cent having a gastric primary tumor.

The sonographic appearance is of an irregular echogenic solid mass with clearly defined tumor margins, often with variable 'moth-eaten' cystic spaces. The appearance is often similar to that of cystadenocarcinoma.

Lymphomatous involvement has a similar sonographic appearance to that of lymphoma, with hypoechoic trans-sonic solid masses.

Transvaginal color flow Doppler in ovarian masses

Technique

The intent is to identify small tumor vessels (arteries) with low-resistance flow which occur within malignant neoplasms. Color flow Doppler is used to direct placement of the pulsed Doppler sample volume to obtain a spectral display. This is used to calculate peak velocity and resistive index (RI). These indices have been found to be helpful in differentiating benign from malignant disease. Resistive index is calculated using the formula:

$$RI = A - (B/A)$$

where A is the systolic peak and B is the minimum diastolic flow velocity.

Patients should be scanned prior to day 8 of their menstrual cycle to avoid confusion with the low-resistance flow of the corpus luteum.

Results

An ovarian or adnexal mass may be highly suggestive of malignancy based on morphological characteristics, RI and peak velocity. Suspicious morphology includes papillary projections, thick vascularized walls or mural nodules, and. an RI of less than 0.40 in a premenopausal women and less than 0.60 in a postmenopausal one. If the RI is >0.40 or 0.50 respectively, the mass is almost always benign. A peak velocity of 20–30 cm/s or more is highly suggestive of malignant neoplasm.

Various studies quote varying degrees of success, even up to 99.5 per cent for differentiating benign from malignant disease.[27] Hemorrhagic luteal cysts and endometriomata may demonstrate high-velocity, low-impedance flow but when followed over 3 months, with or without pharmacological suppression, they regress and the flow characteristics acquire a more benign appearance.

THE FALLOPIAN TUBE

Pelvic Inflammatory Disease (PID)

On TVS there is sonographic spectrum of appearances although TVS demonstrates tubal pathology with a sensitivity of 93 per cent and an overall accuracy of 91 per cent. The sonographic findings include the following:

1. Enlarged tortuous, ill-defined hypoechoic tubular structures extending from the uterine cornua to the adnexa. (Fig. 5.42).
2. The mass may be differentiated from surrounding small bowel by the absence of peristalsis and from distended pelvic veins by the absence of flow.
3. Internal debris suggests the presence of a pyosalpinx rather than hydrosalpinx.

Periovarian inflammation is demonstrated with a sensitivity of 90 per cent and an accuracy of 93 per cent. The sonographic findings include the following:

1. Ovarian enlargement with indistinct margins.
2. The more severe disease results in adnexal masses and distortion of normal anatomical landmarks.

Uterine and periuterine inflammatory abnormalities are identified with a sensitivity of only 25 per cent. In a series by Patten et al[28] the inability of TVS to detect subtle uterine inflammatory changes was not clinically important, because all patients had other sonographic stigmata of PID.

Free fluid is a common normal finding in pre- and postmenopausal patients. Small fluid collections in the posterior cul-de-sac may, however, be missed in patients with PID. Echogenic debris suggests the presence of blood or pus but the lack of these internal echoes does not exclude the presence of pus.

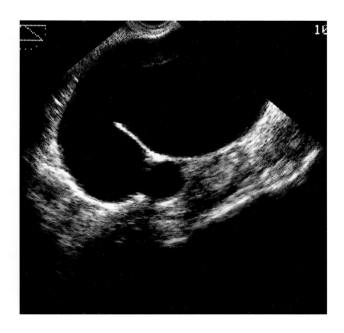

Figure 5.42 *Hydrosalpinx. TVS of dilated tortuous right fallopian tube. No internal debris is seen.*

Abscess drainage

After abscess localization with TVS, drainage may be performed per vagina under ultrasound guidance using either an transvaginal or transvesical probe.

For non-viscous fluid collections, simple needle aspiration with systemic antibiotic therapy may be adequate. More viscous fluid collections require catheter drainage by either direct puncture or the Seldinger guide wire technique.

In a series by vanSonnenberg et al,[29] transvaginal drainage obviated the need for surgery in 86 per cent of patients with pelvic abscesses. The catheters were left in place an average of 6.7 days.

Ectopic Pregnancy

The use of TVS in ectopic pregnancy is one of its most important applications. TVS can see the gestational or chorionic sac within the endometrial canal as early as 36 days of menstrual age. The early diagnosis of ectopic pregnancy is more and more based on a combination of clinical data, levels of beta-HCG and the sonographic findings of an empty uterus. The gestational sac is seen in the tube in only 20 per cent of patients, whereas an echogenic mass is seen in more than 80 per cent of cases (Fig. 5.43). The live embryo per se is seen in only 20 per cent of cases, but when present is 100 per cent positive of an ectopic pregnancy. Transvaginal Doppler and color Doppler of the corpus luteum and the ectopic trophoblast may allow for an increased percentage of positive diagnoses of ectopic pregnancy (Fig. 5.44).

Fluid within the endometrial canal surrounded by an echogenic zone is the decidual cast and is present up to 30 per cent of the time. This may be confused with the gestational sac and is referred to as a pseudogestational sac. The absence of an intrauterine embryo or yolk sac will also indicate a pseudogestational sac.

Free fluid in the posterior cul-de-sac with or without echogenic clots is present in up to 70 per cent of ectopic pregnancies but echogenic fluid is less common and more specific.

Newer methods of treatment of ectopic gestation involve a single intramuscular injection of methotrexate. This is a radical change in the treatment of ectopic pregnancy which may well result in a more natural healing of the tube with a reduction in the incidence of future ectopic pregnancies.

Solid Neoplasms

Solid neoplasms of the fallopian tube are uncommon and are difficult to differentiate from some ovarian or other adnexal masses.

THE POSTERIOR CUL-DE-SAC

Fluid

The presence of small amounts of fluid may be more readily seen transvaginally but more important is the characterization of the fluid. Bloody or purulent fluid is slightly more echogenic than a serous effusion, but the finding of echogenic fluid with a positive beta-HCG and an empty uterus will strongly suggest the diagnosis of ectopic gestation. The volume of fluid may be misleading to the neophyte. Transvaginally, even small amounts of fluid may appear large, and one is cautioned to compare the findings with the transvesical ones.

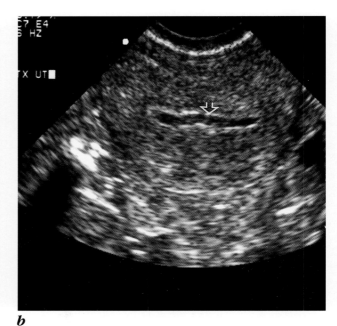

a

b

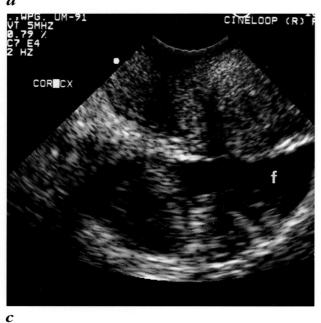

c

Figure 5.43 *TVS of right-sided ectopic pregnancy. (a) Echogenic sac of the ectopic gestation (electronic calipers) medial to the right ovary and corpus luteal cyst (c). (b) Transverse scans of the uterus containing the decidual cast (open arrowhead). (c) Fluid (f) and echogenic clots in the posterior cul-de-sac.*

Masses

Endometriomata and other pelvic masses can be assessed more readily by TVS because of its ability to characterize the contents of the mass. Fluid–debris levels with echogenic material may be seen in endometriomata. In addition, the mobility and degree of tenderness can best be assessed with TVS. Postoperative peritoneal pseudocysts are irregular-shaped fluid collections which are generally echofree and have at least some border with acute angulations (Fig. 5.45). Primary ovarian cysts or dilated fallopian tubes are round or oblong with no acute angulations. They displace structures rather than wrap around them. A pseudocyst will not change in location or in configuration during the scan or with palpation.

Bowel

Bowel with peristalsis is normally seen in the posterior cul-de-sac. There should not be confusion in mistaking bowel loops for mass lesions. Inflamed

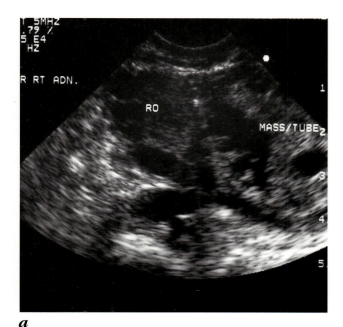

a

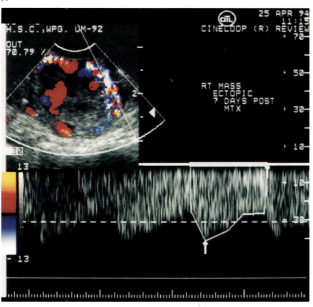

b

Figure 5.44 *Color duplex of right ectopic pregnancy. (a) Echogenic gestational sac ('mass/tube') medial to the right ovary (ro). (b) Color and pulsed Doppler of the ectopic pregnancy demonstrated high-velocity, low-resistance flow.*

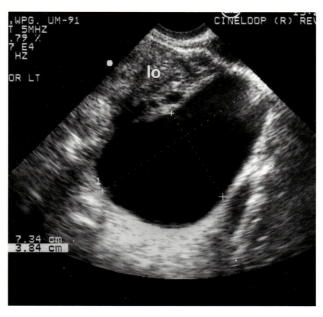

Figure 5.45 *Pelvic or peritoneal pseudocyst. Left adnexal cystic mass adjacent to the ovary (lo). At laparotomy this was a pseudocyst related to previous adhesions from an appendiceal rupture.*

loops of bowel may be seen if they lie in the cul-de-sac. They will lack normal peristalsis, have a thick wall (>4 mm) and may be associated with inflammatory masses (Fig. 5.46).

INTERVENTIONAL PROCEDURES

Follicle Aspiration

The transvaginal approach is by far the most common mode of oocyte retrieval. It requires only mild analgesia and local anesthesia as opposed to general anesthesia used in laparoscopic retrieval. The technique is relatively benign with very low morbidity.

Cyst Aspiration

This is a use which is just starting to gain some consideration particularly in establishing the diagnosis. Fine needle aspiration has been used extensively with relative impunity in all areas of the body. The

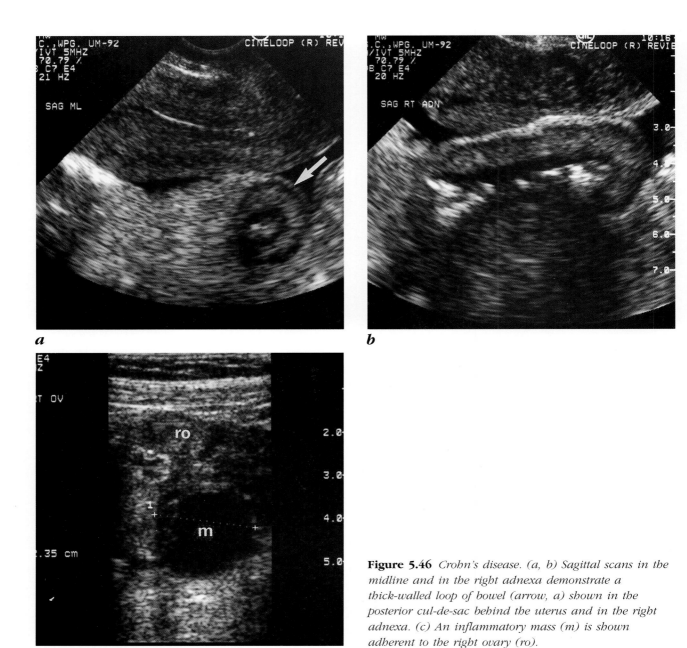

Figure 5.46 *Crohn's disease. (a, b) Sagittal scans in the midline and in the right adnexa demonstrate a thick-walled loop of bowel (arrow, a) shown in the posterior cul-de-sac behind the uterus and in the right adnexa. (c) An inflammatory mass (m) is shown adherent to the right ovary (ro).*

claims of tumor spread have been made elsewhere, but with a 22 gauge needle this may not be the case. The therapeutic uses with complete evacuation of the cyst have not proven to be of much value because of frequent recurrence of 25 per cent in perimenopausal cysts.[30]

REFERENCES

1. Kurjak A, Zaku D, Kupesic-Urek S, Normal pelvic blood flow infertility. In: Kurjak A, ed., *Transvaginal Color Doppler* (The Parthenon Publishing Group: New Jersey 1991) 115.

2. Fleisher A, Pittaway D, Beard L et al, Sonographic depiction of endometrial changes occurring with ovulation induction, *J Ultrasound Med* (1984) **3**:341–6.

3. Callen P, DeMartini W, Filly R, The central uterine cavity echo: a useful anatomic sign in the ultrasonographic evaluation of the female pelvis, *Radiology* (1979) **131**:187.

4. Hall D, Hann L, Ferrucci J et al, Sonographic morphology of the menstrual cycle, *Radiology* (1979) **133**:185.

5. Duffield S, Picker R, Ultrasonic evaluation of the uterus in the normal menstrual cycle, *Med Ultrasound* (1981) **5**:70–4

6. Mendelson EB, Bohm–Velez M, Joseph N et al, Endometrial abnormalities: evaluation with transvaginal sonography, *AJR* (1988) **150**:139–42.

7. Lin MC, Gosink BB, Wolf SI et al, Endometrial thickness after menopause: effect of hormone replacement, *Radiology* (1991) **180**:427–32.

8. Cohen H, Tice H, Mandel F, Ovarian volumes measured by ultrasound: bigger than we think, *Radiology* (1990) **177**:189–92.

9. Goswamy R, Campbell S, Whitehead M, Screening of ovarian cancer, *Clin Obstet Gynecol* (1983) **10**:621–43.

10. Bourne T, Campbell S, Steer C et al, Transvaginal colour flow imaging: a possible new screening technique for ovarian cancer, *Br Med J* (1989) **299**:1367–70.

11. Kurjak A, Zalud I, Alfirevic Z, Evaluation of adnexal masses with transvaginal color ultrasound, *J Ultrasound Med* (1991) **10**:295–7.

12. Timor-Tritsch IE, Rottem S, Transvaginal ultrasonographic study of the fallopian tube, *Obstet Gynecol* (1987) **70**:424–8.

13. Timor-Trisch I, Rottem S, *Transvaginal Sonography*, 2nd edn (London: Elsevier 1990).

14. Hulka CA, Hall DA, Endometrial abnormalities associated with Tamoxifen therapy for breast carcinoma, *AJR* (1993) **160**:809–12.

15. Granberg S, Wikland M, Karlsson B et al, Endometrial thickness as measured by endovaginal ultrasonography for identifying endometrial abnormality, *Am J Obstet Gynecol* (1991) **164**:47—52.

16. VanBogaert LJ, Clinicopathologic findings in endometrial polyps, *Obstet Gynecol* (1988) **71**:771–3.

17. Nelson JR, Corson SL, Longterm management of adenomyosis with gonadotropin-releasing hormone agonist: a case report, *Fertil Steril* (1993) **59**:441–3.

18. Fedele L, Bianchi S, Dorta M et al, Transvaginal ultrasonography in the diagnosis of diffuse adenomyosis, *Fertil Steril* (1992) **58**:94–7.

19. Fedele L, Bianchi S, Dorta M et al, Transvaginal ultrasonography in the differential diagnosis of adenomyoma versus leiomyoma, *Am J Obstet Gynecol* (1992) **167**:603–6.

20. Azziz R, Adenomyosis: current perspectives, *Obstet Gynecol Clin North Am* (1989) **16**:221–35.

21. Ascher SM, Arnold LL, Patt RH et al, Ademyosis: prospective comparison of MR imaging and transvaginal sonography, *Radiology* (1994) **190**:803–6.

22. Ritchie WGM, Sonographic evaluation of normal and induced ovulation, *Radiology* (1986) **161**:1–10.

23. Fleischer AC, Pittaway DE, Wentz AC et al, The uses of sonography for monitoring ovarian follicular development. In: Sanders RC, Hill M, eds, *Ultrasound Annual* (Raven Press, New York 1983) 163.

24. Mendelson EB, Friedman H, Neiman HL et al, The role of imaging in infertility management, *AJR* (1985) **144**:415–20.

25. Pache TD, Wladimiroff JW, Hop WCJ et al, How to discriminate between normal and polycystic ovaries: transvaginal US study, *Radiology* (1992) **183**:421.

26. Wolf SI, Gosink BB, Feldesman MR et al, Prevalence of simple adnexal cysts in postmenopausal women, *Radiology* (1991) **180**:65–71.

27. Taylor KJW, Schwartz PE, Screening for early ovarian cancer, *Radiology* (1994) **192**:1–10.

28. Patten RM, Vincent LM, Wolner–Hanssen P et al, Pelvic inflammatory disease. Endovaginal sonography with laparoscopic correlation, *J Ultrasound Med* (1990) **9**:681–9.

29. vanSonnenberg E, D'Agostino HB, Casola G et al, US–guided transvaginal drainage of pelvic abscesses and fluid collections, *Radiology* (1991) **181**:53–6.

30. Bonilla–Musoles F, Ballester MJ, Simon C et al, Is avoidance of surgery possible in patients with perimenopausal ovarian tumors using transvaginal ultrasound and duplex color doppler sonography? *J Ultrasound Med* (1993) **12**:33–9.

Chapter 6 Transvaginal Ultrasound: Early Pregnancy Failure

Roger Chisholm

INTRODUCTION

Over the last 20 years ultrasound has revolutionized the practice of obstetrics and gynaecology. More recently, transvaginal ultrasound (TVS) has continued an already rapid rate of development and is now the method of choice for follicular monitoring in fertility disorders, the differentiation of the normal and abnormal first trimester pregnancy, and the diagnosis of ectopic pregnancy.

EQUIPMENT

The major advantage of TVS over conventional transabdominal sonography (TAS) is the ability to use higher frequency transducers nearer to the organs of interest, thus facilitating higher resolution imaging of the uterus, adnexae, ovaries and cul de sac (Figs. 6.1 and 6.2). TVS also overcomes inherent disadvantages of TAS such as the obese patient, retroverted uterus or low fetal lie. TVS nevertheless has limitations, both because of more limited beam penetration due to the higher frequency and also because of its more invasive nature, which may make the technique less desirable in certain clinical situations. Thus it is generally desirable that TAS, with its ability to give a more global view, and TVS, with its higher resolution, should be regarded as complementary techniques.

Many ultrasound equipment manufacturers offer mechanically or electronically focused transvaginal transducers, with frequencies usually in the range 5–7.5 MHz. Single, dual and multiple frequencies are available. In general, the highest frequency allowing adequate penetration for most clinical situations is 5 MHz, making this a good general-purpose transducer. The size of the sector image is usually between 90° and 115°, although transducers do exist with scan angles up to 240°. Images may be either symmetric or asymmetric, depending on the angle of the active transducer surface to the axis of the probe. Transducer footprints range from 1.5 to 3.0 cm in diameter, and focal zones from 1 to 8 cm.

Duplex Doppler and colour flow imaging are both widely available through transvaginal transducers, and can be used to identify and assess vessels and other areas of vascularity. These techniques may provide useful information in evaluating infertility, early pregnancy and pregnancy-related complications such as ectopic gestations.

Probes are prepared by applying coupling gel to the end of the probe and then sheathing the probe in a condom. Additional gel is applied to the outside of the condom prior to its insertion. A brief description of the technique and reasons for performing it should be given to the patient. Most women find the examination acceptable and often preferable to the transabdominal approach, where a full bladder is necessary. Unless there are unusual aspects to the case, written consent is unnecessary.

Before the examination the patient must empty her bladder, after which the examination is performed supine, with the thighs abducted and knees flexed, and usually with the buttocks elevated on a pillow. A full examination requires evaluation of the uterus and cervix, both ovaries and adnexae and the cul de sac. Movements of the probe include axial advancement/withdrawal, angling and rotation, which may be performed individually or in combination. Following completion of the examination, the transducer assembly should be immersed in a solution such as Cidex for a minimum of 10 min for adequate disinfection. The

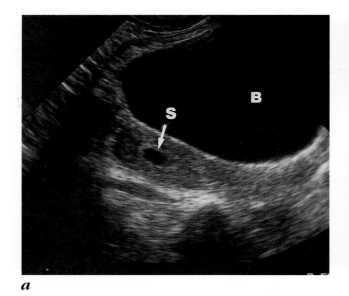

Figure 6.1 *Diagrammatic representation of sagittal transvaginal ultrasound examination. The close proximity of the active transducer end to the uterus (U) is noted. B, bladder; R,rectum.*

manufacturer's recommendations for cleaning should be followed.

SAFETY FACTORS

Although there are potentially harmful side-effects of diagnostic ultrasound, the low acoustic energies involved have never been shown to cause any adverse effect despite many millions of patient examinations. Any potential effect of ultrasound is based on extrapolation from experimental data, where intensities several orders of magnitude greater have been shown to have some bioeffect. The risks of TVS are clearly greater with a relatively high frequency source lying close to the early gestational sac and contents. Likewise, Doppler and colour flow imaging further raise insonation energies, the former technique more so because of its more targeted nature. At present there is little consensus for the use of transvaginal Doppler in early pregnancy. All examinations should apply the principle of the lowest practical energies to achieve diagnostic information (ALARA), thereby minimizing any potentially harmful effects.

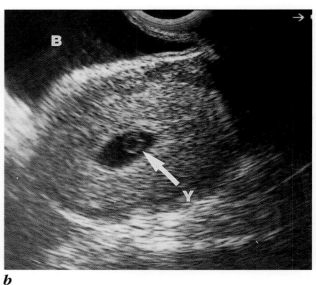

a   *b*

Figure 6.2 *Transabdominal (a) and transvaginal (b) images of an intrauterine pregnancy with a menstrual age of 5 weeks. The yolk sac (Y) is only demonstrated on the transvaginal image. S, gestational sac; B, bladder.*

THE NORMAL FIRST TRIMESTER

An understanding of early embryonic development is essential for anyone performing TVS during early pregnancy. For normal pregnancies, TVS enables the gestational sac, yolk sac and embryo to be viewed in unique detail. For abnormal pregnancies, embryonic demise and ectopic pregnancies may be diagnosed earlier and with greater confidence than is the case with TAS.

NORMAL EMBRYONIC DEVELOPMENT

Fertilization of the oocyte by the sperm usually occurs within the fallopian tube. Cleavage begins on the first day and by day 3 a 16-cell morula enters the uterus. After further differentiation, a blastocyst is formed (around 20 menstrual days) which implants into and invades the endometrium approximately 2 days later (Fig. 6.3). As early chorionic villi develop, human chorionic gonadotrophin (hCG) is produced, with a positive pregnancy test occurring at a menstrual age of 3 weeks. The gestational sac reaches 1 mm at 4 weeks, 3 mm at 32 days, and 5 mm at 35 days.

The inner layer of the blastocyst gives rise to the yolk sac, embryo and umbilical cord, while the outer trophoblastic layer forms the placenta, chorion and amnion. The embryonic disc, consisting of endodermal and ectodermal cell layers, forms along the edge of the blastocyst. Subsequently the amniotic sac develops between the ectodermal germ layer and the adjacent trophoblast in the fourth week of gestation. The primitive yolk sac or cavity of the blastocyst shrinks as the gestation sac grows, eventually forming the secondary yolk sac which is the 'yolk sac' demonstrated by ultrasound. The net result of these changes is the 'double bleb' sign[1] made up of the yolk sac and amnion on either side of the developing embryo. Later development causes a relative decrease in the size of the chorionic cavity, while the amniotic cavity enlarges and becomes the outer covering of the umbilical cord (Fig. 6.4).

The yolk sac develops at approximately 28 days and may be seen within the gestational sac early in the fifth menstrual week (Fig. 6.5). Demonstration of the yolk sac confirms that an intrauterine fluid collection is indeed a true gestational sac and will

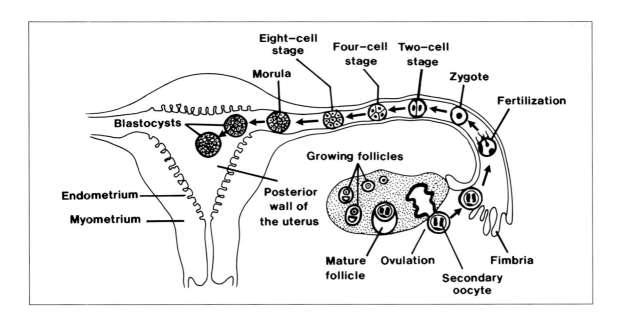

Figure 6.3 *The sequence of ovulation, fertilization and early development of the embryo. (Reproduced with permission from Moore KL, Persaud TVN,* The Developing Human: Clinically Oriented Embryology, *5th edn, Philadelphia, WB Saunders Co., 1993.)*

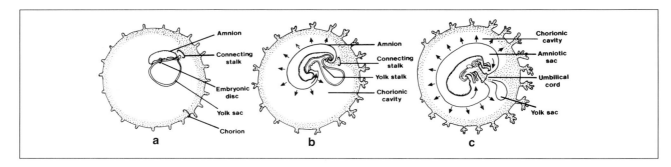

Figure 6.4 *(a) Blastocyst with early development of amnion and yolk sac which lie on either side of the embryonic disc—5 menstrual weeks. (b) The dorsal aspect of the embryo folds into the amnion and the yolk stalk is formed—6 menstrual weeks. (c) The amnion enfolds the umbilical cord and the yolk sac moves further into the chorionic cavity— 12 menstrual weeks.* (Reproduced with permission from Moore KL, Persaud TVN, The Developing Human: Clinically Oriented Embryology, *5th edn, Philadelphia, WB Saunders Co., 1993.)*

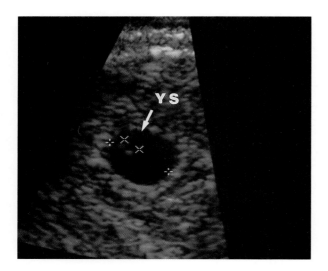

Figure 6.5 *Normal intrauterine gestional sac at 5 menstrual weeks. The yolk sac (YS) measures approximately 2 mm in diameter.*

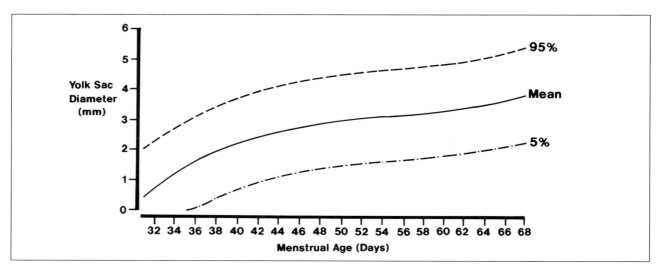

Figure 6.6 *The relationship between yolk sac diameter and menstrual age.* (Reproduced with permission from Lindsay DJ, Lovett IS, Lyons EA et al, Radiology *(1992) **183**:115–18.)*

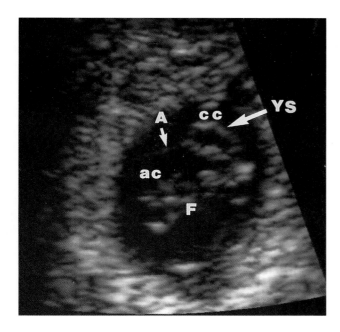

Figure 6.7 *Intrauterine gestational sac at approximately 7 menstrual weeks. The yolk sac (YS) lies outside the amnion (A) and within the chorionic cavity (cc). F, fetus; ac, amniotic cavity.*

commonly precede visualization of the embryo itself. The yolk sac gradually increases in size up to approximately 12 weeks of gestation (Fig. 6.6), coming to lie between the amnion and chorion (Fig. 6.7). After 8 weeks the sac detaches and solidifies and, although it may be found at delivery, it is not usually demonstrated sonographically after the end of the first trimester.

The amnion develops in step with the yolk sac but, being a finer structure, is more difficult to visualize. The amniotic and chorionic membranes fuse during the latter half of the first trimester, the process being completed between 12 and 16 menstrual weeks. The chorionicity of twin pregnancies is established in the first trimester merely by noting the number of gestational sacs. The amnionicity is more difficult to determine, although this is still frequently possible with TVS (Fig. 6.8). Embryonic appearances at various stages through the first trimester are fairly characteristic (Fig. 6.9).

The placenta and umbilical cord may be identified at 8 or 9 weeks (Fig. 6.10). Fetal heart activity has been reported at 40 days and should always be present by 46 menstrual days with TVS.[2] Cardiac motion is generally seen as soon as the embryo is visualized and

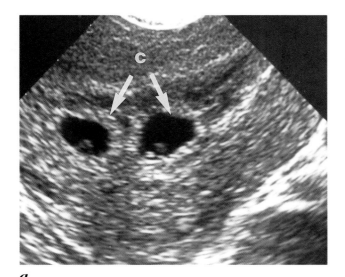

a

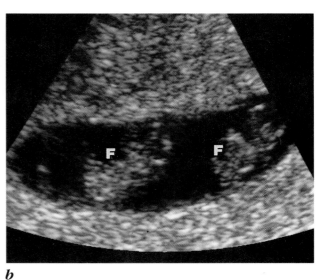

b

Figure 6.8 *(a) Dichorionic twin pregnancy with discrete gestational sacs, each containing a yolk sac. The chorion (C) contributes to the echogenic appearance of the walls. (b) Monochorionic monoamniotic twin pregnancy. TVS showed no amnion between the two fetuses (F).*

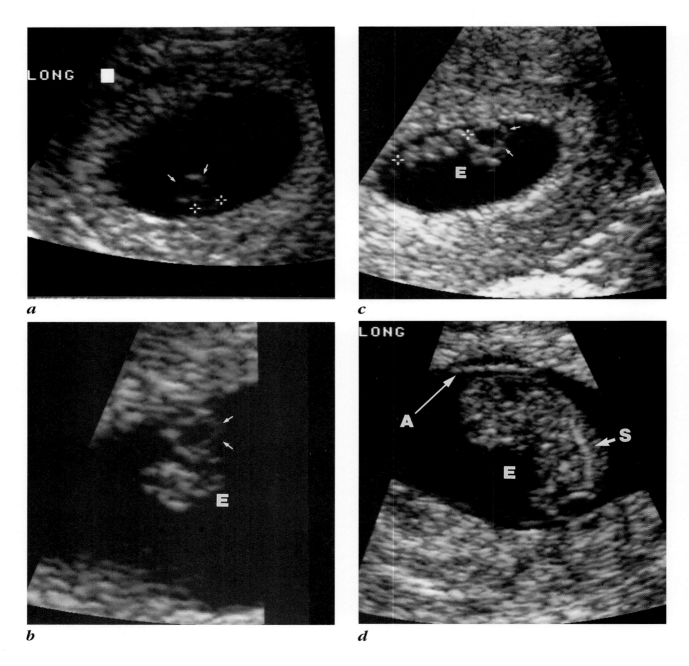

Figure 6.9 *The sonographic appearance of the normally developing embryo: (a) 6-week embryo between cursors; (b) 6-week 4-day embryo; (c) 7-week embryo; (d) 8-week 4-day embryo. Small arrows denote the yolk sac. E, embryo; A, amnion; S, developing spine.*

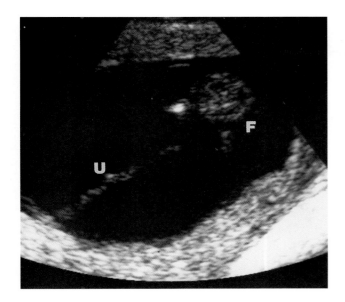

Figure 6.10 *The umbilical cord (U) is shown with a fetus (F) with sonographic and menstrual ages of 10 and 13 weeks respectively. No fetal heart beat was seen.*

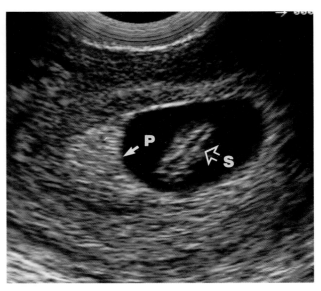

Figure 6.11 *The parallel echogenic lines of the developing spine (S) as well as the placenta (P) are seen in this fetus with a sonographic age of 8 weeks and 2 days.*

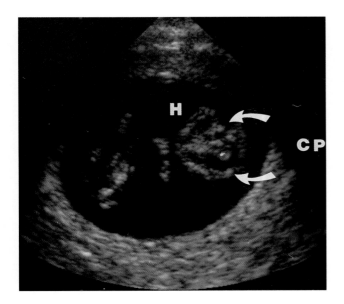

Figure 6.12 *The echogenic choroid plexi (CP) are seen within the head (H) of this normal 10-week fetus.*

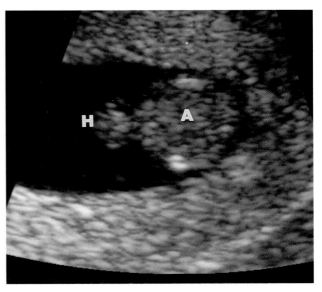

Figure 6.13 *A normal 10-week fetus. The midgut herniation (H) is seen arising from the anterior wall of the abdomen (A).*

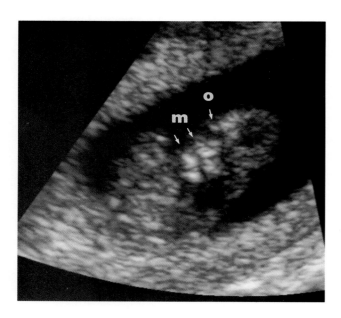

Figure 6.14 *A normal 10-week fetus. The orbits (o), maxilla and mandible (m) are seen on this coronal section through the face.*

always when the crown–rump length is greater than 5 mm.[2] For crown–rump lengths smaller than 5 mm it is important that the examination should be repeated after a time interval, as absent cardiac activity has been noted in a number of such embryos where the pregnancy has subsequently developed normally.[3] Normal cardiac rates vary with menstrual age, with values anywhere between 90 and 128 beats/min at 6 weeks, reaching a peak of up to 174 beats/min at 9 menstrual weeks, and subsequently declining to around 150 beats/min at 14 weeks.

The timing and early appearance of subsequent fetal structures by TVS is now fairly well established.[4] Early limb buds appear during the eighth week, rotating over the following 3 weeks into the normal parasagittal plane. Hands can be seen and fingers counted in the twelfth week. The developing spine can be imaged from the seventh week, with the parallel lines of the developing neural tube seen on coronal sections (Fig. 6.11). At 7 weeks the fetal brain is seen as a single ventricle, and by the ninth week two lateral ventricles largely filled with choroid plexus become apparent (Fig. 6.12). Midgut herniation into the umbilical cord occurs during weeks 9 to 11 (Fig. 6.13), after

which the bowel returns to the abdominal cavity and undergoes its normal rotation. It is not possible to diagnose abdominal wall defects such as omphalocoele or gastroschisis before 14 menstrual weeks.

Significant facial development occurs during the middle of the first trimester, with the bony elements of the mandible, maxilla and orbits being seen by 10 weeks (Fig. 6.14) and soft tissue structures such as the nose and lips by 12 weeks. Although imaging the face may prove difficult before 10 weeks because of the embryonic position, clues may nevertheless be obtained to suggest a fetus at risk of certain genetic disorders.

GESTATIONAL AGE

The menstrual age of a pregnancy may prove unreliable both because of inaccurate or uncertain dates and because of variation in the time of ovulation and fertilization. Gestational age may be established more accurately and objectively from the gestational sac size, embryonic size or hCG levels.

Gestational Sac Size

The mean sac diameter (MSD) correlates well with menstrual age during the early first trimester, with similar confidence limits to the crown–rump length during the first 8 weeks.

Embryonic Size

The embryo is consistently visualized from 6 weeks of gestation. Several published data sets are available for the estimation of gestational age from the crown–rump length[5–7] (Fig. 6.15), generally regarded as the most accurate method of pregnancy dating between 6 and 10 weeks. Most studies show a variability of 4–5 days, although there are pitfalls to accurate measurement, such as erroneous inclusion of the adjacent yolk sac[8] as well as problems common to all sonographic measurements such as beam divergence and side-lobe artifacts.

THE NORMAL GESTATIONAL SAC

A normal sac tends to be round or oval with a smooth contour and is generally located in the fundus or middle uterus. The walls frequently appear as two adjacent concentric echogenic rings, formed by the decidua vera and decidua capsularis, and

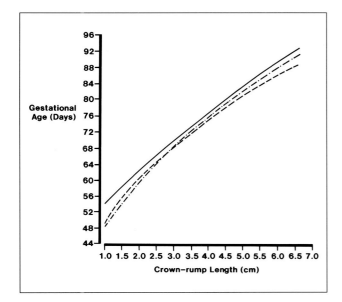

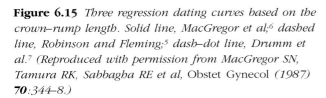

Figure 6.15 *Three regression dating curves based on the crown–rump length. Solid line, MacGregor et al;*[6] *dashed line, Robinson and Fleming;*[5] *dash–dot line, Drumm et al.*[7] *(Reproduced with permission from MacGregor SN, Tamura RK, Sabbagha RE et al,* Obstet Gynecol *(1987)* **70***:344–8.)*

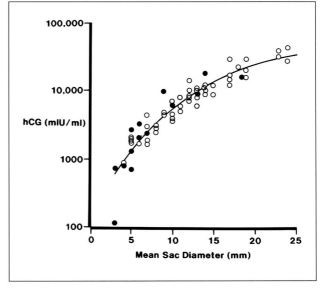

Figure 6.16 *Correlation of log hCG levels (2IS) with mean sac diameter. The data combine measurements from transvaginal sonography (*black circles*) and transabdominal sonography (*open circles*). (Reproduced with permission from Nyberg DA, Mack LA, Laing FC, Jeffrey RB,* Radiology *(1988)* **167***:619–22.)*

described as the double decidual sac sign or DDSS[9] (see Fig. 6.26). Furthermore, the sac is eccentrically positioned relative to the endometrium due to the mechanism of implantation.[10] Any or all of the above features may be lost with an abnormal gestational sac, as detailed below.

Normal sac growth rates have been documented[11] with a range of 0.7–1.5 mm and a mean of around 1 mm/day. With this information, follow-up examinations may be timed with the minimum delay necessary to make a definitive diagnosis.

Discriminatory Gestational Sac Size

The normal yolk sac, amnion and embryo can always be identified at a certain gestational age and therefore, by definition, when the gestational sac has reached a certain *discriminatory* size.

Different researchers have suggested that on TAS a living embryo should be seen once the gestational sac exceeds values ranging from 17 to 30 mm. The corresponding values with TVS again vary from 9 to 18 mm, although a conservative approach would

suggest that 16[12] to 18 mm[13] would be more appropriate values on which to base clinical management.

Values can be established in a similar fashion for the appearance of the yolk sac. Although in theory this should be present as soon as the gestational sac is visible, this is often not the case in practice, presumably because of its small size and eccentric position. Studies with TAS have suggested that the yolk sac should be present when the MSD exceeds 20 mm,[14] and with TVS the corresponding value is anything between 6 and 10 mm.[15] Once again, the larger value is clearly the one on which it is prudent to base clinical practice.

Human Chorionic Hormone and Gestational Age

Human chorionic gonadotrophin, secreted by trophoblasts, shows an exponential rise after implantation, and serum levels can be detected by 3 menstrual weeks. There is close correlation between hCG levels, menstrual age and gestational sac size before sonographic demonstration of the embryo (Fig. 6.16). Thus, as with gestational and yolk sac

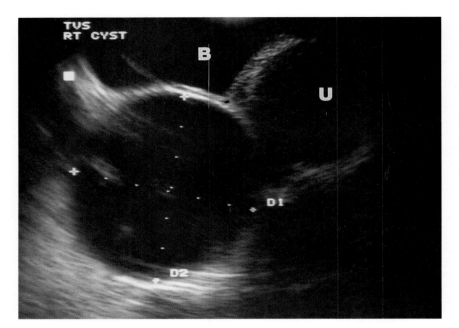

a

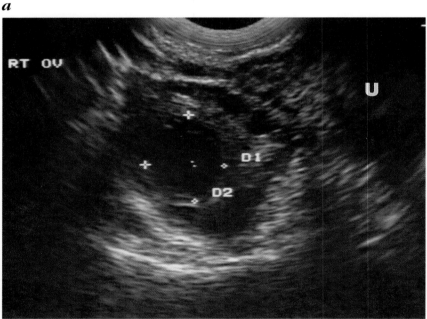

b

Figure 6.17 *Corpus luteum cysts accompanying normal gestations at 6 weeks and 6 days (a) and 8 weeks and 2 days (b). Although the cyst in (a) appears anechoic and could be mistaken for a simple ovarian cyst, that in (b) is more complex and has a wider differential diagnosis. U, uterus; B, bladder.*

visualization, there is a discriminatory hCG level above which an intrauterine gestational sac should always be visualized. Conversely, a level higher than the discriminatory level in the absence of such a sac indicates the presence of an abnormal pregnancy.

There are two methods for measuring and reporting the hormone, the International Reference Preparation (IRP) and the Second International Standard (2IS), the former being approximately twice as sensitive as the latter. Suggested discriminatory levels for visualization of an intrauterine gestational sac are 1800 IU/l (2IS) with TAS[16] and 750 IU/l (2IS) with TVS.[17] In addition, a gestational sac will frequently be seen in patients with hCG levels above 300 IU/l (2IS), and so the

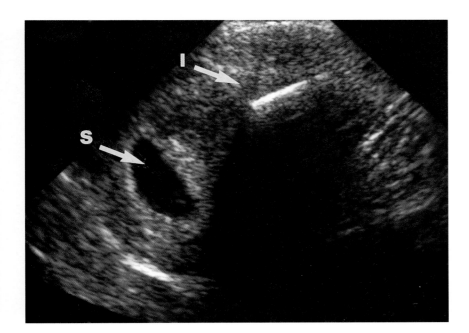

Figure 6.18 *Normal intrauterine gestational sac (S) at 5 weeks and 3 days. An IUCD (I) is noted within the endometrial cavity.*

absence of a sac at levels above this raises the possibility of an abnormal pregnancy. Since the normal hCG doubling time is 2.2 days the logical step with such patients is to rescan after 2–3 days, when the gestational sac should normally be visible. If the sac is still not seen or the hCG fails to rise at the normal rate, an ectopic pregnancy or threatened or inevitable abortion is likely.

Discriminatory levels of hCG have also been published for the appearance of the yolk sac and embryo[18] and can be used in a way similar to that described above. Sequential TVS examinations every 3 days allows progression through the milestones of gestational sac, yolk sac, embryo and heart beat.

MISCELLANEOUS

As with any ultrasound examination a complete gestational assessment by TVS will involve evaluation of the adnexa and cul de sac as well as the uterus. This will be considered in more detail when considering ectopic pregnancy. Nevertheless, normal structures such as corpus luteum cysts will commonly be seen and their widely variable appearance must be appreciated to prevent false-positive pathological diagnoses being made (Fig. 6.17). It may sometimes be necessary to follow up such masses to ensure

resolution and exclude neoplasia. Likewise, other factors relevant to the wellbeing of a normal gestation may be seen (Fig. 6.18).

In summary, TVS provides a unique window through which to view the the first trimester of pregnancy. Gestational age can be determined earlier and with a greater accuracy than with previous techniques. Furthermore, a knowledge of normal development, sonographic findings and hCG correlation allows for earlier diagnosis of the abnormal gestation.

ABNORMAL FIRST TRIMESTER INTRAUTERINE PREGNANCY

Ultrasound has become a fundamental part of the evaluation of women who present with vaginal bleeding during the first trimester of pregnancy. Approximately 25 per cent of women present with a *threatened abortion* during the first trimester and of these up to 50 per cent will subsequently abort.[19] If all pregnancies documented with an elevated hCG are included, loss rates of up to 60 per cent have been reported,[20] many of these being associated with chromosome abnormalities.[21]

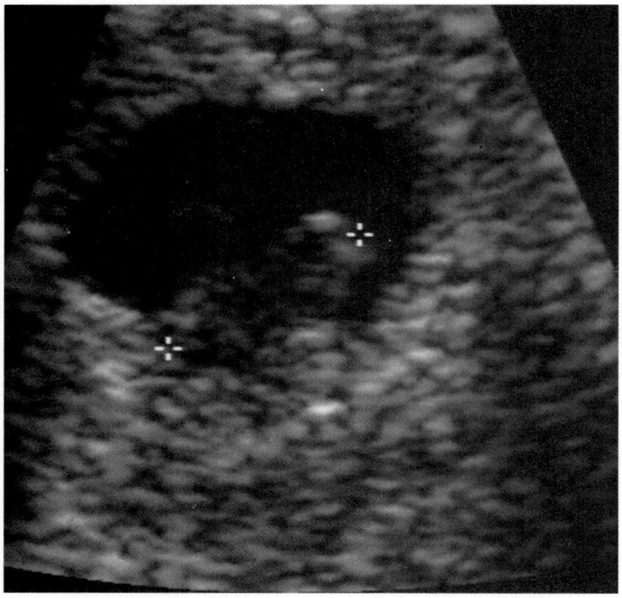

The role of ultrasound in the threatened abortion has traditionally been to demonstrate a living or dead embryo (Fig. 6.19). The establishment of discriminatory zones for sonography and hCG levels as documented above has greatly widened the search to areas other than the presence or absence of a beating heart. These include the uterus and its decidual reaction, the gestational sac and its membranes and the fetal pole and yolk sac. All of these are seen more clearly and earlier with TVS than TAS, and this has therefore become the initial investigation of choice in the evaluation of such patients.

THE ABNORMAL GESTATIONAL SAC

As previously described, there is a linear relationship between embryonic growth and the size of the gestational sac. The discriminatory sac size is the MSD when an embryonic pole should always be visualized, 18 mm being accepted as a conservative value with TVS. Sac diameters between 12 and 18 mm are also suggestive of nonviability but should be correlated with other clinical and sonographic features.

Figure 6.19 *A rather amorphous embryo with sonographic and menstrual ages of 7 and 10 weeks respectively was seen in this patient with vaginal bleeding. No fetal heart beat was seen.*

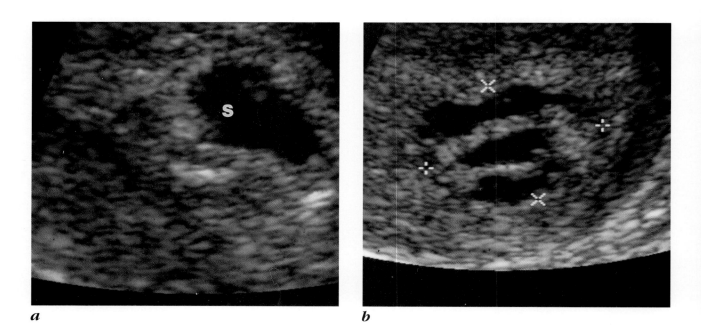

a *b*

Figure 6.20 *Abnormal gestational sacs in patients with vaginal bleeding, both at approximately 7 menstrual weeks. In (a) the wall of the sac (S) has become irregular and faint, while in (b) there is hydropic degeneration with haemorrhage and oedema.*

With an abnormal gestation the normal double decidual ring may become thicker, heterogeneous and irregular due to hydropic degeneration or may conversely become fainter or even disappear with decidual necrosis, adopting an echotexture similar to that of the adjacent myometrium (Fig. 6.20). Haemorrhage within the decidua may cause partial or complete separation. Abnormal perigestational blood flow, clearly seen with duplex or colour flow systems within the trophoblast, is a late finding, often accompanied by other features of an abnormal pregnancy.[22]

Complete, Incomplete and Missed Abortions

If, in addition to the gross morphological abnormalities of sac size, shape and appearance, there is also echogenic debris or fluid present within the endometrial cavity, an *incomplete abortion* is likely. Where there has been a further but still incomplete loss the only sign of retained products of conception may be a thickened endometrium.[23] Colour flow imaging may be helpful when deciding whether curettage is necessary by demonstrating retained trophoblastic tissue.[24]

A completely empty uterus in the presence of a positive pregnancy test indicates either a *complete spontaneous abortion*, a very early normal intrauterine pregnancy or an ectopic pregnancy. Correlation with the menstrual history and ß-hCG levels helps to differentiate these possibilities.

The term *missed abortion* is generally unsatisfactory, being subject to multiple definitions and some inconsistency with clinical presentation, as patients may present with vaginal bleeding. The terms *embryonic demise* or *blighted ovum* (see below), depending on whether or not a fetal pole or remnants are seen within the gestational sac, are preferable.

Blighted Ovum

Although they were previously described as *blighted ova*, *anembryonic* or *empty sacs*, more recent studies[25] have suggested that in many sacs previously thought to be empty on TAS, the majority in fact contain embryonic structures when examined with TVS (Fig. 6.21). It has furthermore been noted that following selective fetal reduction the fetal pole may gradually resolve and disappear without any further intervention. Thus the term *blighted ovum* should perhaps be changed to *early embryonic demise*, the earlier arrest of development frequently being due to chromosome abnormalities.[26]

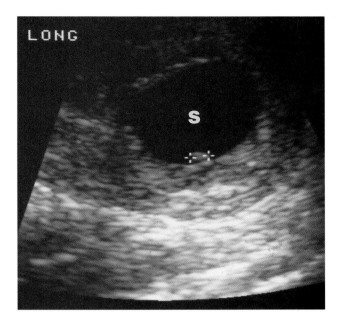

Figure 6.21 *Transvaginal study of a 10-menstrual-week gestational sac (S). A 2-mm embryo (cursors) is seen posteriorly which would almost certainly not have been seen transabdominally. There was no evidence of cardiac activity.*

Oligohydramnios

In pregnancies where a live fetus is demonstrated, a relatively small gestational sac is a poor prognostic sign, with a universally fatal outcome in one study where the MSD was less than 4 mm greater than the crown–rump length[27] (Fig. 6.22).

Subchorionic or Perigestational Haematoma

In normal pregnancies the commonest cause of vaginal bleeding during the first trimester is bleeding from the chorion frondosum, which may also give rise to a subchorionic haematoma. TVS may give some indication as to whether the haemorrhage is causing separation of the early placenta, which carries a poor prognosis[28] (Fig. 6.23), or whether it is away from the placenta and nearer to the internal os, in which case a favourable outcome is more likely (Fig. 6.24). Most small haemorrhages resolve without clinical sequelae,[29] although there may sometimes be a higher incidence of further bleeding and preterm labour.

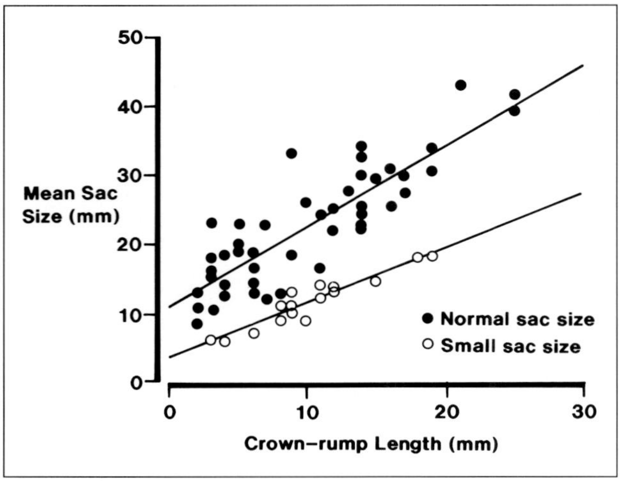

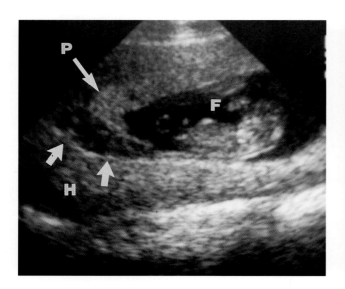

Figure 6.22 *The association of first trimester oligohydramnios with pregnancy outcome. Mean gestational sac size has been compared with crown–rump length in 16 embryos with small gestational sacs (open circles) and 52 control embryos with normal-size gestational sacs (black circles). Spontaneous abortions occurred in 15 of 16 embryos with small sacs compared with 4 of 52 control embryos. (Reproduced with permission from Bromley B, Harlow BL, Laboda LA, Benacerraf BR, Radiology (1991)* **178***:375–7.)*

Of note, is the fact that the amnion and chorion may occasionally separate later in the second trimester and subsequent to their initial fusion. This *chorioamniotic separation* is often the result of needle puncture of the membranes during amniocentesis and does not represent haemorrhage. It is generally of no consequence to the fetus.

THE YOLK SAC AND AMNION

As with the appearance of the embryo, there is a discriminatory gestational sac size for the appearance of the yolk sac. The values suggested above are 8 and 10 mm for gestations which are usually and always abnormal. The presence of a normal yolk sac does not, of course, necessarily indicate a normal gestation.

Large, calcified or free-floating yolk sacs[30] may also be associated with a poor pregnancy outcome, as may an unusually thickened amniotic membrane.[31]

THE FETUS

The presence of a beating fetal heart clearly confirms that an embryo is alive and should be seen in all

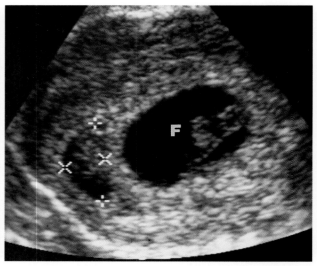

Figure 6.23 *Subchorionic haematoma (H) which is tracking behind the placenta (P). The fetus (F) was alive, with a sonographic age of 10 weeks.*

Figure 6.24 *Subchorionic haematoma (cursors) not related to the placenta. The fetus (F) was alive.*

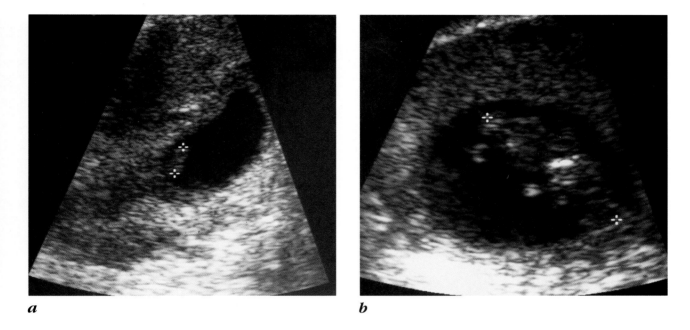

a   *b*

Figure 6.25 *Twin pregnancy as a result of in vitro fertilization. Menstrual age 10 weeks. Following vaginal bleeding, twin 1 (a) was noted to have a sonographic age of only 7 weeks and no heart beat was seen. In comparison, twin 2 (b) had an appropriate 10-week sonographic age and a normal heart.*

normal gestations by 46 menstrual days using TVS[13] or a week or more later with TAS. Conversely, a pregnancy may still be entirely normal when an apparently empty gestational sac is seen between 5 and 6.5 menstrual weeks or even when no gestational sac is seen before 5 weeks. A knowledge of normal fetal growth rates allows reassessment at a time when the status of the pregnancy can be reliably confirmed.

Fetal bradycardia (less than 90 beats/min) is a poor prognostic sign,[32] frequently being associated with an embryo which is small compared with the menstrual age. Early follow-up is advisable in these patients.

Multiple gestations are prone to a significant fetal loss rate in the first trimester, with estimates ranging up to 78 per cent for the loss of one of a twin pregnancy.[33] Fetal loss may be associated with vaginal bleeding, sonography showing either an empty sac or persisting fetal pole on the affected side (Fig. 6.25). In many cases the blighted twin will be resorbed and is thus not seen later in pregnancy.

Hydatidiform Mole

Hydatidiform mole is the commonest and most benign form of gestational trophoblastic disease, occurring in up to 1 per 1200 pregnancies.[34] In the first trimester a molar pregnancy may be sonographically indistinguishable from an incomplete or missed abortion or a hydropic placenta. The endometrium generally takes on a complex appearance, with areas of increased and decreased echogenicity around and within the endometrium, representing trophoblastic tumour and blood respectively. The characteristic 'snowstorm' appearance described in the second trimester is often not seen at this earlier stage. Human chorionic gonadotrophin levels may be disproportionately high compared with the size of the gestational sac, the converse of the finding with other abnormal first trimester gestations. The combination of TVS and colour flow imaging may demonstrate both trophoblastic invasion and residual trophoblastic tissue after treatment.[35]

ECTOPIC PREGNANCY

In recent years there has been a worldwide increase in the incidence of ectopic pregnancies.[36] The reported incidence is up to 1 per cent of all pregnancies in the USA, where the condition accounts for approximately 25 per cent of all maternal deaths and considerable maternal morbidity. Up to 18 per cent of subsequent pregnancies will also result in an ectopic gestation and less than 50 per cent of women will carry a subsequently normal pregnancy to term. Furthermore, early treatment before rupture may decrease morbidity and preserve reproductive capabilities. Making the diagnosis accurately and early is thus of crucial importance and in achieving this the role of sonography is fundamental.[37]

Patients at risk include:

- those with history of a previous ectopic pregnancy;
- those with history of pelvic inflammatory disease;
- pregnant women with an IUCD in situ;
- those who had in vitro fertilization or tubal micro-surgery;
- those who have had laparoscopic tubal coagulation.

PRESENTING SYMPTOMS

The classic clinical triad of pelvic pain, abnormal vaginal bleeding and a palpable adnexal mass occurs in less than 50 per cent of patients.[38] Other clinical signs may be amenorrhoea, an enlarged soft uterus, shoulder tip pain and fainting or shock. Despite this the overall clinical diagnosis of ectopic pregnancy is correct in less than 50 per cent of cases.[39]

DIAGNOSIS

Pregnancy Testing

With the advent of ß-hCG testing, pregnancy may now be confirmed at a menstrual age of only 3½ weeks. Normal intrauterine gestations show an hCG doubling time of approximately 2 days, a rate not usually achieved by an ectopic pregnancy. Likewise, at any given gestational age, ß-hCG levels tend to be lower for an ectopic than an intrauterine gestation. Nevertheless, there is a considerable overlap of values for the two conditions at a given gestational age so that serial measurements are generally of greater value than a single assay. Subnormal increases generally indicate an ectopic or nonviable intrauterine pregnancy, while very low values may indicate an ectopic which is already dead and which may possibly resolve spontaneously.[40]

Ultrasonography

Many studies have evaluated various aspects of the sonographic diagnosis of ectopic pregnancy. Traditionally, the diagnosis was made by TAS when an enlarged uterus was seen with an adnexal mass and fluid in the cul de sac.[41] These findings are frequently not present, however, and, despite the significant contribution made by discriminatory hCG levels,[16] TAS reaches diagnostic accuracy only in the seventh menstrual week, too late for making the diagnosis in the majority of cases. TVS, with its earlier visualization of anatomical structures and correspondingly lower discriminatory levels of hCG, has proved to be a major step forward in the diagnosis of ectopic pregnancy.[42,43]

The sonographic findings of ectopic pregnancy are variable and a systematic approach must be taken to the evaluation of the uterus, adnexa and cul de sac. TAS is still a valuable technique for searching for the small minority of ectopic gestations beyond the reach of the transvaginal probe and also in cases where more extensive pelvic pathology, including the ruptured ectopic pregnancy, may be confusing with the relatively limited field of view provided by the vaginal transducer. It may be performed either before or after TVS, depending on local protocols and whether or not the patient presents with a full urinary bladder.

The uterus

Intrauterine pregnancies
As discussed earlier, an intrauterine pregnancy can be reliably diagnosed with TVS from 5 menstrual weeks by demonstrating a yolk sac, cardiac activity or an embryo itself within an intrauterine gestational sac. Coexistent intra- and extrauterine pregnancies are very uncommon, with estimates varying from 1 in 30 000 to 1 in 6000, depending on the patient's risk factors.[44,45] The demonstration of an intrauterine pregnancy thus makes an additional ectopic gestation highly unlikely.

Extrauterine gestations
An empty uterus may be seen either with an early intrauterine pregnancy, a recent abortion or an

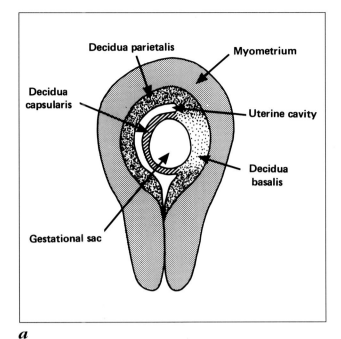
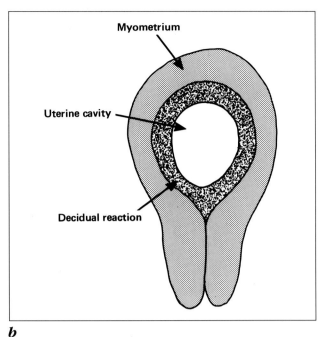

a

b

Figure 6.26 *(a) Diagrammatic representation of a normal intrauterine gestational sac with close apposition of the decidua capsularis and decidua parietalis forming the double decidual sac sign. (b) Widely separated uterine walls are present in patients with pseudogestational sacs of ectopic pregnancy. (Reproduced with permission from Nyberg DA, Laing FC, Filly RA et al, Ultrasonographic differentiation of the gestational sac of early intrauterine pregnancy from the pseudogestational sac of ectopic pregnancy,* Radiology *(1983)* **146***:755–9.)*

ectopic pregnancy. In this last case the endometrium tends to be thickened to a variable extent, indicating hormonal stimulation from the extrauterine gestation.

A pseudogestational sac may develop as a result of decidual degeneration in up to 20 per cent of patients with an ectopic pregnancy.[46] These structures are located centrally within the endometrium, rather than eccentrically, as with a true gestational sac[10] (Fig. 6.26). The wall is thinner and poorly defined compared with the double decidual sac usually seen with a normal gestation. With TVS it is also possible to determine that the contents of the pseudogestational sac are more echogenic than the virtually anechoic contents seen with a normal gestational sac (Fig. 6.27).

Correlation with serum ß-hCG levels is necessary where there is persisting doubt about whether the uterine contents represent a true or pseudogestational sac. As previously discussed, there is a linear relationship between the size of a normal intrauterine gestational sac and hCG levels. A significant discrepancy raises the possibility of either an abnormal intrauterine pregnancy or an ectopic pregnancy. Once a normal pregnancy has been confidently excluded, uterine curettage may, if necessary, be performed. The presence or absence of chorionic tissue will distinguish between these two possibilities and indicate to the obstetrician whether further, more invasive, investigation is required. Doppler ultrasound has also been shown to be helpful in assessing peritrophoblastic blood flow, with one study[47] showing high-velocity low-impedance flow in all normal gestations over 36 menstrual days. No false-positive diagnoses of a normal intrauterine gestation were made using the Doppler criteria stated by these authors.

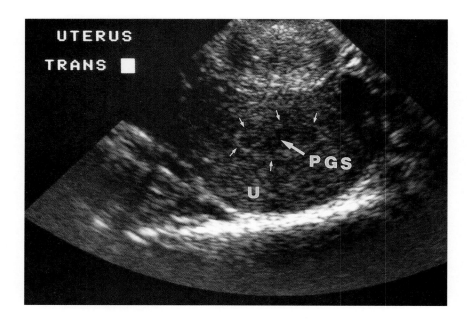

Figure 6.27 *Pseudogestational sac (PGS) within the uterus (U) of a patient with an ectopic pregnancy. The central location of the sac can be seen, along with the faint wall (small arrows) and rather echogenic contents.*

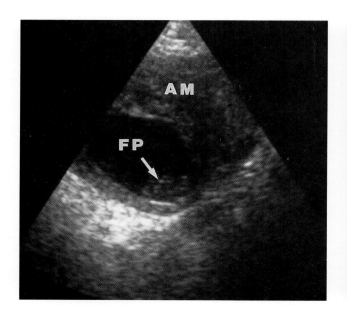

Figure 6.28 *Ectopic pregnancy: an adnexal mass (AM) containing a gestational sac and fetal pole (FP) was detected (no cardiac motion seen).*

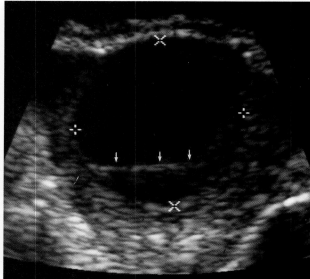

Figure 6.29 *Corpus luteum cyst (cursors) containing a debris/fluid level (small arrows), the result of haemorrhage. There was a normal 6-week intrauterine pregnancy.*

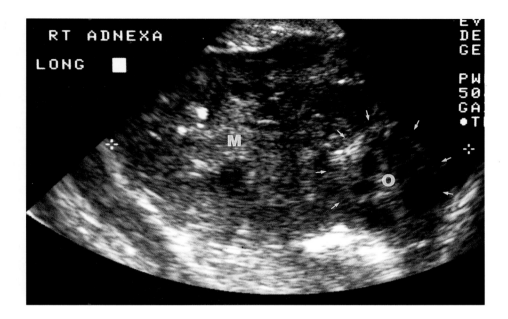

Figure 6.30 *Ectopic pregnancy: complex adnexal mass (M) in a patient found at surgery to have a ruptured fallopian tube. The normal ovary (O) containing follicles is seen contiguous with the mass.*

The adnexa

With TVS a live embryo may be seen in the adnexa in up to a quarter of patients with an ectopic pregnancy, significantly more than with TAS.[48] In these cases the diagnosis is established without doubt. Almost as significant is the presence of an adnexal gestational sac seen in up to 70 per cent[48,49] of patients with an ectopic pregnancy. These are usually small and thick-walled and may be empty or may contain a yolk sac or embryo (Fig. 6.28). They may sometimes be confused with a haemorrhagic corpus luteum cyst (Fig. 6.29), although it should be noted that these may coexist in up to one quarter of patients with an ectopic pregnancy.[50]

Complex adnexal masses are seen with TVS in up to 91 per cent of patients with an ectopic pregnancy[51] (Fig. 6.30), although rather less often if the mass is predominantly cystic rather than solid.[52] Pelvic inflammatory disease with tubovarian abscesses is clearly one important differential diagnosis and, as before, the ability to characterize trophoblastic tissue with duplex Doppler anaysis may prove useful.[53]

Fluid may be seen within the cul de sac and elsewhere within the peritoneum in over two thirds of patients with an ectopic gestation and may be either simple or particulate (bloody). Depending on the age of the collection there may be varying amounts of clotted and unclotted blood present and septae may develop. Blood may leak from the ends of the fallopian tubes or, less commonly, there may be tubal rupture and massive haemorrhage. The relative risk of an ectopic pregnancy rises with the volume of blood seen and the presence of any associated features such as an adnexal mass. Lesser amounts of fluid may also be seen with a ruptured or haemorrhagic corpus luteum cyst or pelvic inflammatory disease.

Other sites

Although 95 per cent of ectopic pregnancies originate in the fallopian tubes, there are other relatively rare sites including the ovary (3 per cent), the interstitial portions of the tubes (2 per cent) and even less commonly the cervix or peritoneum.

CLINICAL MANAGEMENT

Traditionally, failure to make the diagnosis of an ectopic gestation by the combination of TAS and hCG analysis resulted in further investigations, including uterine curettage, culdocentesis and laparoscopy. The developments outlined above, and in particular the greater and more informed use of TVS, have substantially reduced the need for these more invasive procedures although they may still occasionally be necessary.

Once the diagnosis has been made, surgery with salpingectomy used to be the almost inevitable result. More recently the advances in diagnosis made by TVS have allowed a more conservative approach to be taken in a proportion of patients.

Recently it has been shown that between a quarter and two thirds of ectopic pregnancies may resolve spontaneously,[54,55] in particular where the ß-hCG level is relatively low, the size of the gestation is small and the vascularity of the adnexal mass is limited. Further work[49] has shown that an intact adnexal gestational sac is frequently associated with an intact fallopian tube, while a complex adnexal mass is associated with tubal haematoma, an incomplete tubal abortion or a ruptured fallopian tube.

This more detailed characterization of an ectopic pregnancy by TVS provides some potential for allowing clinicians to choose specific therapies for different patients[56] within the appropriate clinical context. Apart from expectant management, possibilities include systemic methotrexate, local injection of methotrexate or potassium into the ectopic gestation, laparoscopic removal of the gestation or, finally, laparotomy.

Clearly, expectant management is only practical where the patient is clinically stable with low hCG levels and a small adnexal mass. TVS has been used both to aspirate an ectopic sac and also for local methotrexate injection.[57,58] Systemic methotrexate has proved successful in the medical management of a high proportion of unruptured ectopic pregnancies,

individual doses being determined by serial hCG levels. In one study[59] hysterosalpingography demonstrated patent ipsilateral fallopian tubes in a high proportion of patients following such treatment and approximately half of these subsequently achieved a normal intrauterine pregnancy.

Although salpingectomy is the common surgical treatment at laparotomy when the tube has ruptured or there is major haemorrhage, a more conservative salpingostomy with expression of the ectopic from a tubal incision may be appropriate in some patients. While this procedure has the advantage of frequently being performed laparoscopically, there is a small risk that a further operation may become necessary as determined by either clinical status or persistently elevated hCG values.[60]

SUMMARY

TVS has cast new light on the development of the normal first trimester pregnancy and has played a fundamental role in the diagnosis and management of both the abnormal intrauterine and ectopic pregnancy. Not only can the diagnosis of an intrauterine pregnancy be made significantly earlier with the combination of TVS and ß-hCG assays, but the discriminatory levels of hCG in combination with TVS allow earlier definition of an abnormal pregnancy, whether inside or outside the uterus. Furthermore, in a high proportion of cases TVS will make the diagnosis of an ectopic pregnancy by demonstrating the ectopic embryo or gestational sac or the slightly less specific adnexal mass. In all cases appropriate management decisions can be made about the abnormal pregnancy significantly earlier than was the case with TAS.

REFERENCES

1. Yeh H, Rabinowitz JG, Amniotic sac development: ultrasound features of early pregnancy—the double bleb sign, *Radiology* (1988) **166**:97–103.

2. Howe RS, Isaacson HJ, Albert JL, Coutifaris CB, Embryonic heart rate in human pregnancy, *J Ultrasound Med* (1991) **10**:367–71.

3. Levi CS, Lyons EA, Zheng XH et al, Endovaginal US: demonstration of cardiac activity in embryos of less than 5 mm in crown rump length, *Radiology* (1990) **176**:71–4.

4. Timor–Tritsch IE, Farine D, Rosen MG, A close look at early embryonic development with the high frequency transvaginal transducer, *Am J Obstet Gynecol* (1988) **159**:676–81.

5. Robinson HP, Fleming JEE, A critical evaluation of sonar crown–rump length measurement, *Br J Obstet Gynecol* (1975) **82**:702–10.

6. MacGregor SN, Tamura RK, Sabbagha RE et al, Underestimation of gestational age by conventional crown–rump length dating curves, *Obstet Gynecol* (1987) **70**:344–8.

7. Drumm JE, Clinch J, MacKenzie G, The ultrasonic measurement of the fetal crown–rump length as a method of assessing gestational age, *Br J Obstet Gynecol* (1976) **83**:417–21.

8. Sauerbrei E, Cooperberg PL, Poland JB, Ultrasound demonstration of the normal fetal yolk sac, *J Clin Ultrasound* (1980) **8**:217–19.

9. Nyberg DA, Laing FC, Filly et al, Ultrasonographic differentiation of the gestational sac of early intrauterine pregnancy from the pseudogestational sac of ectopic pregnancy, *Radiology* (1983) **146**:755–9.

10. Yeh HC, Goodman JD, Carr L, Rabinowitz JG, Intradecidual sign: a US criterion of early intrauterine pregnancy, *Radiology* (1986) **161**:463–7.

11. Nyberg DA, Mack LA, Laing FC, Patten RM, Distinguishing normal from abnormal gestational sac growth in early pregnancy, *J Ultrasound Med* (1987) **6**:23–7.

12. Levi CS, Lyons EA, Lindsay DJ, Early diagnosis of nonviable pregnancy with endovaginal US, *Radiology* (1988) **167**:383–5.

13. Rempen A, Diagnosis of viability in early pregnancy with vaginal sonography, *J Ultrasound Med* (1990) **9**:717–24.

14. Nyberg DA, Laing FC, Filly RA, Threatened abortion: sonographic distinction of normal and abnormal gestational sacs, *Radiology* (1986) **158**:397–400.

15. Cacciatore B, Titinen A, Stenman U, Ylostalo P, Normal early pregnancy: serum hCG levels and vaginal ultrasonography findings, *Br J Obstet Gynecol* (1990) **97**:889–903.

16. Nyberg DA, Filly RA, Mahony BS et al, Early gestation: correlation of hCG levels and sonographic identification, *AJR* (1985) **144**:951–4.

17. Bernaschek G, Rudelstorfer R, Csaicsich P, Vaginal sonography versus serum human chorionic gonadotrophin in early detection of pregnancy, *Am J Obstet Gynecol* (1988) **158**:608–12.

18. Bree RL, Marn CS, Transvaginal sonography in the first trimester, *Semin Ultrasound, CT MR* (1990) **11**:17.

19. Filly RA, The first trimester. In: Callen PW, ed. *Ultrasonography in Obstetrics and Gynecology*, 2nd edn (Saunders: Philadelphia, 1988) 19–46.

20. Roberts CJ, Lowe CR, Where have all the conceptions gone? *Lancet* (1973) **1**:498–9.

21. Guerneri S, Bettio D, Simoni G et al, Prevalence and distribution of chromosome abnormalities in a sample of first trimester internal abortions, *Hum Reprod* (1987) **2**:735–9.

22. Schaaps JP, Soyeur D, Pulsed Doppler on a vaginal probe: necessity, convenience or luxury? *J Ultrasound Med* (1989) **8**:315–20.

23. Kurtz AB, Schlansky–Goldberg RD, Choi HY et al, Detection of retained products of conception following spontaneous abortion in the first trimester, *J Ultrasound Med* (1991) **10**:387–95.

24. Dillon EH, Case CQ, Ramos IM et al, Endovaginal US and Doppler findings after first trimester abortion, *Radiology* (1993) **186**:87–91.

25. Pirrone EC, Monteagudo A, Timor Tritsch IE, Does 'Blighted Ovum' really exist? *J Ultrasound Med* (1990) **9**:41.

26. Ruchelli ED, Shen–Schqarz S, Martim J, Surti U, Correlation between pathological and ultrasound findings in first trimester spontaneous abortions, *Pediatr Pathol* (1990) **10**:743–56.

27. Bromley B, Harlow BL, Laboda LA, Benacerraf BR, Small sac size in the first trimester: a predictor of poor fetal outcome, *Radiology* (1991) **178**:375–7.

28. Goldstein SR, Subrumanyan BR, Raghavendra BN et al, Subchorionic bleeding in threatened abortion: sonographic findings and significance, *AJR* (1983) **141**:975–8.

29. Sauerbrei EE, Pham DH, Placental abruption and subchorionic hemorrhage in the first half of pregnancy: US appearance and clinical outcome, *Radiology* (1986) **160**:109–12.

30. Lindsay DJ, Lovett IS, Lyons EA et al, Yolk sac diameter and shape at endovaginal US: predictors of pregnancy outcome in the first trimester, *Radiology* (1992) **183**:115–18.

31. Horrow MM, Enlarged amniotic cavity: a new sonographic sign of early embryonic demise, *AJR* (1992) **158**:359–62.

32. Laboda LA, Estroff JA, Benacerraf BR, First trimester bradycardia: a sign of impending fetal loss, *J Ultrasound Med* (1989) **8**:561–3.

33. Landy HJ, Weiner S, Corson SL et al, The 'vanishing twin': ultrasonographic assessment of fetal disappearance in the first trimester, *Am J Obstet Gynecol* (1986) **155**:14–19.

34. Callen PW, Ultrasound evaluation of gestational trophoblastic disease. In: Callen PW, ed., *Ultrasonography in Obstetrics and Gynecology*, 2nd edn (Saunders: Philadelphia, 1988) 412.

35. Desai RK, Desberg AL, Diagnosis of gestational trophoblastic disease: value of endovaginal colour flow Doppler sonography, *AJR* (1991) **157**:787–8.

36. Stabile I, Grudzinskas JG, Ectopic pregnancy: a review of incidence, etiology, and diagnostic aspects, *Obstet Gynecol Surv* (1990) **45**:335–47.

37. Filly R, Ectopic pregnancy: the role of sonography, *Radiology* (1987) **162**:661–8.

38. Schwartz RD, DiPietro DL, ß-hCG as a diagnostic aid for suspected ectopic pregnancy, *Obstet Gynecol* (1980) **56**:197–201.

39. Weckstein LN, Clinical diagnosis of ectopic pregnancy, *Clin Obstet Gynecol* (1987) **30**:236–44.

40. Fernandez H, Rainhorn JD, Papiernik E et al, Spontaneous resolution of ectopic pregnancy, *Obstet Gynecol* (1988) **71**:171–4.

41. Lawson TL, Ectopic pregnancy, criteria and accuracy of ultrasonic diagnosis, *AJR* (1978) **131**:153–8.

42. Nyberg DA, Mack LA, Jeffrey RB, Laing FC, Endovaginal sonographic evaluation of ectopic pregnancy: a prospective study, *AJR* (1987) **149**:1181–6.

43. Thorsen MK, Lawson TL, Airman EJ et al, Diagnosis of ectopic pregnancy: endovaginal vs. transabdominal sonography, *AJR* (1990) **155**:307–10.

44. Hann LE, Bachman DM, McArdle CR, Coexistent intrauterine and ectopic pregnancy: a re–evaluation, *Radiology* (1984) **152**:151–4.

45. Reece EA, Petrie RH, Simans MF, Combined intrauterine and extrauterine gestations – a review, *Am J Obstet Gynecol* (1983) **146**:323–30.

46. Marks WM, Filly RA, Callen PW, Laing FC, The decidual cast of ectopic pregnancy: a confusing ultrasonographic appearance, *Radiology* (1979) **133**:451–4.

47. Dillon EH, Feyock AL, Taylor KJW, Pseudogestational sacs: Doppler US differentiation from normal or abnormal intrauterine pregnancies, *Radiology* (1990) **176**:359–64.

48. Rempen A, Vaginal sonography in ectopic pregnancy: a prospective evaluation, *J Ultrasound Med* (1988) **7**:381–7.

49. Cacciatore B, Can the status of tubal pregnancy be predicted with transvaginal sonography? A prospective comparison of sonographic, surgical and serum hCG findings, *Radiology* (1990) **177**:481–4.

50. Simons ME, Cooperberg PL, Graham MF, Ultrasound findings in ectopic gestation, *J Can Assoc Radiol* (1986) **37**:9–12.

51. Newton J, Ectopic pregnancy review article. *Br Med J* (1988) **649**:633–5.

52. Romero R, Kadar N, Castro D et al, The value of adnexal sonographic findings in the diagnosis of ectopic pregnancy, *Am J Obstet Gynecol* (1988) **158**:52–5.

53. Taylor KJW, Ramos IM, Feyock AL et al, Ectopic pregnancy: duplex doppler evaluation, *Radiology* (1989) **173**:93–7.

54. Atri M, Bret PM, Tulandi T, Spontaneous resolution of ectopic pregnancy: initial appearance and evolution at transvaginal US, *Radiology* (1993) **186**:83–6.

55. Fernandez H, Rainhorn J, Papiernik E et al, Spontaneous resolution of ectopic pregnancy, *Obstet Gynecol* (1988) **71**:171–4.

56. Laing FC, Sonographic determination of tubal rupture in patients with ectopic pregnancy: is it feasible? *Radiology* (1990) **177**:330–1.

57. Venezia R, Zangara C, Comparetto G, Cittadini E, Conservative treatment of ectopic pregnancies using a single echo guided injection of methotrexate into the gestational sac, *Ultrasound Obstet Gynecol* (1991) **1**:132–5.

58. Atri M, Bret PM, Tulandi T, Senterman MK, Ectopic pregnancy: evolution after treatment with transvaginal methotrexate, *Radiology* (1992) **185**:749–53.

59. Stovall TG, Ling FW, Gray LA et al, Methotrexate treatment of unruptured ectopic pregnancy: a report of 100 cases, *Obstet Gynecol* (1991) **77**:749–53.

60 Lundorff P, Hahlin M, Sjoblom P, Lindblom B, Persistent trophoblast after conservative treatment of tubal pregnancy: prediction and detection, *Obstet Gynecol* (1991) **77**:129–33.

Chapter 7 The Upper GI Tract: The Oesophagus

Jonathan R Glover

There is an ever increasing literature attesting to the great accuracy of endoscopic ultrasound (EUS) in staging oesophageal cancer and delineating benign diseases. The use of high-frequency transducers combined with balloon stand-off allows resolution of five distinct layers in the oesophageal wall which correspond to the levels seen on histology.[1] It is also possible to image beyond the oesophageal wall and see local lymph nodes, as well as invasion of, or adherence to, surrounding structures. Thus the technique has proved to provide far more accurate information than any other imaging modality, including computed tomography (CT) and magnetic resonance imaging (MRI).

EQUIPMENT

The standard equipment used for oesophageal ultrasound is the fibreoptic Endoscopic Ultrasound probe made by Olympus (EU-M1, M2 and M3). This has a mechanically driven rotating ultrasound probe mounted on the end of a side-viewing endoscope (Figs. 7.1 and 7.2). The transducer is covered by a tubular balloon which is filled up with water to provide a stand-off and create good acoustic coupling with the mucosa. The transducer rotates continually, producing a real-time 360° image of the oesophageal wall and surrounding structures. Recent models of this equipment allow switching between two frequencies, 7.5 MHz and 10 or 12 MHz, to give the best combination of resolution of the oesophageal wall and visualization of the surrounding structures, as well as incorporating a biopsy channel for ultrasound guided biopsy. However, these probes are beginning to be superseded by thinner 10-mm side-viewing videoecho-endoscopes (e.g. VU-M2, Olympus), and 3-mm catheter echoprobes which will pass down the biopsy channel of large-calibre forward-viewing endoscopes.

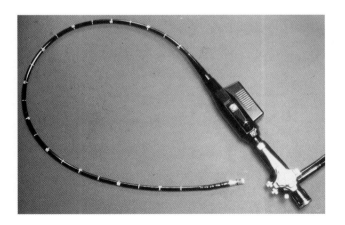

Figure 7.1 *Olympus EU-M1 Echo-probe.*

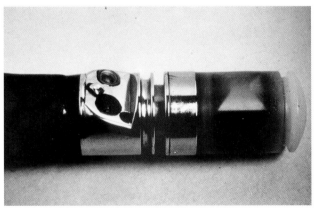

Figure 7.2 *Close-up view of the rigid tip of the EUS probe with the ultrasound transducer to the right.*

TECHNIQUE

The echo-endoscope is passed in the same way as a standard endoscope, with the same requirements for local anaesthesia, patient preparation, position, sedation and monitoring. Although useful to confirm position within the stomach, a light source and the other equipment needed for standard endoscopy are not strictly essential for oesophageal scanning. The standard endoscope is rather bulky (13 mm diameter) and has a longer rigid portion at the end than normal endoscopes which incorporates the transducer. This can make it a little more difficult to pass into the oesophagus, but there is seldom much problem for an experienced endoscopist. It is possible for the endoscopy and ultrasonography to be performed by the same operator, but this author finds it easier to have different operators for the endoscope and the ultrasound console.

The endoscope is passed into the oesophagus and down into the stomach, or as far as possible when there is a stenosing lesion, by gentle pressure and manipulation; as the endoscope is side-viewing, direct vision cannot be used. The balloon is then blown up with water (Fig. 7.3) and the endoscope slowly withdrawn while scanning the oesophagus. If the endoscope can be passed into the stomach, the left lobe of the liver and the perigastric and retroperitoneal lymph nodes can be imaged after aspirating air from the stomach, and/or filling the gastric lumen with water. The balloon should be kept just full enough to maintain good contact with the oesophageal wall: if it is overfilled the anatomical detail of the wall may be obscured due to compression, and only three layers seen instead of five. It is useful to record the investigation on videotape for later reference, but the sonographic image may be frozen to allow acquisition of still images on film etc. The procedure can be repeated as necessary. It must be recognized that where there is significant oesophageal stenosis, it may not be possible to pass the scope beyond the tumour, and over-vigorous attempts to do so carry the risk of oesophageal rupture.

THE NORMAL OESOPHAGUS

The normal oesophageal wall is seen as a series of concentric circles of hyperechoic and hypoechoic layers alternating bright and dark. The innermost layer is bright and corresponds to the mucosa–balloon interface. The next layer, which is dark, is made up of mucosa and inner submucosa, and is followed by a third bright layer, the outer submucosa. The fourth dark layer corresponds to muscularis propria, and the outer, fifth bright and dark layers are formed by the adventitia and peri-oesophageal fat (Figs. 7.4 and 7.5).

THE ABNORMAL OESOPHAGUS

Abnormalities of the oesophagus are shown as distortions or destruction of the normal sonographic layers seen on ultrasound. Malignant and inflammatory lesions both show as hypoechoic areas altering this pattern. It is not possible to distinguish between malignancy and inflammation on sonographic criteria alone, and therefore the sonographic findings must always be combined with biopsy results. Most pathological processes are hypoechoic, but some benign pathologies may show up as hyperechoic areas – see below.

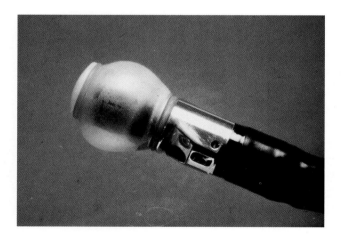

Figure 7.3 *Ultrasound transducer covered with water-filled balloon.*

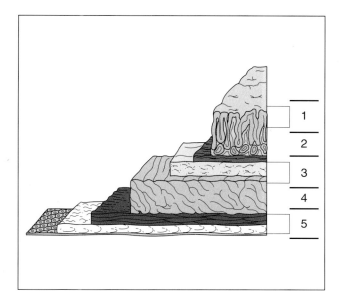

Figure 7.4 *Diagram demonstrating the correlation between the layers seen on EUS with histological structure of the oesophageal wall (see text).*

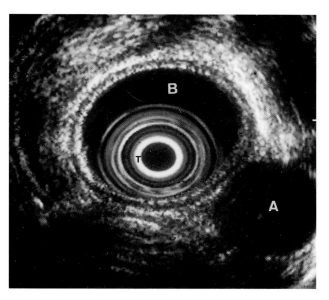

Figure 7.5 *Normal oesophageal wall on endoscopic ultrasound. T, transducer; B, balloon; A, aorta.*

OESOPHAGEAL CANCER

The most widespread use of EUS of the oesophagus has been in the staging of oesophageal cancer. There are now numerous papers attesting to the great accuracy of the technique in staging the depth of tumour infiltration through the oesophageal wall. Accuracy figures for T staging from various centres vary from 59 per cent to 92 per cent, but most papers give accuracy figures greater than 80 per cent, which is much better than figures for CT or MRI.

Oesophageal cancer appears as an ill-defined amorphous hypoechoic thickening of the oesophageal wall with destruction of the normal layered architecture which may penetrate through the wall into surrounding structures. The maximum normal thickness for each layer as measured by EUS is 2 mm.

The depth of penetration seen on EUS corresponds closely to the depth of penetration found at histology, and this has led to the adoption of a new TNM staging for oesophageal cancer[2] (Tables 7.1, 7.2 and 7.3).

Thus the T staging can be assessed on EUS by destruction of the sonographic layers of the oesophageal wall (see Figs. 7.6 and 7.7) as shown in Table 7.4.

The ability of EUS to image small peri-oesophageal lymph nodes is also unique. Lymph nodes as small as 5 mm can be seen reliably and distinguished from the oesophageal tumour, normal wall and surrounding tissues. If the endoscope can be manoeuvred past the tumour and into the stomach, the coeliac, left gastric and paracardial lymph node groups can also be assessed.

Criteria for distinguishing benign from malignant nodes (Fig. 7.8) have been described. Benign nodes are less than 5 mm in diameter, hyperechoic, and ellipsoid or triangular. Malignancy is indicated by one or more of the following: diameter greater than 10 mm, local depression of the adventitia, hypo-echogenicity, well-defined margins or round contour.[3] These features should be regarded as guide lines, but quite accurate figures have been obtained using them. Similar changes are also seen in lymph nodes in response to simple inflammation, and microscopic metastases may be found on histological examination

Table 7.1 T – Primary tumour.

Tx	Cannot be assessed
To	No evidence
TIS	In situ
T1	Invades lamina propria or submucosa
T2	Invades muscularis propria
T3	Invades adventitia
T4	Invades adjacent structures

Table 7.2 N – Lymph nodes.

Nx	Not assessed
N0	No nodal involvement
N1	Nodes involved with tumour

Table 7.3 M – Metastases.

M0	No evidence of liver metastases or nodal metastases in perigastric or coeliac node groups
M1	Liver metastases or nodal spread below diaphragm

Table 7.4

T stage	EUS finding
<TIS	Normal appearance on EUS
T1	Disease confined to the inner three layers
T2	Fourth, hypoechoic layer involved
T3	Tumour into fifth hyper- and hypoechoic layers
T4	Extension beyond hyperechoic peri-oesophageal fat into adjacent organs

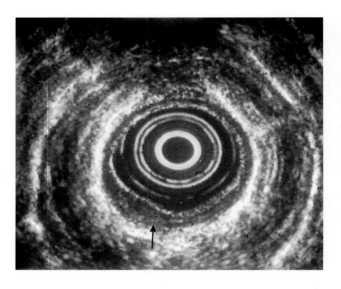

Figure 7.6 *Early carcinoma of the oesophagus (arrow) confined to the inner three layers of the oesophageal wall (stage T1).*

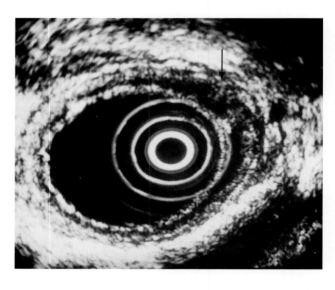

Figure 7.7 *More advanced oesophageal cancer penetrating through the oesophageal wall to the fourth hypoechoic layer, arrowed (stage T2).*

of apparently 'normal' nodes on EUS. However, the demonstration of direct extension of tumour mass into a node is regarded as pathognomonic for N1 staging. There is no N2 stage in the new classification – evidence of metastatic disease in distant node groups is classified as M1, along with liver metastases, under the new TNM system.

PROBLEMS WITH STAGING ON EUS

Virtually all patients are able to tolerate the 13-mm endoscope. However, the vast majority of oesophageal carcinomas in the Western world present with severe or near total dysphagia due to advanced stenosing disease. Thus the lesion is frequently T3 or

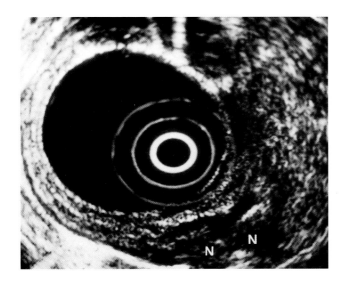

Figure 7.8 *Stage T3 N1 oesophageal cancer extending out into peri-oesophageal fat, and into some local lymph nodes (N).*

ACCURACY OF STAGING

Several centres have now published their results from EUS staging of oesophageal cancer. Accuracy figures vary from 59 per cent[5] to over 90 per cent[6] for T staging. There is a tendency to overstage T1 and T2 tumours, and understage T3 and T4 tumours, but the accuracy figures show that this is not a great problem. The accuracy is lower in cases where the stenosis is too tight to allow the endoscope to pass, since a full assessment cannot be performed, but one paper reports an accuracy of 77 per cent even in those non-traversable tumours.[7]

Sugimachi et al[8] analysed visualization rates of mediastinal lymph nodes with respect to size; they found a visualization rate of 92.9 per cent for nodes of 10 mm or more, 53.1 per cent for nodes 5–9 mm and 1 per cent for nodes less than 5 mm. For N staging accuracy figures range from 70 per cent[7,9] to 94 per cent.[10] These figures use the criteria of malignancy detailed above. N staging refers to local nodes, since distant node groups now fall into the M category, and overall accuracy for M staging (which includes lung and liver metastases, as well as coeliac and other remote node groups) is approximately 70 per cent[10,11] using EUS and this is significantly worse than the results using CT – 90 per cent accuracy.[11]

UTILIZATION OF EUS INFORMATION

The great accuracy of EUS in staging oesophageal carcinoma begs the question of how the information should be employed. There is currently no widely accepted stage-related treatment regime for this disease, and whereas the accuracy of the data is impressive, the data may not assist in treatment decisions.[12] Opinions vary considerably between centres, physicians, radiotherapists and surgeons as to the best treatment at each stage of the disease. Some clinicians refer virtually all patients for radiotherapy or simple palliative measures, while some surgeons will operate on any patient fit enough for surgery in the belief that surgery is the best palliation and the only hope of cure. However, the information provided by EUS is beginning to be used in deciding patient management and patient selection for surgery, presurgical radiotherapy, or radiotherapy alone, but given the many various regimes of radiotherapy and chemotherapy, and different surgical techniques, comparison between centres is difficult, and few centres have large enough study populations to produce meaningful results. As a result, very

T4 at presentation, and it may be difficult or impossible to traverse the lesion with the EUS endoscope. This reduces the information available from EUS and reduces the accuracy of T and N staging, while making it virtually impossible for EUS to make any contribution to M staging (see above). The proportion of patients in whom the lesion cannot be passed will undoubtedly fall as narrower probes become available but these are mostly still at the prototype stage. The modality will still be unable to assess the liver fully, as the right lobe cannot be imaged on EUS, and lung and other remote metastases will remain impossible to assess.[4] As mentioned above, EUS cannot distinguish between malignancy and inflammation – radiotherapy causes inflammatory changes which cannot be distinguished from tumour, and therefore it is advisable to postpone radiotherapy until after initial EUS examination.

Therefore, EUS should not be considered as the sole modality for comprehensively assessing the stage of oesophageal cancers, but its strengths of staging local disease should be combined with information from other imaging modalities better at diagnosing distant spread, e.g. CT and transabdominal ultrasound, to give the most accurate overall staging.

rigorous trials will have to be performed before the value of the accurate staging becomes apparent.

FOLLOWING TREATMENT AND DIAGNOSING RECURRENCE

A further function of this accuracy is the ability to detect residual disease after radiotherapy, and detection of recurrent tumour before there is any endoscopic evidence.

Nosbaum et al[13] investigated 34 patients with inoperable carcinoma of the oesophagus, before and after treatment with a combination of chemotherapy and radiotherapy. They found that in those 10 patients with no evidence of residual disease on endoscopy or CT scanning, where there was evidence on EUS of residual disease, local recurrence or distant metastases developed within a few months, whereas those patients with no evidence of residual disease on EUS after treatment showed no evidence of tumoral recurrence or progression within 8 months. They also observed that residual or recurrent tumour was hypoechoic, but radiation fibrosis was hyperechoic.

EUS is also capable of diagnosing locally recurrent cancer at the sites of surgical anastomoses[14] with an accuracy of 88 per cent and a negative predictive accuracy of 92 per cent. The site of anastomosis normally appears as a three-layered area with a maximum thickness of 6 mm – occasionally it may appear more complex due to overlapping of walls. However, recurrent cancer shows as nodularity and irregular thickening of the anastomosis site to more than 7 mm. Locally involved lymph nodes may also be seen with similar characteristics to those described above for nodes involved with primary disease. It is possible that these figures may be even further improved if EUS guided biopsy of suspected recurrence is used.

In a study of the effectiveness of preoperative chemotherapy[9] it was found that although there was apparent improvement of symptomatology, and/or regression of disease on endoscopy, EUS did not show any reduction on T staging following chemotherapy. In fact, there was progression of N staging in two patients (confirmed histologically).

Radiotherapy changes cause an inflammatory response in the short term which cannot be distinguished from malignant disease, but later these are replaced by fibrosis, which is hyperechoic. It has been suggested[15] that 3 months is a suitable period to allow for the initial radiotherapy changes to subside before rescanning.

EUS IN BENIGN OESOPHAGEAL DISEASE

The role of EUS is now being extended into the investigation of an increasing number of benign pathologies.

PORTAL HYPERTENSION

Because EUS can image outside the oesophageal wall it can be used to assess extraluminal varices in patients with portal hypertension.[16] The varices are seen as anechoic structures in continuity with each other. The EUS findings have confirmed that intramural oesophageal varices are fed by the short gastric and left gastric venous systems and that these could be assessed without resort to angiography. Abnormal para-oesophageal vessels can be visualized coalescing with intramural varices, which in severe cases are seen to have a two-layered structure. The procedure can be performed intraoperatively, allowing the effectiveness of devascularization procedures to be monitored 'on table'. Post-operative assessment initially shows an intraluminal hyperechoic pattern, probably corresponding to thrombus formation, followed later by a disappearance (Fig. 7.9) of the vessel lumen into the oesophageal wall in effectively devascularized patients.

SMOOTH MUSCLE TUMOURS

Smooth muscle tumours are infrequently encountered in the upper gastrointestinal tract. Although most commonly benign (leiomyomas), they may be malignant (leiomyosarcomas). Like oesophageal carcinomas, they are not well demonstrated by conventional imaging modalities, but they are amenable to imaging by EUS. In one study EUS was compared with CT, barium studies and endoscopy in 42 cases of suspected smooth muscle tumours.[17] Twelve oesophageal lesions were reported – with seven leiomyomas, two leiomyosarcomas, one carcinoma of the bronchus, and one case each of varices and metastatic carcinoid. Only EUS was able to determine the relationship of the lesion to the oesophageal wall, and give any useful characterization of the lesion. Leiomyomas were shown as homogeneous, sharply demarcated, hypoechoic tumours with no evidence of extension into the surrounding tissues, or of nodal metastases (Fig. 7.10). Leiomyosarcomas had an

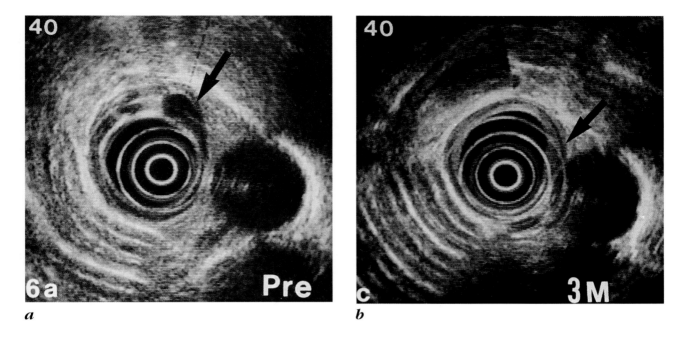

Figure 7.9 *(a) Preoperative appearance of oesophageal varices at 40 cm from the incisors (arrowed varix). (Taken from Nakamura et al,[16] Copyright Springer-Verlag.) (b) Same patient and same level as (a), 3 months after operation, with no evidence of any residual varices. (From Nakamura et al[16].)*

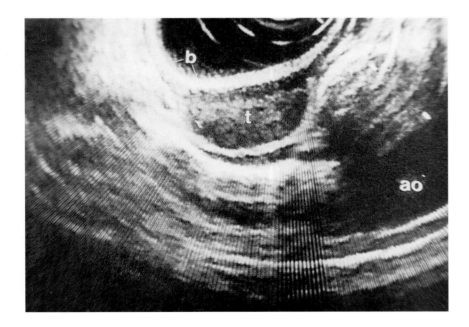

Figure 7.10 *Well-demarcated hypoechoic appearance of a leiomyoma, marked 't'. b, balloon; ao, aorta. (Taken from Tio et al,[17] Copyright Mosby Yearbook.)*

inhomogeneous, hypoechoic appearance with ill-defined margins and penetration of the surrounding tissues and/or destruction of the normal oesophageal wall architecture. However, leiomyomas greater than 4 cm with central ulceration also developed an inhomogeneous echo pattern, throwing doubt on their benignity. On sonographic criteria alone it was not possible to distinguish between leiomyosarcoma and invading bronchial carcinoma, carcinoid, or (in the stomach) non-Hodgkins lymphoma and adenocarcinoma. However, para-oesophageal metastases could be diagnosed by location, varices by their serpiginous hypoechoic pattern and mural lipoma (in the stomach) by a hyperechoic echo pattern.

GRANULAR CELL TUMOUR

A case of submucosal oesophageal location of this strange tumour was reported from Japan.[18] Endoscopy showed a sessile tumour, but EUS was able to demonstrate that the lesion was confined to the mucosa and submucosa, with no extension into the muscularis propria (Fig. 7.11). This knowledge allowed the 2-cm tumour to be resected safely via the endoscope, eliminating the need for major surgery. On EUS the lesion appeared as a hypoechoic tumour surrounded by the hyperechoic submucosal layer.

OESOPHAGEAL MOTILITY DISORDERS

The investigation of non-obstructive dysphagia has relied heavily on fluoroscopy during barium swallow, and oesophageal manometry. EUS has now been introduced into the field with interesting early results.[19] Scleroderma patients with dysphagia may have normal manometry studies, but demonstrable structural changes on EUS. In the early stages of the disease, there is thickening of the wall, although the normal layered architecture is preserved, with increased echogenicity of the outer hyperechoic layer at the junction with the peri-oesophageal fat. Later in the disease, the wall may be thickened up to 4 mm with replacement of the normal layered structure by an amorphous hyperechoic band (Fig. 7.12). If malignancy develops, it should be easily distinguishable as a hypoechoic change, but this remains to be proven.

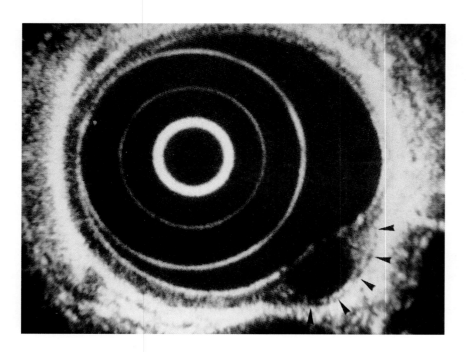

Figure 7.11 *A smooth and well-defined hypoechoic lesion confined to the mucosa and submucosa (arrowheads) was found to be a granulosa cell tumour. (Taken from Tada et al,[18] Copyright Williams and Wilkins.)*

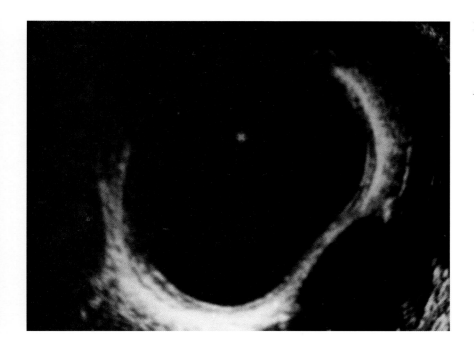

Figure 7.12 *Greatly increased echogenicity of the outer hyperechoic layer at the junction with the peri-oesophageal fat in this patient with advanced scleroderma. (Taken from Ziegler and Zimmer[19] Copyright Georg Thieme Verlag.)*

Achalasia is a benign disease caused by failure of the lower oesophageal sphincter to relax but it does have malignant associations. EUS is able to show hypertrophy of the muscularis propria at the cardia in this condition, and apparently is able to demonstrate a decrease in this hypertrophy when there is good response to drug therapy. As detailed above, it is very sensitive at detecting any associated malignancy.

NEW DEVELOPMENTS IN OESOPHAGEAL ULTRASOUND

The development of the technique has been slow because of two major factors – principally the expense of EUS machines, and limitations in applicability of the technique due to the wide diameter of the endoscope. Narrower video endoscopes and non-optic transducers are beginning to be introduced, and very narrow 3-mm probes which will pass down the biopsy channel of conventional endoscopes[17] have been developed. These will have the advantage of being able to traverse much tighter strictures than conventional echo-endoscopes, and

the 'blind' probes should be considerably less expensive. However, they will need to be combined with a water balloon stand-off to allow adequate assessment of the non-stenosed oesophagus.

Conventional EUS machines remain very expensive, but lower frequency ultrasound probes designed for echocardiography which attach to a standard ultrasound console have been shown to have some value in evaluating advanced oesophageal cancer.[20] Gross local disease can be assessed, although these probes do not have the resolution necessary for T staging, and peri-oesophageal lymph nodes are well seen. While limited in their use for oesophageal imaging, these probes are available as relatively inexpensive add-ons to most ultrasound machines (at less than one-tenth the cost of a conventional EUS machine) and therefore may find favour in certain situations.

Further technical developments in the probes, such as colour Doppler, may enhance the accuracy of the technique further, and may begin to distinguish between inflammation and malignancy, but no such facilities are available yet. Three-dimensional reconstruction is already available using sophisticated imaging workstations, but in future it may become a feature incorporated into the machine console to allow better evaluation of the extent of disease.

CONCLUSION

Endoscopic ultrasound is a highly accurate tool in staging oesophageal malignancy, but at the moment the information it provides is rarely utilized in management of the disease. The technique is still in its infancy, but it should be recognized that it has great potential in investigation of all oesophageal diseases, including benign pathologies.

REFERENCES

1. Aibe T, Fuji T, Okita K et al, A fundamental study of normal layer structure of the gastrointestinal wall visualized by endoscopic ultrasonography, *Scand J Gastroenterol* (1986) **21**(Suppl. 123):6–15.

2. Hermanek P, Sobin LH, eds, *TNM Classification of Malignant Tumours*, 4th edn (Springer Verlag: Heidelberg, 1988).

3. Vilgrain V, Mompoint D, Palazzo L et al, Staging of esophageal carcinoma: comparison of the results with endoscopic sonography and CT, *Am J Roentgenol* (1990) **155**:277–81.

4. Lightdale CJ, Endoscopic ultrasonography in the diagnosis, staging and follow-up of esophageal and gastric cancer, *Endoscopy* (1992) **24**(Suppl. 1):297–303.

5. Rice TW, Boyce GA, Sivak MV, Esophageal ultrasound and the preoperative staging of carcinoma of the esophagus, *J Thorac Cardiovasc Surg* (1991) **101**:536–44.

6. Tio TL, Coene PPL, Schouwink MH, Tytgat GN, Esophagogastric carcinoma: preoperative TNM classification with endosonography, *Radiology* (1989) **173**:411–17.

7. Rosch T, Lorenz R, Zenker K et al, Local staging and assessment of respectability in carcinoma of the esophagus, stomach, and duodenum by endoscopic ultrasonography. *Gastrointest Endosc* (1992) **38**:460–7.

8. Sugimachi K, Ohno S, Fujishima H et al, Endoscopic ultrasonographic detection of carcinomatous invasion of lymph nodes in the thoracic esophagus, *Surgery* (1990) **107**:366–71.

9. Rice TW, Boyce GA, Sivak MV et al, Esophageal carcinoma: esophageal ultrasound assessment of preoperative chemotherapy, *Ann Thorac Surg* (1992) **53**:972–7.

10. Tio TL, Coene PPL, Den Hartog Jeger FCA, Tytgat GNJ, Preoperative TNM classification of esophageal carcinoma by endosonography, *Hepato–gastroenterology* (1990) **37**:376–81.

11. Botet JF, Lightdale CJ, Zauber AG et al, Preoperative staging of esophageal cancer: comaprison of endoscopic US and dynamic CT, *Radiology* (1991) **181**:419–25.

12. Fok M, Cheng SWK, Wong J, Endosonography in patient selection for surgical treatment of esophageal carcinoma, *World J Surg* (1992) **16**:1098–103.

13. Nosbaum JB, Robaszkiewicz M, Cauvin JM et al, Endosonography can detect residual tumour infiltration after medical treatment of oesophageal cancer in the absence of endoscopic lesions, *Gut* (1992) **33**:1459–61.

14. Lightdale CJ, Botet JF, Kelsen DP et al, Diagnosis of recurrent upper gastrointestinal cancer at the surgical anastomosis by endoscopic ultrasound, *Gastrointest Endosc* (1989) **35**:407–12.

15. Souquet JC, Napoleon B, Pujol B et al, Endosonography-guided treatment of esophageal carcinoma, *Endoscopy* (1992) **24** (Suppl. 1):324–8.

16. Nakamura H, Endo M, Shimojuu K et al, Esophageal varices evaluated by endoscopic ultrasonography: observation of collateral circulation during non-shunting operations. *Surg Endosc* (1990); **4**:69–75.

17. Tio TL, Tytgat GNJ, den Hartog Jager FCA, Endoscopic ultrasonography for the evaluation of smooth muscle tumors in the upper gastrointestinal tract: an experience with 42 cases, *Gastrointest Endosc* (1990) **36**:342–50.

18. Tada S, Iida M, Takashi Y et al, Granular cell tumor of the esophagus: endoscopic ultrasonographic demonstration and endoscopic removal, *Am J Gastroenterol* (1990) **85**:1507–11.

19. Ziegler K, Zimmer T, The role of endoscopic ultrasonography in esophageal motility disorders, *Endoscopy* (1992) **24** (Suppl. 1):338–41.

20. Glover JR, Sargeant IR, Bown SG, Lees WR, Non-optic endosonography in advanced carcinoma of the esophagus, *Gastrointest Endosc* (1994) **40**:194–8.

Chapter 8 Endoscopic Ultrasonography of the Stomach

Fotini Laoudi
William R Lees

The stomach is divided into the fundus, body and antrum. The thickness of the gastric wall varies in different parts of the stomach, and according to the degree of gastric distension. In a stomach full of water the maximum thickness of the body is 3 mm and the antrum is that of 4 mm.

The endoscopy literature describes seven anatomical levels (I, II, III, IV, V, VI and VII) for examining the upper gastrointestinal tract by endoscopic ultrasonography.[1] The most common positions of the endosonography probe for visualizing the gastric wall and surrounding organs and tissues are: position IV (antrum), position V (body) and position VI (fundus).

From position IV, the liver, body of the pancreas, common bile duct, gall bladder, portal vein and superior mesenteric artery are examined; in position V, the body and tail of the pancreas, aorta, splenic vein, left renal vein, left adrenal, liver and spleen are visualized, and from position VI the left lobe of the liver, spleen, diaphragm and inferior vena cava are the most important landmarks.

ENDOSCOPIC ULTRASOUND (EUS) TECHNIQUE

At present, the instruments of EUS consist of an endoscope, which can be side-viewing or blind, combined with an ultrasound probe or with a miniature probe with frequencies ranging from 5 MHz to 20 MHz.

These echo instruments include a small biopsy channel to allow fine-needle aspiration under direct ultrasound guidance. A practical large-calibre cutting needle has not yet been designed for these instruments.

SCANNING TECHNIQUE

1. Direct contact of the probe with the gastric wall.
2. Using a water-filled balloon for the best contact between the echoprobe and the stomach wall.
3. Filling the stomach with deaerated water.

The water-filled balloon technique is the most appropriate for the stomach and duodenum, particularly for the study of submucosal lesions.[2] 500–600 ml of water can be used safely provided care is taken to minimize aspiration.

Five layers of normal gastric wall can be visualized by EUS (Fig. 8.1). The first is the junction between lumen and mucosa, which is hyperechoic, and the second layer is hypoechoic, corresponding to the base of the mucosa and the muscularis mucosae. The

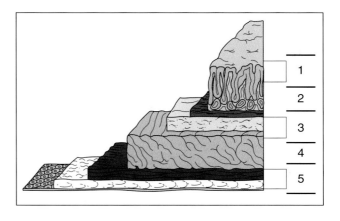

Figure 8.1 *The five layers of the gastric wall: 1, mucosa; 2, muscularis mucosae; 3, submucosa; 4, muscularis propria; 5, serosa.*

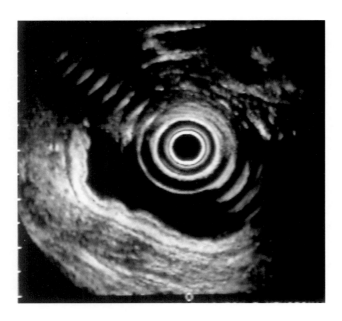

Figure 8.2 *The normal gastric wall seen by EUS.*

DIAGNOSIS OF SUBMUCOSAL LESIONS

Differentiation of submucosal lesions from extrinsic compression is difficult by conventional endoscopy or barium studies. The accurate delineation of the layered pattern of the gastric wall makes location of such lesions easy. The differential diagnosis then depends mainly on the layer in which the lesion originates. Carcinoid and heterotopic pancreatic tissue are mucosal processes. Lipomas, cysts, granulomas and varices arise within the submucosa, and leiomyomas within the muscularis propria.

The diagnostic accuracy of EUS for differentiation of intrinsic from extrinsic lesions is 94 per cent. Although it is accurate in describing submucosal lesions, diagnosis of solid lesions still requires biopsy. The most common intrinsic lesions are leiomyomas/sarcomas, aberrant pancreatic tissue and varices. All other lesions are rare.

third layer is submucosa, which is a complex structure histologically and generates a hyperechoic zone. The main bulk of the gastric wall is the muscle layer, which is hypoechoic. The fifth hyperechoic layer corresponds to the interface between the muscle layer and the surrounding tissue (serosa) (Fig. 8.2).

GASTRIC CANCER

Although gastric cancer has a characteristic appearance at EUS, the diagnostic accuracy for early cancer versus benign ulceration (Fig. 8.3) is approximately 80–90 per cent and hence biopsy is mandatory.

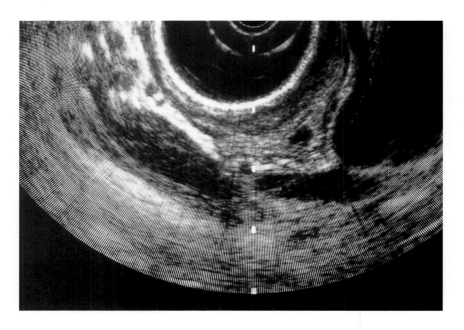

Figure 8.3 *A benign gastric ulcer. The layers are thickened but preserved, although the base of the ulcer crater is seen as a defect in the submucosa. The Japanese groups with great experience of early gastric cancer can differentiate benign from malignant on the basis of the EUS with approximately 85 per cent accuracy.*

In Western Europe the majority of gastric cancers are advanced at the time of presentation, with poor prognosis (Figs. 8.4, 8.5, 8.6 and 8.7). EUS is less accurate in staging gastric than oesophageal cancer (80–90 per cent), mainly due to the higher incidence of liver and distant lymph node metastases. Computed tomography (CT) is no more accurate, but the two techniques combined will have a staging accuracy of 85–95 per cent and will allow accurate assessment of operability for curative resection or palliation.

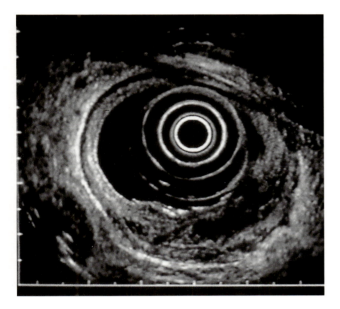

Figure 8.4 *T2 gastric cancer. There is disruption of the normal layered pattern of the stomach wall with poorly echogenic tumour infiltrating throught the submucosa into the muscularis propria.*

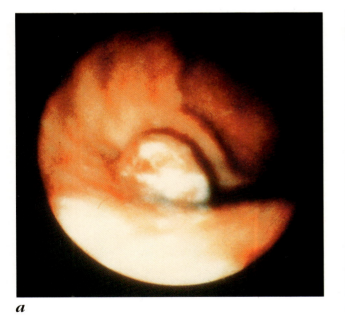

a

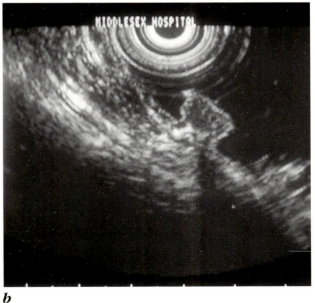

b

Figure 8.5 *(a) Mucosal polyp. (b) EUS shows that the lesion is confined to the deep part of the mucosa, which gives a differential diagnosis of carcinoid tumour or heterotopic pancreatic tissue. (The diagnosis was carcinoid.)*

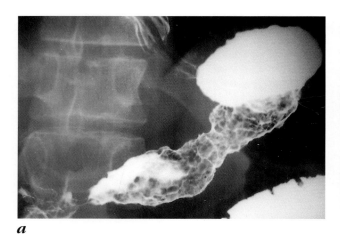

a

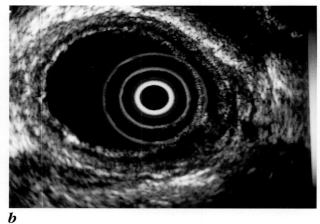

b

Figure 8.6 *(a) Lymphoma of the stomach. (b) EUS shows thickening of all the layers to the serosa but with only patchy areas of boundary loss.*

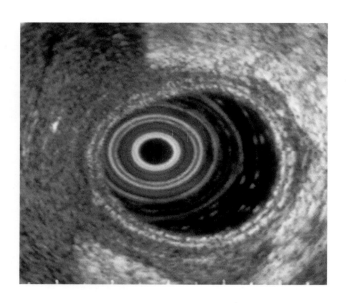

Figure 8.7 *Eosinophilic gastritis. There is thickening of all the layers as with the lymphoma but this is mostly of the mucosal and submucosal layers. The echogenicity of the thickened layers is only slightly reduced from the normal.*

LOCAL RECURRENCE OF GASTRIC CANCER

The EUS appearances of recurrent disease are identical to those of the primary process, with the exception that recurrence is usually in the submucosal or muscularis propria layers or in local nodes (Figs. 8.8 and 8.9). The mucosa may well be intact.

Node recurrence is recognized by enlargement (>2 cm = 100 per cent involved; 0.5–2.0 cm = 66 per cent involved; <5 mm = <10 per cent involved), low echogenicity and loss of normal structure.[3]

EUS has been described as a method of evaluating endoscopic laser ablation of early gastric cancer, but even in T1 cancers up to 10 per cent may have nodal metastases at the time of presentation.

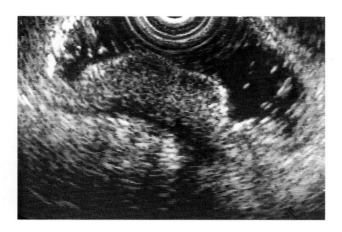

Figure 8.8 *Anastamotic recurrence of a gastric cancer. The poorly echogenic tumour is most prominent at the serosal surface although tumour nodules can be seen in the submucosa also. The mucosal surface was intact.*

5. Evaluation of interventional procedures under EUS control (e.g. treatment of pancreatic pseudocysts, sclerotherapy of submucosal varices etc.) (Fig. 8.10).

The diagnosis of a visible lesion at endoscopy is always by biopsy. EUS can be very helpful where the mucosa is intact or superficial biopsies are unhelpful.[4-11] The technique is currently handicapped by the lack of a good histology needle for use via the biopsy channel of the EUS scope. Some of the newer instruments using limited field of view phased array transducers are better adapted to biopsy than the 360° radial viewing instruments but although cytological biopsy is readily performed it is still difficult to get deep histological biopsies (Fig. 8.11).

Miniprobe EUS can be very useful at the pylorus, where the larger endoscopes will not pass a stricture.

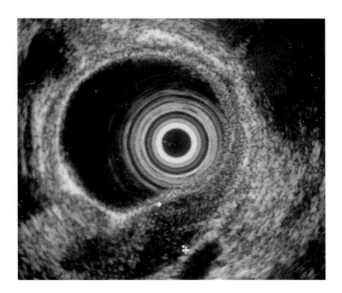

Figure 8.9 *Perigastric lymph node metastases.*

INDICATIONS FOR GASTRIC EUS

1. Diagnosis and staging of gastric tumours.
2. Diagnosis of submucosal lesions and differentiation from extragastric compression.
3. Determination of local recurrence in patients with resected gastric cancer.
4. Diagnosis of early gastric cancer.

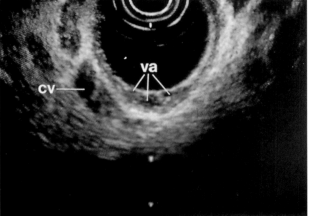

Figure 8.10 *Gastric varices (va).*

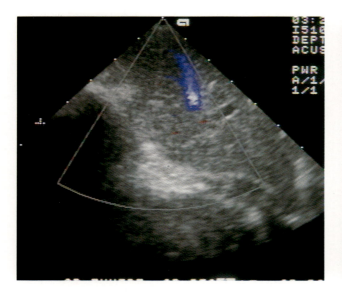

Figure 8.11 *A phased array EUS image. The angle of view is only 90° but is somewhat compensated by the electronic focusing of these devices, giving better tissue penetration and depth resolution. Most of these instruments also allow full duplex and colour Doppler studies.*

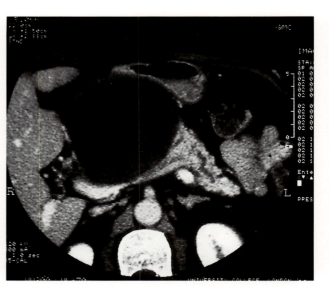

Figure 8.12 *Helical CT of a pseudocyst arising from the head of the pancreas showing the relationship with the stomach and duodenum.*

We are now using EUS to guide endoscopic drainage of pseudocysts. EUS is used to determine the closest point of the pseudocyst to the gastric or duodenal wall, and to identify the portal varices frequently associated with pancreatitis (Fig. 8.12). The wall can then be incised or punctured with confidence.

The usefulness of EUS in gastric cancer remains debatable. In the West a surgical resection for cure of an early gastric cancer is a rare event. For most patients the best palliation will be by surgery, and determination of which patients are unsuitable even

for a palliative resection, e.g. because of spread into the oesophagus, can be done very easily by endoscopy, barium studies and conventional ultrasound and CT. The main role of EUS in these circumstances is to enhance the conventional endoscopy study.

EUS remains invaluable in the follow-up of the patient treated by surgery or chemotherapy, and in detection of local recurrence, which usually occurs in the deep layers of the anastamosis or in contiguous nodes and spreads to the mucosa much later.

REFERENCES

1. Lux G, Heyder N, Lutz H, EUS-technique orientation and diagnosis, *Endoscopy* (1982) **14**:220–5.

2. Lees WR, Endoscopic ultrasound, *BMUS Bull* (1993) **1**:21–4.

3. Tohnosu N, Onoda S, Isono K, Ultrasonographic evaluation of cervical lymph node metastases in oesophageal cancer, *J Clin Ultrasound* (1989) **17**:101–6.

4. Botet JF, Lightdale CJ, Zauber AG, Preoperative staging of gastric cancer: comparison of endoscopic US and dynamic CT, *Radiology* (1991) **181**:426–32.

5. Kalantzis N, Laoudi F, Kallimanis G, Gabriel P, Farmakis N, The role of endoscopic ultrasonography in diagnosis of benign lesions of the upper GI tract, *Eur J Surg Oncol* (1993) **19**:449–54.

6. Wang KK, Dimagno EP, Endoscopic ultrasonography: high technology and cost containment, *Gastroenterology* (1993) **105**:283–5.

7. Tio TL, Coene PP, Schouwink MH, Tytgat GN, Esophagogastric carcinoma: preoperative TNM classification with endosonography, *Radiology* (1989) **173**:411–17.

8. Tio TL, Ben Hartog Jager FC, Tytgart GN, Endoscopic ultrasonography in detection and staging of gastric non-Hodgkin lymphoma. Comparison with gastroscopy, barium meal, and computerized tomography scan, *Scand J Gastroenterol* (1986) **123**:52–8.

9. Takemoto T, Okito K, Aibe T, Advances in tumour diagnosis: endoscopic ultrasonography. In: Krasner N, ed, *Lasers in Gastroenterology* (Chapman and Hall Medical: London, 1991) 301–12.

10. Miller LS, Liu JB, Klenn PJ et al, Endoluminal ultrasonograhy of the distal esophagus in systemic sclerosis, *Gastroenterol* (1993) **105**:31–9.

11. Liu JB, Miller LS, Feld RI et al, Gastric and esophageal varices: 20-MHz transnasal endoluminal US, *Radiology* (1993) **187**(2):363–6.

Chapter 9 Endoscopic Ultrasonography of the Pancreas and Biliary Tract

Andreas Müller
Adrian RW Hatfield
William R Lees

Imaging evaluation of patients with pancreatobiliary tract diseases has greatly improved in the last two decades. Abdominal ultrasound, endoscopic retrograde cholangiopancreatography (ERCP) and computed tomography (CT) have widely replaced the older imaging modalities. However, there are still difficulties, mainly in imaging small tumours of the pancreas, ampullary region and biliary tree. Endoscopic ultrasound (EUS) has now been shown to be an imaging method with a high accuracy for detecting and staging these tumours. Recently, significant competition has arisen from helical CT with high-speed volume imaging coupled with good control of contrast opacification. Therefore the established role of EUS is changing and needs to be defined by controlled comparative studies.

tumour staging.[1] The main advantage of the linear scanner is that, unlike with the radial scanners, it is possible to perform ultrasound-guided fine-needle aspiration and localize the tip of the needle in the ultrasound image. This is helpful in pancreatic lesions or suspicious lymph nodes which cannot be visualized or punctured under guidance by other imaging methods.

In addition, intraductal ultrasonography is under clinical evaluation using miniature ultrasound probes that can be advanced through the biopsy channel of conventional endoscopes (see Chapter 13). These probes provide high-frequency ultrasound with high-resolution imaging, but their limited depth of penetration prevents their use for staging most tumours.

EQUIPMENT

The most widely used EUS instrument is the Olympus side-viewing instrument. Its radial scan format ensures easier anatomical orientation. The newest instrument, the EUM-20, is completely water submersible and is therefore much easier to clean. In addition, the transducer has a diameter of less than 13 mm which is much better tolerated by the patients. However, no forward-viewing instrument is yet available. With the existing forward-oblique optic system, the view is still limited and conventional endoscopy must be performed separately. However, when examining the pancreatobiliary tract this forward-oblique system is advantageous for viewing the ampulla.

Linear scanning with other probes is currently under clinical trial, and preliminary results comparing the two scanning types reveal similar accuracy in

TECHNIQUE

The technique of EUS is unfortunately difficult and requires a skilled endoscopist who has experience with side-viewing instruments. In addition, ultrasound interpretative skills are mandatory. Anatomical orientation during EUS is very difficult in the pancreatobiliary tract due to the different viewing angles of the transducer (Table 9.1) from various positions in the stomach and around the duodenal loop. Before ultrasound scanning can be performed, the endoscope has to be introduced through the pylorus into the duodenum. This can be difficult and occasionally impossible because of tumour infiltration into the duodenal wall and consequent obstruction. However, in these patients, scanning from the duodenal cap, or at least from the antrum, can provide a view of most of the pancreatic head, although not of the ampullary region.

Table 9.1 Different anatomical structures that can be observed from the different ultrasound transducer positions (see Figure 9.1).

Position of ultrasound probe	Visualized structure
Position I: Horizontal duodenum	Kidney vessels Aorta Inferior vena cava
Position II: Descending duodenum	Right kidney Papilla vater Distal common bile duct Distal main pancreatic duct Pancreatic head and uncinatus Superior mesenteric artery/vein
Position III: Duodenal bulb	Pancreatic head Common bile duct Portal vein Hepatic artery Gall bladder
Position IV: Gastric antrum	Pancreatic body Gall bladder Portal vein Splenic vein
Position V: Gastric body	Pancreatic body Main pancreatic duct Splenic vein Coeliac axis
Position VI: Gastric fundus	Pancreatic tail Spleen Left kidney Splenic and renal vessels

Otherwise, scanning can be started as soon as deep cannulation of the duodenum has been achieved. We prefer to visualize first the right kidney or the aorta and inferior vena cava from the third part of the duodenum. Other authors recommend endoscopic visualization of the ampulla first. In either case, the endoscope is slowly withdrawn and scanning is performed while slightly altering the tip of the endoscope to observe the various anatomical structures from different angles. Small adjustments of the position of the endoscopic tip may dramatically improve the image by bringing the structure into focus. Because of the limited depth of penetration, the liver, hilum of liver and intrahepatic ducts can only partly be imaged and are the 'problem spots' of EUS.

Within the duodenum the water-filled balloon method is used most commonly. The exceptions are lesions protruding into the duodenal lumen, e.g. ampullary and duodenal tumours – these can be compressed and distorted by the balloon. Distension of the stomach and duodenum by deaerated water is preferred. The examination rarely takes more than 20 min and should not exceed 30 min.

There are no reports on the side-effects and complication rate of EUS, but it is estimated that the risk of EUS is comparable to that of standard upper gastrointestinal endoscopy.

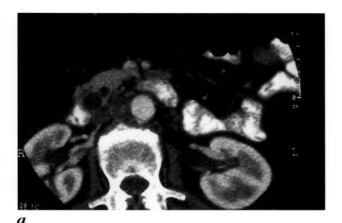
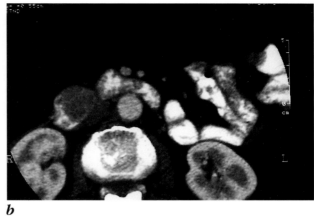

a *b*

Figure 9.3 *(a) Helical CT. Dilated CBD and MPD seen within normal pancreas. (b) The ampullary tumour is seen as a rounded filling defect within the contrast-enhanced duodenum.*

become important in assessing disease progress (Figs. 9.3–9.6).

PANCREATIC ENDOCRINE TUMOURS

Small pancreatic endocrine tumours can be detected by EUS with an accuracy rate of over 80 per cent in patients with negative ultrasound and/or CT.[9] It is open for debate whether CT should be performed before EUS (Fig. 9.7).

The EUS features for endocrine tumours of different histological types are similar. In patients with multiple endocrine neoplasia type 1, EUS has been shown to be a very accurate imaging method.[10] Extrapancreatic endocrine tumours are difficult to detect. Duodenal wall lesions can be predicted by endoscopy more accurately than with EUS.[11] However, when clinically indicated, we recommend performing both imaging methods, because small lesions can easily be overlooked by endoscopy.

In ampullary carcinoma (Fig. 9.8) EUS is superior to ultrasound and CT in evaluation of both tumour size and extent. The balloon cannot be inflated at the site of the ampulla because the papilla will be compressed. Therefore the water-fill method is preferred.[12] Most of the patients from our unit have a biliary stent in place. Due to the consecutive decompression of the common bile duct and artifacts due to the stents, some technical difficulties arise in scanning the tumours. In addition, the stent causes

air interference and local inflammation around the stent, observed as a hypoechogenic concentric ring of about 2–3 mm. On the other hand, the stent is also helpful in marking the CBD and hence simplifying EUS. Crucial for resectability is tumour infiltration into the peripancreatic vessels. Due to the relatively slow growth of ampullary tumours, this is rarely the case and therefore if vessels are involved the tumour is already at a T4 stage in the TNM classification.

EUS cannot differentiate between ampullary T1 carcinoma and benign adenoma.[13] Therefore histology is still mandatory.

PANCREATITIS

EUS has no role in acute pancreatitis except in those cases with the possibility of an underlying tumour or stone in failed ERCPs.

Chronic pancreatitis is still a big challenge for the various imaging methods. For judgement of peripancreatic involvement due to chronic pancreatitis, CT scanning is superior to ultrasound. For the pancreatic parenchyma, however, EUS appears to be a very promising imaging modality. In our own clinical experience, if the poorly echogenic ventral segment can be visualized, diffuse chronic pancreatitis can be excluded. Logistic regression analysis of parenchymal abnormalities (focal regions of reduced or increased echogenicity, cysts, accentuation of lobular pattern) and ductal abnormalities (narrowing, dilatation, irregular contour,

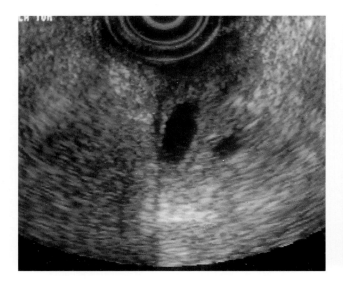

Figure 9.4 *Invasive ampullary tumour (T3). Poorly echogenic tumour infiltrates the distal CBD and muscularis propria of the duodenum.*

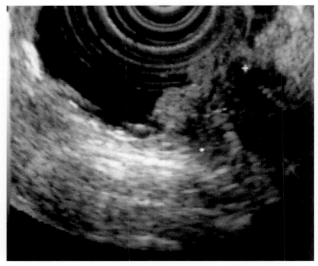

Figure 9.5 *Typical pancreatic ductal adenocarcinoma. The poorly echogenic mass infiltrates and destroys the layers of the duodenum, but even at only 3 cm in size the deeper aspects of the mass are not visualized by EUS. Staging of this type of tumour is best performed by helical CT.*

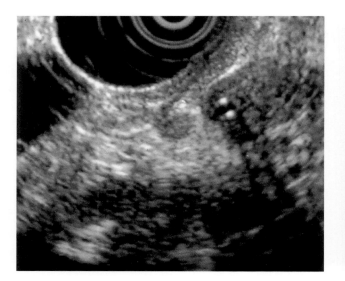

Figure 9.6 *Cholangiocarcinoma of the distal CBD (position III). An endobiliary stent defines the lumen of the duct. The mass is smoothly marginated and potentially operable. A small contiguous lymph node is seen. This is so common after intervention that lymphadenopathy cannot be used as a staging factor.*

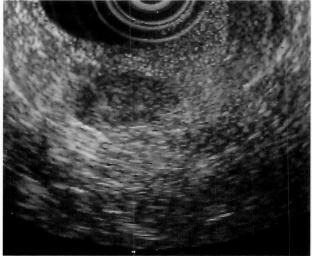

Figure 9.7 *Insulinoma (seen from position V). Most functioning islet cell tumours are seen as rounded or slightly lobulated masses with a uniform echogenicity less than that of normal pancreatic tissue. The difference in echogenicity may be subtle.*

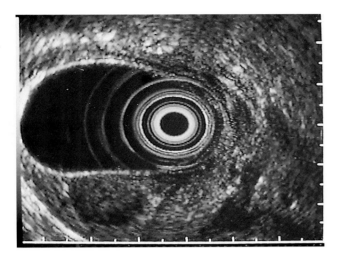

Figure 9.8 *Adenoma of the ampulla of Vater. The uniformly echogenic mass lies within the line of the muscularis propria of the duodenum.*

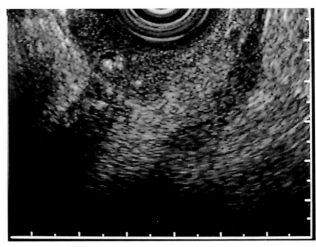

Figure 9.9 *Chronic pancreatitis (viewed from position II). The poorly echogenic fibrous tissue around the ampulla is indistinguishable from pancreatic adenocarcinoma but shows well-defined smooth margins. The calculi are clearly seen to lie within the duct system.*

increased duct wall echogenicity, calculi, side branch dilatation) on EUS were found to be indicative of chronic pancreatitis.[14] Interestingly enough, EUS reveals some of these abnormalities in patients with a clinical episode of pancreatic inflammation but normal ERCP, most likely corresponding to an early stage of chronic pancreatitis. We therefore recommend performing EUS in addition to ERCP in patients with no apparent abnormalities on CT scanning. With positive CT scans, EUS rarely provides additional information. We have performed an EUS in 58 patients with severe pain of possible pancreatic origin and few or equivocal changes on conventional imaging. At EUS 27 showed unequivocal changes of chronic pancreatitis which was confirmed histologically in 14 cases (unpublished data).

EUS has difficulties in distinguishing inflammatory from malignant tumours (Fig. 9.9), like other imaging methods. Fibrosis of chronic pancreatitis may be as homogeneous as that within a desmoplastic carcinoma and may even infiltrate the duodenal wall or invade the retroperitoneum.

Despite these problems, EUS is the most reliable imaging method. However, we recommend that to ensure the diagnosis a percutaneous ultrasound or CT-guided trucut biopsy should be done. In lesions which cannot be visualized by transabdominal imaging methods, fine-needle aspiration performed

with linear EUS is now available.[15] Further studies are needed to prove the diagnostic value of this method.

EUS might improve safety in performing drainage of pseudocysts.[16] EUS-guided drainage is now performed routinely in many medical centres. In the rare case of vascular or intestinal loops interposed between the stomach or duodenal site of puncture and pseudocyst, EUS can detect this and thereby prevent possible complications. After EUS-guided puncture of the cyst, insertion of a guide wire and enlargement of the puncture site by sphincterotomy knife, stenting can be performed safely.

BILIARY TREE MALIGNANCIES

Despite limited experience, EUS of biliary tree malignancies has been reported to be accurate in staging.[17,18] It is, however, not possible to differentiate between a primary gall bladder carcinoma infiltrating into the biliary ducts and a biliary duct carcinoma infiltrating into the gall bladder. Overall accuracy in assessing the depth of tumour infiltration is over 85 per cent. EUS has a tendency to overstage T2 cholangiocarcinomas, possibly due to compression of blood vessels, simulating penetration by tumour on ultrasound examination.[19] However, the liver hilum and the right intrahepatic duct tumours are difficult to access with conventional EUS due to the distance between transducer and lesions. For these cases the newest generation of miniature high-frequency ultrasound probes that can be introduced through a conventional duodenoscope into the biliary tree show promising results (Figs. 9.10, 9.11). In our own preliminary experience, cholangiocarcinomas can be well visualized (Fig. 9.12), but on occasions these tumours may cause strictures that have to be dilated before insertion of even a 2–4 mm probe is possible. They are hyperechogenic and irregular if compared to the thickened wall in sclerosing cholangitis (Fig. 9.13). Staging of the transmural extent is easy; the longitudinal extent has to be determined by combined EUS and fluoroscopy combined. Distant metastases cannot be observed by EUS. Therefore, as in pancreatic cancer, this method has to be used as a complementary method to other imaging methods. EUS is not accurate in staging metastatic lymph nodes, particularly after endoscopic or percutaneous stenting, where reactive hyperplasia is common.[18]

Of course, cholangiography is still the imaging method of first choice in the patient with obstructive jaundice, not least because therapeutic procedures may be necessary. However, in patients at high risk for ERCP, EUS may be an alternative because of its higher accuracy compared with ERCP and CT, and because of the additional possibility of tumour staging that is not possible with ERCP.[19,20] The miniature ultrasound probes that can be introduced through conventional endoscopes into the biliary tree show, according to preliminary results, the ability to differentiate inflammatory from malignant strictures,[21–23] but although this method is unable to stage larger tumours, conventional ultrasound or helical CT is unusually effective in staging tumours of >2 cm diameter. In patients with bile and duct stones EUS is very reliable,[24,25] and in our limited experience with intraductal EUS it appears that this method is even more sensitive than ERCP and can be performed in most cases via the transampullary route without previous sphincter-sphincterotomy.[26] In patients who can be predicted to have a small risk of common bile duct stones, conventional EUS may be justified as a primary diagnostic tool in order to select the patients who will require a therapeutic procedure (Figs. 9.14, 9.15).[27]

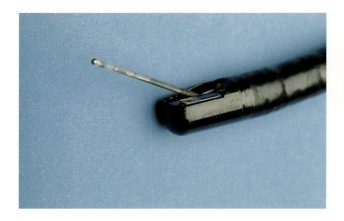

Figure 9.10 *Miniature endoscopic ultrasound probe (EUS).*

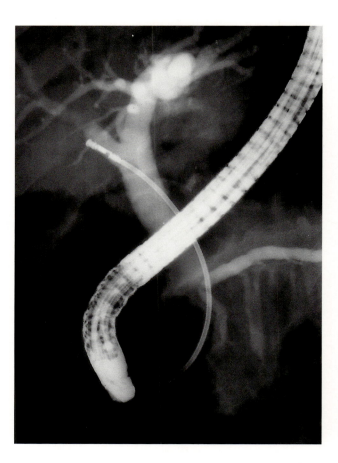

Figure 9.11 *The 20-MHz probe is readily passed into the CBD and MPD.*

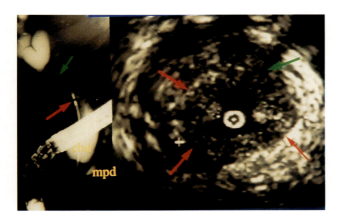

Figure 9.12 *Miniature endoscopic ultrasound (MEUS). Typical cholangiocarcinoma. mpd, main pancreatic duct; arrows, tumour margin.*

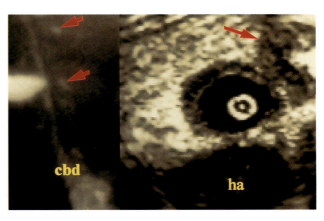

Figure 9.13 *Primary sclerosing cholangitis. Subtle bile duct wall thickening is easily seen. Pseudodivertica have been shown to be microabscesses related to CBD perforation. ha, hepatic artery; arrows, pseudodiverticulum.*

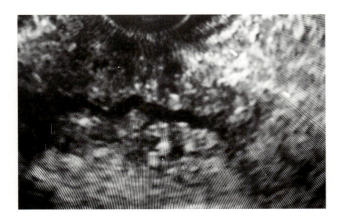

Figure 9.14 *Chronic pancreatitis seen by EUS (position V). Note dilated MPD and side branches and echogenic foci in the parenchyma.*

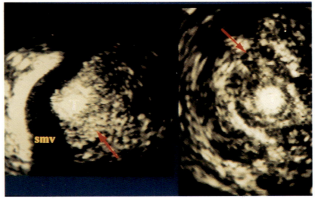

Figure 9.15 *Chronic pancreatitis seen by MEUS. Most chronic pancreatitis presents too much disruption of architecture to be well resolved by MEUS. Subtle changes around MPD strictures are difficult to interpret at the present time. smv, superior mesenteric vein.*

For the diagnosis of gall bladder stones, conventional transabdominal ultrasound is the method of choice because of the high accuracy. However, in difficult patients (e.g. obesity, contracted atropic gall bladder) EUS might be helpful. In 38 patients with strong clinical suspicion of symptomatic gall bladder stones, EUS in 28 patients found small stones ($n = 5$), sludge ($n = 7$) or microlithiasis ($n = 13$), confirmed by cholecystectomy and/or bile crystal analysis.[28] Whether EUS can differentiate cholesterol polyps from small adenomas is not yet known. The crucial endosonographic feature of gall bladder carcinoma is its transmural tumour growth,[29] which cannot be observed in adenomas.

CONCLUSIONS

In conclusion, the pancreatobiliary tract is a major target for EUS today and reveals high accuracy in tumour staging. The difference in accuracy between EUS and other imaging methods is becoming less pronounced. The crucial question is whether this difference makes a difference to the outcome for the patient, e.g. whether it prevents an unnecessary laparotomy. Further studies have to clarify this. Meanwhile all potentially operable ampullary and pancreatic tumour patients must be staged by EUS if abdominal ultrasound and/or CT have not yet excluded resectability.

However, the EUS purchase price and repair costs remain a problem. It is hoped that costs may decrease as a result of the above mentioned miniature probe technique, which potentially enables EUS to be performed at the same time as endoscopy.

Three-dimensional reconstruction is under current trial for introduction to EUS. It promises easier spatial understanding of the anatomy and pathology and at the same time high-resolution pictures. EUS remains in competition with improving methods like CT and MRI. As therapeutic medical possibilities are increasing, assessment of success by any imaging method become more important. However, even with the newest high-frequency probes, which reveal more than five layers of wall structure, final diagnosis should always be by biopsy.

ACKNOWLEDGEMENT

This study was supported by the Sassella Foundation, Zürich. Switzerland.

REFERENCES

1. Roesch T, Dittler HJ, Kunte M et al, Comparison of a sector-type with a linear-type echoendoscope in the staging of GI cancer, *Gastroenterology* (1994), **106**:A3 (abstract).

2. Rösch T, Braig C, Gain T, Staging of pancreatic and ampullary carcinoma by endoscopic ultrasonography, *Gastroenterology* (1992) **102**:188–99.

3. Kaneko T, Nakao A, Inoue S et al, Portal venous invasion by pancreatobiliary carcinoma: diagnosis with intraportal endovascular US, *Radiology* (1994) **192**:681–6.

4. Palazzo L, Roseau G, Gayet B, Endoscopic ultrasonography in the diagnosis and staging of pancreatic adenocarcinoma, *Endoscopy* (1993) **25**:143–50.

5. Müller M, Meyenberger C, Bertschinger P, Pancreatic tumors: evaluation with endoscopic US, CT, and MR imaging, *Radiology* (1994) **190**:745–51.

6. Yasuda K, Mukai H, Nakajima M, Staging pancreatic carcinoma by endoscopic ultrasonography, *Endoscopy* (1993) **25**:151–5.

7. Snady H, Bruckner H, Siegel J, Endoscopic ultrasonography criteria of vascular invasion by potentially resectable pancreatic tumors, *Gastrointest Endosc* (1994) **40**:326–33.

8. Furukawa T, Tsukamoto Y, Naitoh Y et al, Evaluation of intraductal ultrasonography in the diagnosis of pancreatic cancer, *Endoscopy* (1993) **25**:577–81.

9. Glover JR, Shorvon PJ, Lees WR, Endoscopic ultrasound for localisation of islet cell tumours, *Gut* (1992) **33**:108–10.

10. Palazzo L, Borotto E, Napoleon B et al, Is endoscopic ultrasonography accurate for the localisation of pancreatic and duodenal tumours in patients with multiple endocrine neoplasia type 1? *Gastroenterology* (1994) **106**:A313 (abstract).

11. Ruszniewski P, Amouyal P, Amouyal G et al, Diagnostic value of endoscopic ultrasonography (EUS) for the localisation of gastrinomas, *Gastroenterology* (1993) **104**:A331 (abstract).

12. Mitake M, Nakazawa S, Tsukamoto Y, Endoscopic ultrasonography in the diagnosis of depth invasion and lymph node metastasis of carcinoma of the papilla vater, *J Ultrasound Med* (1990) **9**:645–50.

13. Roesch T, Dittlker HJ, Lorenz T et al, The role of endoscopic ultrasonography in the diagnosis and staging of tumours of the papilla of Vater, *Gastrointest Endosc* (1992) **38**:259–60 (abstract).

14. Wiersema MJ, Hawe RH, Lehman GA, Prospective evaluation of endoscopic ultrasonography and endoscopic retrograde cholangiopancreatography in patients with chronic abdominal pain of suspected pancreatic origin, *Endoscopy* (1993) **25**:555–64.

15. Vilman P, Hancke S, Henriksen FW, Endosonographically-guided fine needle aspiration biopsy of malignant lesions in the upper gastrointestinal tract, *Endoscopy* (1993) **25**:523–7.

16. Binmoeller KGF, Walter A, Seifert H et al, Endoscopic stenting for pancreatic pseudocysts in 53 patients, *Gastrointest Endosc* (1993) **39**:A308 (abstract).

17. Tio T, Cheng J, Wijers O et al, Endosonographic TNM staging of extrahepatic bile duct cancer: comparison with pathological staging, *Gastroenterology* (1991) **100**:1351–61.

18. Tio TL, Reeders JWA, Sie LH et al, Endosonography in the clinical staging of Klatskin Tumor, *Endoscopy* (1993) **25**:81–5.

19. Snady H, Cooperman A, Siegel J, Endoscopic ultrasonography compared with computed tomography with ERCP in patients with obstructive jaundice or small peripancreatic mass, *Gastrointest Endosc* (1992) **38**:27–34.

20. Meyenberger C, Bertschinger P, Marincek B et al, Dilatation of the common bile duct: what is the role of endoscopic ultrasound? *Gastroenterology* (1994) **106**:A797 (abstract).

21. Müller A, Hatfield ARW, The use of high frequency ultrasound miniprobes in routine ERCP, *GUT* (1994) (abstract) (in press).

22. Ponchon T, Hedelius F, Soquet JC et al, Echoendoscopy of bile duct strictures with miniprobes, *Gut* (1994) **35**(S4):A91 (abstract).

23. Buscail L, Escourrou J, Pradines C et al, Evaluation of intraductal ultrasonography of the biliary system during ERCP, *Gut* (1994) **35**(S4):A88 (abstract).

24. Edmundowicz SA, Aliperti G, Middleton WD, Preliminary experience using endoscopic ultrasonography in the diagnosis of choledocholithiasis, *Endoscopy* (1992) **24**:774–8.

25. Salmeron M, Simon JF, Houdart F et al, Endoscopic ultrasonography (EUS) versus invasive methods for the diagnosis of common bile duct stones (cbds), *Gastroenterology* (1994) **106**:A357 (abstract).

26. Müller A, Hatfield A, Fairclough P et al, The use of high frequency ultrasound miniprobes in the biliary tree and pancreatic duct, *Gastroenterology* (1994) **106**:A351 (abstract).

27. Marty O, Amouyal P, Amouyal G, Proportion of common bile duct lithiasis in cholecystectomized patients with normal biliary ultrasound, *Gastroenterology* (1994) **106**:A349 (abstract).

28. Dahan P, Amouyal P, Amouyal G et al, Is endoscopic ultrasonography (EUS) helpful in patients with suspicion of complicated gallstones and normal ultrasonography (US)? *Gastroenterology* (1993) **104**:A358 (abstract).

29. Morita K, Nakazawa S, Naitoh Y et al, *Endoscopic Ultrasonography in Gastroenterology* (Igaku-Shoin: New York, 1988).

Chapter 10 Intraoperative and Laparoscopic Ultrasonography

Timothy G John
Paul Allan
O James Garden

INTRODUCTION

The access to the organs of the abdomen provided during laparotomy or laparoscopy affords a unique opportunity for contact ultrasound scanning. The availability of sterilizable, ultracompact, high-frequency ultrasound probes which may be placed directly upon the viscera provides the surgeon or radiologist with the means to obtain high-resolution real-time images of the intra-abdominal structures. The visual and tactile feedback obtained in this way is enhanced by the operator's intimate knowledge of the three-dimensional regional anatomy, such that the information obtained is often superior to that derived from conventional transcutaneous scanning. There is now a well-established literature documenting the evolution of intraoperative ultrasound over the last decade, with the major contribution reflecting the interests of those specializing in hepatobiliary and pancreatic surgery. Many surgeons now consider intraoperative ultrasound (IOUS) to be invaluable for decision-making during a variety of upper abdominal operations, and, by consensus, it is regarded as the 'gold standard' for detecting 'occult' liver metastases at the time of colorectal cancer surgery.

Technological advances associated with the recent 'revolution' in minimal access surgery have renewed interest in laparoscopic ultrasound (LapUS) – the logical extension of IOUS. LapUS takes advantage of the access to the peritoneal cavity afforded by diagnostic or staging laparoscopy, and the high-resolution ultrasound images obtained using contemporary LapUS probes provide detailed information on solid and retroperitoneal organs that cannot be assessed adequately by laparoscopy alone. LapUS has yet to achieve widespread popularity in general surgical practice, but continues to be evaluated in a variety of clinical settings. The current indications for its use are mainly confined to hepatobiliary and pancreatic disorders, and this chapter is based primarily upon this experience. We believe that this technique will become indispensable to radiologists and surgeons wishing to improve existing investigative protocols for the evaluation of intra-abdominal malignancy.

THE LIVER

INTRAOPERATIVE ULTRASOUND

The liver is a large solid organ with few external markings to guide the surgeon. Its evaluation during abdominal exploration is therefore limited to inspection of the visible surface and careful palpation. However, small intrahepatic tumours are frequently impalpable and there are few external clues as to their precise relationship to the intrahepatic vascular and biliary structures upon which many operations on the liver are based. These limitations can, of course, be overcome using intraoperative contact ultrasound which renders the liver 'transparent' to the surgeon.

Background and Current Indications

The common indications for undertaking IOUS of the liver may be separated broadly into those situations where (1) the surgeon has undertaken abdominal exploration intending to resect one or more focal hepatic lesions, and (2) those operations where surgery is directed at primary tumours in other locations, but where accurate disease staging demands the reliable detection of liver metastases.

Assessment of resectability of liver tumours

Careful patient selection is important if resection of primary or secondary malignant liver tumours is to be justified. Early recurrence of liver tumour has been associated with the presence of extrahepatic tumour spread (including regional lymph node invasion) and residual intrahepatic tumour not recognized at the time of liver resection. Resectability depends upon the site, size, number and intrahepatic vascular relationships of the tumours, and the surgeon's ability to perform a 'typical' liver resection along the

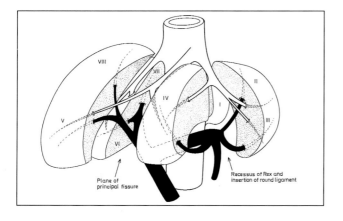

Figure 10.1 *Couinaud's hepatic segmental anatomy. The liver is viewed from its anterior aspect and lies in its correct anatomical orientation. The right hemiliver comprises the paramedian sector (segments V and VIII supplied by the anterior sectoral branch of the right portal vein), which is separated from the posterolateral sector (segments VI and VII supplied by the posterior sectoral branch of the right portal vein) by the right hepatic vein. The left hemiliver comprises the quadrate lobe (segment IV), the left hepatic lobe (segments II and III) and the caudate lobe (segment I). Reproduced from Garden OJ,* Intraoperative and Laparoscopic Ultrasonography, *Blackwell Scientific Publications, Edinburgh, 1995, with the kind permission of the publishers.*

recognized anatomical planes originally defined by Couinaud[1] and later popularized by Bismuth and colleagues[2,3] (Fig. 10.1). Ideally, at least 1 cm of normal liver should remain between the resection margin and tumour. A variety of preoperative staging investigations are usually undertaken to assess these factors, although the ultimate determinant of tumour resectability is bimanual palpation of the liver by the surgeon and IOUS. Only IOUS can provide the hepatic surgeon with precise information of the resection margin and avoid inadvertent breach of the tumour capsule during dissection of the liver. The precise three-dimensional relationships of tumours with the vascular and biliary anatomy of the liver can be defined so as to delineate the planes of resection required in order to achieve tumour extirpation with curative intent. Small intrahepatic lesions beyond the resolution of conventional imaging techniques (usually ≤10 mm) may be detected by IOUS, thereby enabling avoidance of inappropriate resection in the face of more extensive tumour involvement of the liver.

The reported usefulness of such a technique can be difficult to quantify, and its proponents have frequently relied upon anecdote. In reporting an extensive experience with IOUS in hepatobiliary and pancreatic operations, Machi and co-workers[4] have attempted to classify its benefits in terms of: (1) acquiring diagnostic information otherwise not available; (2) replacing or complementing intraoperative radiography; and (3) guiding surgical procedures. Thus, 'beneficial information' was reported as having been provided by IOUS during 73 out of 82 (89 per cent) hepatic operations. The previously planned surgical procedure was altered in 32 cases (39 per cent) and IOUS was useful as a guide to surgery in a total of 88 operations on the liver.[4]

Clarke and colleagues compared the findings of IOUS with those of preoperative ultrasonography and dynamic computed tomography (CT) scanning in 54 patients with a variety of hepatic tumours.[5] They reported that additional liver lesions were defined by IOUS in 25 per cent and 35 per cent of examinations respectively, and that 40 per cent of liver tumours detected by IOUS in this way had neither been visible nor palpable at operation. Of the total 167 lesions defined by IOUS, transcutaneous ultrasonography had detected 127 (76 per cent), whereas CT had demonstrated 91 out of a possible 150 (61 per cent). Parker and colleagues utilized IOUS during 45 exploratory operations in patients with liver tumours and reported its sensitivity in the detection of intrahepatic lesions as 98 per cent compared with 77 per cent for preoperative CT scanning.[6] Furthermore, operative management was altered as a consequence of the IOUS findings in 49 per cent of these operations. In a prospective study of 37 patients with liver metastases recently reported by Soyer and colleagues, 96 per cent of lesions were detected by IOUS compared with 89 per cent following a combination of preoperative transabdominal ultrasonography, dynamic CT scanning and CT portography.[7]

Reports from surgeons in the Far East and France have dominated the literature on the use of IOUS in the surgery of primary liver tumours. Coexisting hepatic cirrhosis may render small intrahepatic lesions especially difficult to palpate at operation, and the diminished functional reserve of the remaining liver makes the full extent of planned resection critical. In describing their experience with IOUS in the operative assessment of 47 patients with small hepatomas (<5 cm), Sheu and co-workers[8] described how IOUS was frequently able to demonstrate tumours which were otherwise impalpable (46 per cent of lesions <3 cm; 14 per cent of lesions 3–5 cm), thus justifying their claim that routine IOUS is 'indispensable' during such operations. Bismuth and colleagues reported that supplementary information was yielded by IOUS in 33 per cent of such patients, this information resulting in a modification of the planned surgical approach in 26 per cent of operations.[9] Thus, major liver resections were modified to subsegmental resections, made possible by the novel manoeuvre of ultrasound guided cannulation of portal venous branches with occlusion or injection of dye into the portal venous territory occupied by the hepatoma.[9,10] This technique, described earlier by Makuuchi's group,[11] may also be extended to include temporary occlusion of the hepatic arterial inflow and hepatic venous outflow, thus permitting liver resection to proceed under relatively avascular conditions.[12]

Lau and colleagues recently compared the outcome following 'curative' resection of hepatocellular carcinomas in patients in whom surgery had been guided by IOUS with the outcomes of a historical group of patients operated upon before the adoption of this technique.[13] They observed a significant reduction in the rate of tumour involvement of the resection margin (0 per cent versus 16 per cent). Although it is obviously impossible to attribute a survival advantage to the use of IOUS alone, this technique has undoubtedly played a major part in the refinement of hepatic surgery witnessed during the last decade.

Detection of occult liver metastases

Accurate staging of malignant intra-abdominal tumours is important for a number of reasons: evidence of liver metastases may contraindicate attempts at curative resection of the primary tumour, e.g. carcinoma of the head of the pancreas; it is desirable to achieve full disease staging in order to assess the patient's prognosis, and to make informed decisions regarding the need for adjuvant therapies and/or further surgery. Finlay and McArdle[14] demonstrated that at least 20 per cent of patients with colorectal carcinoma, in whom an apparently curative bowel resection had been undertaken, concealed occult liver metastases at the time of their initial surgery, and that this was the single most important factor in determining long-term survival. IOUS of the liver at the time of primary colorectal surgery has been shown to be the most sensitive method for detecting these impalpable tumours, which often measure less than 10 mm, and occult liver metastases have been demonstrated by IOUS, where both intraoperative palpation and preoperative investigations have previously failed in up to 10 per cent of laparotomies.[4,15–19] Machi and colleagues also report the IOUS detection of previously unsuspected liver metastases in 12 per cent of laparotomies performed upon patients with a variety of other intra-abdominal malignancies.[4]

Equipment

A variety of versatile ultrasound machines suitable for intraoperative work are commercially available, most of which may also be used for conventional real-time scanning and for which a wide range of probes are available. The transducer is usually a 5- or 7.5-MHz T-shaped linear array and must be both waterproof and sterilizable (either by ethylene oxide or by immersion in glutaraldehyde solution), although it is possible to undertake IOUS with the probe placed within a sterilized plastic bag (the system with which the authors are familiar is the portable Aloka SSD 500 machine employing a UST-587T-5 probe which gives a 7 cm 'footprint', and the Aloka SSD-680 system with a 7.5-MHz intraoperative T-probe with the facility for colour Doppler flow assessment). The equipment is placed on a trolley alongside the operating table (Fig. 10.2), and adjustment of the machine controls requires an unscrubbed assistant 'on the floor' to follow the operator's directions.

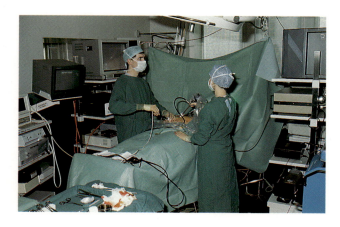

Figure 10.2 *The arrangement of IOUS and LapUS equipment in the operating theatre. A sterile LapUS probe has been inserted through the umbilical port in the patient's abdomen and is connected to a portable ultrasound machine (left), while the 'cameraman' (right) operates the laparoscope through the subxiphoid port. Ultrasound and camera images are viewed on the monitors positioned either side of the operating table.*

Anatomy and Basic Technique

An anatomical survey of the liver is performed by sliding the probe over the liver capsule as part of the initial laparotomy, and following a full mobilization of the liver, dividing its ligaments and revealing the bare area if greater exposure is desired. The moist film which covers the intra-abdominal organs usually establishes excellent transducer contact without the need for an interposed water balloon or instilled fluid, although these manoeuvres may be required if the liver surface is deformed and irregular because of cirrhosis or malignant infiltration. Although descriptions of the segmental liver anatomy may at first appear complicated to those familiar with other conventional anatomical classifications (Fig. 10.1), they are based upon fundamentally simple principles as described in Couinaud's seminal article[1] and later popularized by Bismuth and colleagues.[2,3,20] A good working knowledge of the segmental liver anatomy

may be rapidly acquired through the systematic use of IOUS in examinations of the liver and is indispensable to the surgeon and radiologist in transmitting accurate information on pre- and intraoperative investigations.

The anatomical survey starts with the T-probe placed upon the diaphragmatic surface of the quadrate lobe (segment IV), between the imaginary line which connects the gall bladder fossa with the inferior vena cava (principal fissure) and the falciform ligament (Fig. 10.3a). The transverse 'cut' of the liver obtained from this position with the beam angled cephalad identifies the hepatic venous confluence with the inferior vena cava (Fig. 10.4a), while slight rotation of the probe caudally demonstrates the structures traversing the porta hepatis (Fig. 10.4b). Hepatic veins are recognized by their characteristic suprahepatic venous pulsation and the absence of an identifiable vein wall, whereas hyperechoic fascial sheaths derived from Glisson's capsule characterize the portal venous radicles. The intrahepatic arterial and biliary structures are not normally identifiable, although the characteristic 'double-barrel shotgun' sign is apparent in the presence of intrahepatic bile duct dilatation in cases of extrahepatic biliary obstruction.

The left portal vein passes from the portal bifurcation transversely to the left supplying segmental branches to the left hemiliver (segments II, III and IV), and terminates abruptly in the recessus of Rex adjacent to the insertion of the round ligament (Fig. 10.4b) The right portal vein bifurcates almost immediately into anterior and posterior divisions, supplying the segments of the paramedian (segments V and VIII) and posterolateral (segments VI and VII) sectors of the right hemiliver respectively. These portal venous radicles may be traced with slow sweeps of the probe over the right liver, altering the orientation of the probe to obtain a range of oblique and parasagittal scanning planes. The right hepatic vein is identified bisecting the plane formed by the bifurcation of the right portal vein and separates the paramedian from the posterolateral sectors of the right liver. In this way, the segmental hepatic architecture can be determined from the three-dimensional spatial relationships of the portal venous branches with the interdigitating hepatic veins (Fig. 10.5)

An inferior right hepatic vein may be demonstrated entering the inferior vena cava in up to 24 per cent of patients[21] by inclining the probe to an angle which traverses the porta hepatis. The recognition of this common anatomical variant may have important implications for surgical decision-making in permitting novel segmental resections involving the sacrifice of the main right hepatic vein.[22] Furthermore, the

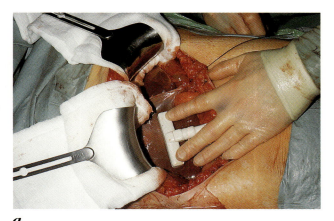

a

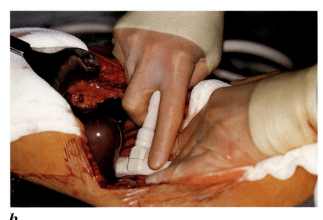

b

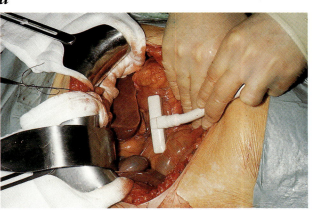

c

Figure 10.3 *(a) IOUS examination of the liver with the T-probe placed upon the inferior diaphragmatic surface of the liver (segments IV and V). (b) IOUS examination of the bile duct and associated vascular structures with the T-probe placed longitudinally upon the hepatoduodenal ligament. (c) IOUS of the pancreas in its longitudinal axis with the T-probe placed transversely upon the stomach.*

surgeon alerted to the existence of an inferior right hepatic vein may avoid troublesome haemorrhage following its inadvertent transection during right-sided liver resections. The middle hepatic vein lies along the plane marking the functional division of the left and right sides of the liver (principal fissure), and is often an important landmark for determining whether resectability may be achieved, e.g. by means of right hepatectomy or extended right hepatectomy (i.e. including segment IV) (Fig. 10.4a). Examination of the left lobe of the liver (segments II and III) reveals the left hepatic vein and the hyperechoic fissure formed by the fascial extension of the lesser omentum insertion which separates the left lobe from the underlying caudate lobe (segment I), posterior to which lie the inferior vena cava, aorta and vertebral column (Fig. 10.6).

The way in which IOUS influences the decision to undertake liver resection will vary from case to case and many permutations may be encountered.

Bismuth et al[23] have usefully summarized the possible ways in which IOUS may influence the surgical management of a palpable and apparently solitary tumour within the right hemiliver: (1) the detection of unsuspected bilobar tumour, thus precluding resection; (2) precise segmental localization of tumour, making segmentectomy feasible; (3) involvement of right hepatic vein, indicating that right hepatectomy is required; (4) involvement of middle hepatic vein necessitating extended right hepatectomy; (5) involvement of all three hepatic veins, rendering the tumour non-resectable. There are many other variations on this theme.

Intraoperative Ultrasound Guidance During Liver Surgery

Intraoperative ultrasound guided needle biopsy of intrahepatic lesions may be performed with precision,

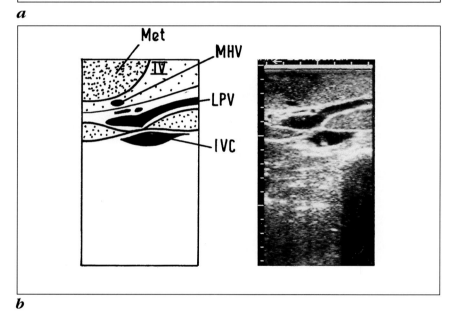

Figure 10.4 *(a) Transverse IOUS scan angled cephalad through the liver identifying the hepatic venous confluence. Note how the right hepatic vein (RHV) separates segments VII (posterolateral sector) and VIII (anteromedial sector). The hypoechoic metastatic tumour (Met) encroaches across the functional midline of the liver identified by the middle hepatic vein (MHV). An extended right hepatectomy (resection of segments IV–VIII) will consequently be required to achieve complete resection along anatomical lines. (b) Transverse IOUS scan angled more caudally than in (a) traverses the porta hepatis. Note the proximity of the tumour (Met) to the portal venous bifurcation, anterior to which lies the left hepatic artery. MHV, middle hepatic vein; LPV, left portal vein; IVC, inferior vena cava.* Reproduced from Garden OJ, Intraoperative and Laparoscopic Ultrasonography, *Blackwell Scientific Publications, Edinburgh, 1995, with the kind permission of the publishers.*

allowing the operator to avoid major vascular structures, and the procedure can be facilitated by the use of an accessory puncture adapter. The passage of the needle tip can be defined better if it is lightly abraded beforehand. Guided biopsy is of particular value in patients with cirrhosis, in whom a small hepatocellular carcinoma may be difficult to differentiate from a regenerating cirrhotic nodule. Guidance of liver resections may be facilitated by placing a small sheet of nylon mesh into the resection plane,[24] or the insertion of an array of needles has been described in order to direct accurately the hepatic transection without resort to repeated IOUS examinations.[25] We have not found these particular manoeuvres necessary, as the loss of contact between liver capsule and transducer at the resection line usually serves to define the plane of dissection and its relations to the underlying tumour.

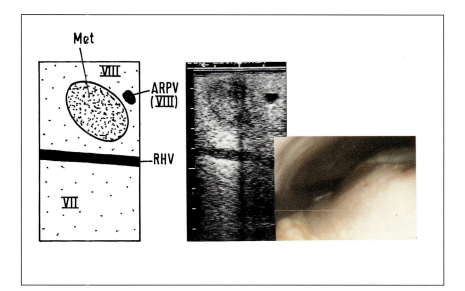

Figure 10.5 *Linear array laparoscopic sonogram obtained with the probe inserted obliquely via the right lateral port and scanning the right hepatic vein (RHV) in its long axis. A 3-cm-diameter hypoechoic tumour (Met) lies above this in the anteromedial sector adjacent to the twig to segment VIII from the anterior sectoral branch of the right portal vein (ARPV(VIII)). Note the large superficial umbilicated tumour identified laparoscopically (insert).*

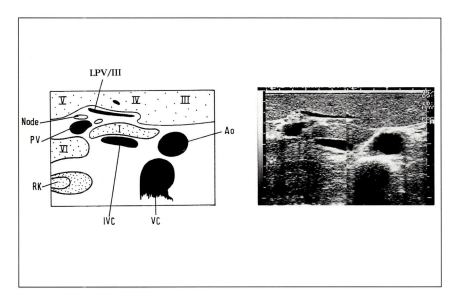

Figure 10.6 *Transverse IOUS scan of the liver at the level of the porta hepatis. Two small hilar lymph nodes have been identified alongside the portal vein (PV), biopsy of which revealed metastatic carcinoma. Note the transverse course of the structures in the left hepatic pedicle, and how the caudate lobe (segment I) separates the portal vein from the inferior vena cava (IVC). The right kidney (RK) lies posterior to segment VI, while the aorta (Ao) lies behind segments I and III. LPV/III, portal venous radicle to segment III; VC, vertebral column.*

LAPAROSCOPIC ULTRASOUND

Background

Laparoscopy is an effective means of obtaining valuable diagnostic and staging information in patients with liver disease. The greatly magnified view of the visceral surfaces obtained by the laparoscopist allows the detection of small superficial liver lesions and peritoneal tumour seedlings which are beyond the resolution of any current radiological imaging technique. The laparoscopic detection of previously unsuspected factors such as multifocal liver deposits, peritoneal and serosal metastases and hepatic cirrhosis in a substantial proportion of patients under investigation for primary liver tumours was highlighted in reports by Lightdale[26] and Jeffers.[27] In the authors' experience with 50 consecutive

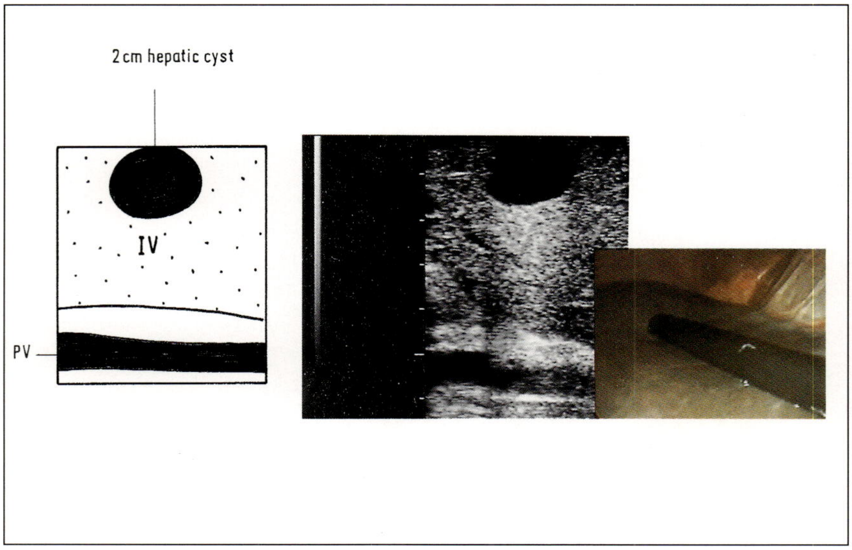

Figure 10.7 *A parasagittal laparoscopic sonogram through segment IV with the probe operated from the umbilical port. A 2-cm-diameter simple intrahepatic cyst has been identified, and, although lying superficially, it could not be identified laparoscopically. PV, portal vein.*

staging laparoscopies in patients thought to have potentially resectable liver tumours, factors contraindicating further operative intervention were demonstrated in 46 per cent of examinations.[28] Previously unsuspected extrahepatic malignant dissemination was observed in 18 cases and a non-resectable bilobar pattern of disease in 11.[28] The information derived from laparoscopy is, however, limited to situations where the disease process affects the surface or contour of the organ. Indeed, laparoscopic visualization of liver tumours was achieved in just 34 out of 50 cases (68 per cent) in the latter study, thus corroborating the findings of other workers.[29]

Accordingly, the incorporation of the principles of IOUS with those of laparoscopy was inevitable, their combination representing an innovative and exciting development. Early reports in the evolution of LapUS testified to the feasibility of this new technology in providing recognizable B-mode images of both the normal and diseased hepatic parenchyma, and of focal liver tumours. Descriptions in the Japanese literature focused on the use of 'echolaparoscopes' which variously incorporated 90°[30] and 360°[31] sector scanning and linear array[32,33] ultrasound transducers within the shaft of the telescope. Later accounts stressed the improved ability of LapUS over trans-abdominal ultrasound in differentiating benign from malignant liver lesions, guiding needle biopsy of 'occult' intrahepatic tumours and determining the resectability of liver tumours.[34–39] The recent trend towards laparoscopic deroofing and drainage of intrahepatic cysts represents another useful application for LapUS,[40] in the same way that IOUS is used to localize and fully assess liver cysts at open operation. The cyst wall and luminal contents may be examined in detail for solid components, and its relations with adjacent vascular and biliary structures defined. Incisions of the cyst may be safely guided in this way, avoiding areas where its wall comprises a thicker layer of liver parenchyma (Fig. 10.7).

The development of LapUS in our department initially involved the use of a commercially available 5-MHz linear array probe designed specifically for endoluminal transrectal ultrasound. This large probe was inserted into the abdomen via a purpose-built 20-mm large port assembly whose introduction first required the use of a guide rod and dilator.[41] Of seven patients examined in this way, LapUS provided diagnostic information which would otherwise have been revealed only during surgical exploration in four. Thereafter, the routine use of staging laparoscopy with LapUS in the assessment of patients thought to have potentially resectable liver tumours had a dramatic effect on patient management. We observed a significant decrease in the number of

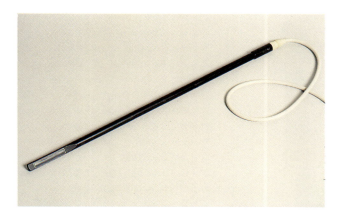

Figure 10.8 *A rigid 7.5-MHz linear array LapUS probe (Aloka UST-5521-7.5).*

'non-therapeutic' laparotomies, and a corresponding increase in the resectability rate from 58 per cent to 93 per cent in patients under consideration for liver resection with curative intent.[28]

Technique

LapUS assessment of the liver is best performed using a linear array probe which may be alternated with the laparoscope between two lower abdominal ports. These should ideally be sited at the umbilicus and laterally in the right flank, although the presence of intra-abdominal adhesions associated with previous surgery may restrict access and require the insertion of cannulae well away from the previous incision. Access to the peritoneal cavity failed in two of 52 patients (4 per cent failure rate) undergoing staging LapUS in our study, of whom 73 per cent bore the scars of previous surgery, reflecting the preponderance of patients with secondary liver tumours in this population.[28] This success is attributable to the liberal use of a direct cutdown technique in achieving abdominal insufflation, and we have experienced no intra-abdominal complications using this technique.

The following description of technique pertains to our use of a 7.5-MHz multi-element linear array

probe (Aloka UST-5521-7.5, KeyMed Ltd, Southend-on-Sea, UK) linked to the same portable ultrasound machine as described for IOUS (Aloka SSD-500) (Figs. 10.2 and 10.8). Alternatively, a similar probe for use with colour flow Doppler facilities was used (Aloka, UST-5523L-7.5/SSD-680). The 9-mm-diameter rigid ultrasound probe has a 3.8-mm transducer 'footprint' at its flattened end, and may be inserted via standard 10/11-mm disposable laparoscopic ports (Endopath, Ethicon Ltd, Edinburgh, UK), which the authors favour in order to minimize the risk of trauma to the transducer from the spring-loaded metal trumpet valves of non-disposable cannulae. The simultaneous demonstration of both laparoscopic and ultrasound images on the operating theatre monitors by 'picture-in-picture' video mixing facilitates the placement of the probe, and may be achieved using any commercially available audio-visual mixing desk.

A laparoscopic inspection of the peritoneal cavity is performed in which the rigid ultrasound probe is useful in 'palpating' the liver for mass lesions, for displacing omentum and bowel loops, for lifting the liver to inspect its undersurface and for tamponade of bleeding biopsy sites. LapUS commences with the anatomical survey of the liver in much the same way as for IOUS, except that the scans are necessarily orientated in parasagittal and oblique planes. The 'trifurcation' of the hepatic veins with the inferior vena cava can be demonstrated with the probe placed alongside the falciform ligament upon hepatic segment IV (Fig. 10.9). Using the middle hepatic vein as a landmark, slight anticlockwise rotation of the shaft scans through the parenchyma of segment IV, whereas movement of the probe towards the right or a clockwise rotation allows the right hemiliver to be examined in detail. Withdrawal of the probe demonstrates the hilar structures entering the liver beneath hepatic segment IV with the caudate lobe behind (Fig. 10.10a), and the right and left branches of the portal vein, hepatic duct and hepatic artery proper can be followed by rotation of the probe clockwise or anticlockwise respectively. Examination of the right hemiliver may be facilitated by moving the probe to the right lateral port, whereby the right hepatic vein is identified in its long axis separating the anterior and posterior branches of the right portal vein (Fig. 10.5). In this way, the anteromedial and posterolateral sectors of the right liver may be delineated, noting that the gall bladder fossa identifies the medial limit of segment V (Fig. 10.10b), while the right kidney normally lies posterior to segment VI (Fig. 10.6). A full examination of the posteriorly

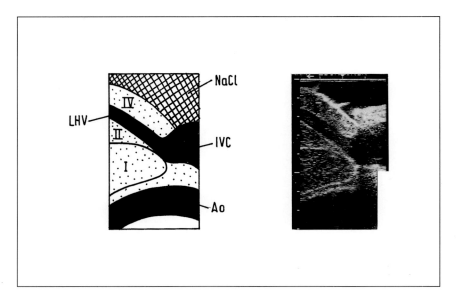

Figure 10.9 *The instillation of warm saline (NaCl) into the peritoneal cavity maintains acoustic contact despite loss of transducer contact with the superior aspect of the liver. With the probe placed in a parasagittal orientation upon hepatic segment IV (via an umbilical port), slight rotation to the left identifies the confluence of the left hepatic vein (LHV) with the suprahepatic inferior vena cava (IVC), which is separated from the supracoeliac aorta (Ao) by the caudate lobe (segment I).*

situated segments (VII and VIII) can be achieved by advancing the transducer over the dome of the liver. Loss of transducer contact with any area of the liver can easily be remedied by the introduction of warm crystalloid solution into the abdomen, and the authors have not found it necessary to replace the rigid probe with one of the new generation of linear array LapUS probes equipped with flexible tips (Fig. 10.9). LapUS guided needle biopsy may be undertaken in much the same way as described for IOUS, albeit without a puncture adapter, having carefully aligned the skin puncture site and needle in the same plane as the transducer beam.

The left hepatic lobe (including the posteriorly situated caudate lobe) should be examined by transferring the probe to the left of the falciform ligament (Fig. 10.11a). From this position it is possible to inspect the aortocaval region of the retroperitoneum for lymphadenopathy to the level of the coeliac axis (Fig. 10.11b). The probe should then be placed directly upon the hepatoduodenal ligament, specifically searching for enlarged portocaval and hilar lymph nodes, and assessing the main portal vein for evidence of direct invasion or involvement with tumour thrombus, especially in cases of hepatocellular carcinoma (Fig. 10.12).

Staging laparoscopy with LapUS was performed using this technique in 43 patients, who, on the basis of preoperative CT scans, were thought to be candidates for curative resection of malignant liver tumours.[28] Staging information which affected the decision to proceed to operative assessment of tumour resectability was obtained in 18 patients (42 per cent). A non-resectable bilobar or multifocal pattern of intrahepatic tumour was confirmed in 14 patients, and malignant hilar lymphadenopathy and main portal vein invasion were each demonstrated in five cases.[28] LapUS was the only investigation to have demonstrated factors contraindicating liver resection in seven patients (16 per cent). In addition, focal malignancy was excluded on the basis of LapUS in two patients who were accordingly also spared operative intervention.[28] Our early experience in assessing patients with hepatic malignancy therefore suggests that the adoption of laparoscopy and LapUS provides additional important information which helps to avoid unnecessary laparotomy and enables more appropriate planning of treatment.

THE BILIARY SYSTEM

Operative imaging of the biliary tree has traditionally been achieved by cholangiography and/or

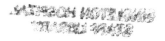

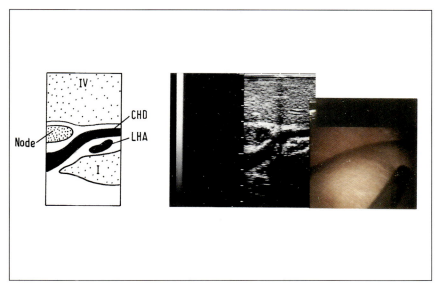
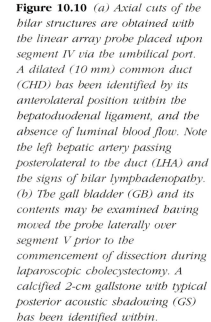

a

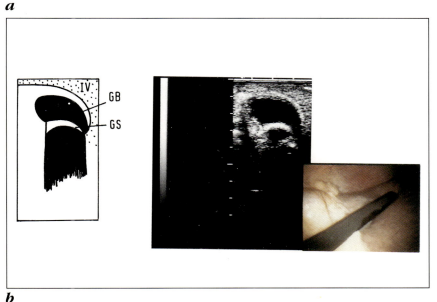

b

Figure 10.10 *(a) Axial cuts of the hilar structures are obtained with the linear array probe placed upon segment IV via the umbilical port. A dilated (10 mm) common duct (CHD) has been identified by its anterolateral position within the hepatoduodenal ligament, and the absence of luminal blood flow. Note the left hepatic artery passing posterolateral to the duct (LHA) and the signs of hilar lymphadenopathy. (b) The gall bladder (GB) and its contents may be examined having moved the probe laterally over segment V prior to the commencement of dissection during laparoscopic cholecystectomy. A calcified 2-cm gallstone with typical posterior acoustic shadowing (GS) has been identified within.*

fibreoptic cholangioscopy, and these invasive procedures have become firmly established as routine techniques in the armamentarium of the biliary surgeon. However, the potential of invasive ultrasound imaging of the biliary tree was recognized more than 30 years ago when both British[42] and American[43] workers described the feasibility of contact ultrasound using A-mode scanners in the operative detection of choledocholithiasis. With subsequent refinements in ultrasound technology, a number of enthusiasts reported impressive results for B-mode IOUS in this role by demonstrating that, in the hands of experts, IOUS could be at least as accurate as intraoperative cholangiography in alerting the surgeon to the presence of common duct stones[4,44–49] (Table 10.1). Although the use of routine intraoperative cholangiography continued to attract considerable debate, IOUS failed to achieve wider

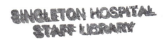

SINGLETON HOSPITAL
STAFF LIBRARY

Table 10.1 IOUS and the detection of choledocholithiasis.

Reference	Sensitivity	Specificity	PPV	NPV	Accuracy
48 (n = 50)	100	97	–	–	–
47 (n = 100)	96	93	–	–	–
49 (n = 449)	94	99	96	98	98
4 (n = 666)	92	99	95*	99	99

* Statistically significantly superior result compared with operative cholangiography.

PPV = Post predictive value.

NPV = Negative predictive value.

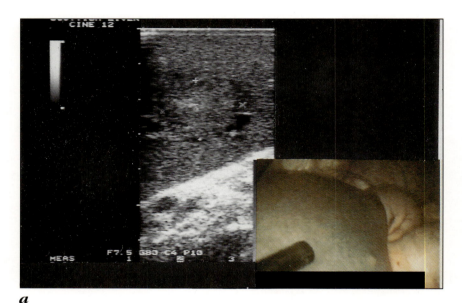

a

b

Figure 10.11 *(a) Examination of the left hepatic lobe during staging LapUS, in a patient thought to have a solitary right liver metastasis, has defined a previously unsuspected 17 × 23 mm metastasis (demonstrating the typical 'anechoic halo'). This patient, therefore, has a non-resectable bilobar pattern of disease and unnecessary laparotomy was avoided. (b) A parasagittal cut throught the left hepatic lobe enables scrutiny of the retroperitoneum. Para-aortic lymphadenopathy was identified in this patient with a solitary colorectal metastasis who was later confirmed to have malignant regional lymphadenopathy at laparotomy.*

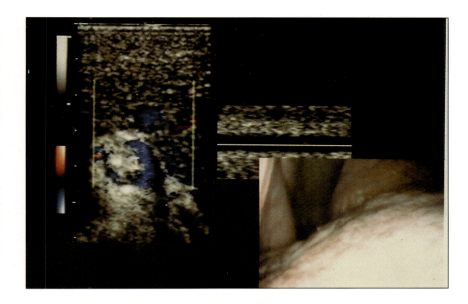

Figure 10.12 *Diagnostic laparoscopy with biopsy confirmed diffuse hepatocellular carcinoma on a background of cirrhosis in this patient (see insert). Doppler sampling with colour flow during LapUS identified tumour thrombus occluding the main portal vein. Reproduced from Garden OJ,* Intraoperative and Laparoscopic Ultrasonography, *Blackwell Scientific Publications, Edinburgh, 1995, with the kind permission of the publishers.*

popularity in the pre-laparoscopic cholecystectomy era. The advent, in the 1990s, of laparoscopic cholecystectomy as the preferred method for removal of the diseased gall bladder has served not only to resurrect controversy regarding the need for intraoperative cholangiography, but also to renew interest in LapUS as a viable alternative.

INTRAOPERATIVE ULTRASOUND EXAMINATION OF THE BILIARY SYSTEM

The indications for IOUS in assessing the biliary tree include its use during cholecystectomy, and during hepatobiliary procedures for benign biliary strictures or malignant biliary obstruction. Imaging of the intrahepatic biliary tree, the gall bladder and proximal common duct may be performed with the T probe placed upon hepatic segment IV as described above (Fig. 10.3a). The gall bladder wall and luminal contents can easily be assessed prior to the division of adhesions in the subhepatic space. The intrahepatic and common hepatic ducts are frequently small, collapsed and not easily visualized, and this of itself may be sufficient to exclude more distal bile duct pathology. Scanning in the transverse plane allows the extrahepatic course of the left hepatic duct as it lies immediately anterior to the left portal vein to be

traced from the hilar region to its termination as segment II and III branches in the recess of Rex (Figs. 10.4b and 10.6). This aspect of the examination may be particularly useful in planning biliary reconstructions based upon the extrahepatic course of the left hepatic duct, or for palliative cholangioenteric bypass procedures which utilize distended intrahepatic ducts in cases of obstructing hilar malignancy. The extent of infiltration of the liver and the structures entering the porta hepatis by tumours arising from the bile duct confluence can be assessed in detail with the probe placed upon the overlying liver (Fig. 10.13). Preoperative investigations often underestimate the extent of local invasion in such cases, and operative decisions can be made regarding tumour resectability based upon the patency of hilar vascular structures and the extent of tumour infiltration proximally into the intrahepatic biliary tree.

The extrahepatic common bile duct may be traced distally in the free edge of the lesser omentum using the standard T-shaped linear array probe in both transverse and parasagittal planes (Fig. 10.3b), although some find the use of an I-shaped linear array or end-viewing curvilinear array probe better adapted for this manoeuvre. Extrahepatic biliary obstruction makes it easy to identify the common duct and to trace it to the level of the obstructing lesion. Alternatively, the presence of a biliary stent

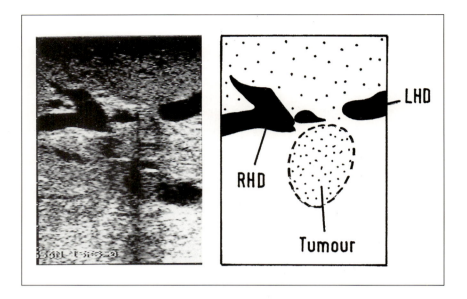

Figure 10.13 *Transverse IOUS scan through the porta hepatis in a patient undergoing operative assessment of resectability of a hilar cholangiocarcinoma. A 4-cm tumour mass was identified which had infiltrated the liver with right portal vein occlusion. Note separation of the distended right (RHD) and left (LHD) duct systems, with patent secondary biliary confluences (Bismuth type II stricture). A palliative segment III cholangiojejunostomy was performed having identified the dilated segment III biliary radicle. Reproduced from Garden OJ,* Intraoperative and Laparoscopic Ultrasonography, *Blackwell Scientific Publications, Edinburgh, 1995, with the kind permission of the publishers.*

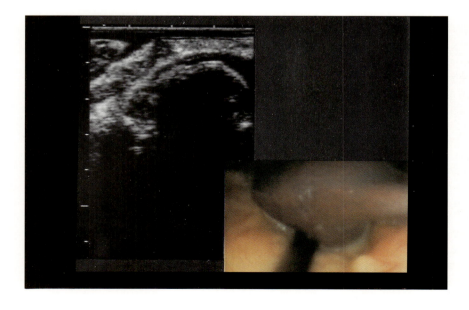

Figure 10.14 *Laparoscopic cholecystectomy. Examination of the distal common bile duct with the linear array probe upon the hepatoduodenal ligament has identified the classical appearances of a large obstructing gallstone.*

may also help to identify the duct and obstructing lesion, although air in a collapsed biliary tree may degrade the image under these circumstances. Calcified gallstones can be identified by their characteristic echogenic borders and dense posterior acoustic shadows (Fig. 10.14).

LAPAROSCOPIC ULTRASOUND AND THE BILIARY TREE

The dramatic proliferation in the practice of laparoscopic cholecystectomy witnessed in recent years has been accompanied by a number of reports describing the use of a variety of LapUS probe configurations in both human and animal subjects. These describe the use of 90–360° mechanical sector scanning probes,[50-53] and curvilinear[54] and linear array probes[53,55-59] operating with transducer frequencies of 7.5–12.5 MHz, and in some cases incorporating Doppler technology. The authors have been involved in the development and preliminary evaluation of two types of LapUS system (linear array and 90° mechanical sector probes) for the assessment of the biliary system during laparoscopic cholecystectomy.[52,59]

Technique

LapUS may be performed without modification of the conventional four-port arrangement for laparoscopic cholecystectomy, and the camera may be alternated with the ultrasound probe between the 10/11-mm diameter epigastric and umbilical ports (Fig. 10.2). The authors' preference is to perform LapUS at the outset of the procedure and prior to surgical dissection in order to minimize acoustic interference associated with surgical clips and the introduction of gas into the underlying tissues. Retraction of the gall bladder, and the instillation of a crystalloid solution into the peritoneal cavity to act as a 'stand-off', are ploys which may improve transducer contact. However, we have not found these manoeuvres to be routinely necessary.

Laparoscopic ultrasound examination of the biliary tree using a linear array probe
The examination commences with the transducer placed upon the liver overlying the gall bladder and porta hepatis, having introduced the probe via the umbilical port. With the interposed hepatic parenchyma acting as an acoustic window, scans of the underlying structures are obtained in a variety of parasagittal and oblique planes. Having observed the degree of fibrosis, oedema or distension affecting the gall bladder, the number and size of calculi within and the presence or absence of intrahepatic bile duct dilatation, the probe position should be adjusted slightly so as to identify the structures passing through the liver hilum. The hepatic artery proper (anteromedial) and common hepatic duct (anterolateral) may be identified within the hepatoduodenal ligament, and multiple longitudinal and oblique views of these structures are obtained by slight rotation of the probe anticlockwise and clockwise respectively. The bile duct is traced distally through a slow, smooth withdrawal of the probe until the transducer loses contact with the liver, whereupon the probe is repositioned upon the free edge of the hepatoduodenal ligament. The normal common bile duct usually measures no greater than 8 mm maximum diameter and care must be taken not to compress and obliterate the hilar structures. The bile duct is characterized by its position relative to the other structures within the lesser omentum, its hyperechoic wall and lack of pulsation or visible luminal blood flow, and this may usefully be confirmed by Doppler sampling where this facility is available. The distal portion of the common bile duct takes a divergent lateral course away from the portal vein and posterior to the duodenum (Fig. 10.15), and slow clockwise rotation of the probe is required to trace its oblique course to the papilla of Vater. The bile duct lumen is scrutinized throughout the examination for the classical sonographic appearances of calculi (Fig. 10.14). Gas within the gastric antrum or duodenum may interfere with the images obtained during this part of the procedure, although this may be displaced by downward pressure with the probe. An alternative strategy which allows imaging of the hilar structures in a transverse plane involves the placement of the probe through the subxiphoid port so that the transducer may be placed perpendicularly alongside the hepatoduodenal ligament (Fig. 10.16). Other workers have recommended this manoeuvre in order to obtain multiple views of the biliary structures.[57]

The authors' initial experience with this technique using a 9-mm-diameter, 7.5-MHz linear array probe was compared with both intraoperative cholangiography and preoperative clinical and biochemical risk factors in 54 patients undergoing laparoscopic cholecystectomy.[59] The accuracy of LapUS was similar to

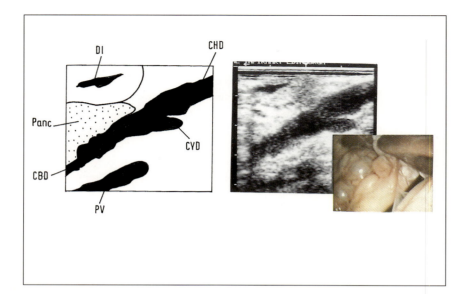

Figure 10.15 *Laparoscopic cholecystectomy. Withdrawal of the linear array probe along the common duct delineates its confluence with the cystic duct (CYD) and its course behind the first part of the duodenum (D1) and head of the pancreas (Panc). PV, portal vein; CHD, common hepatic duct; CBD, common bile duct.*

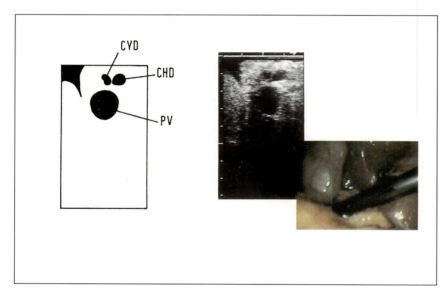

Figure 10.16 *The hepatoduodenal ligament may be examined transversely with the linear array probe placed perpendicularly alongside having been inserted through the subxiphoid port ('Mickey Mouse' appearance). PV, portal vein; CHD, common hepatic duct; CYD, cystic duct.*

that of operative cholangiography in the detection of choledocholithiasis (93 per cent) and superior to that predicted from preoperative risk factors (63 per cent). Using criteria defined by LapUS alone (common duct ≥7 mm diameter; gall bladder stones ≤3 mm diameter), our results suggested that a policy of 'super-selective' operative cholangiography could feasibly have been undertaken in just 19 per cent of patients without prejudicing the accuracy of detection of common duct stones.[59]

Laparoscopic ultrasound examination of the biliary tree using a 90° mechanical sector probe

LapUS examination of the biliary tree utilizing a sector scanning probe is based upon similar principles. The authors are familiar with a commercially available system which provides 90° sectoral images by means of a 7.5-MHz mechanically oscillating transducer situated at the tip of the probe (LaparoScan Intraoperative Diagnostic Ultrasound System U4000, Endomedix Corporation, Irvine, CA,

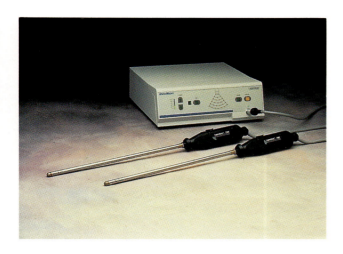

Figure 10.17 *The Endomedix LaparoScan 7.5-MHz 90 ° mechanical sector scanning LapUS system. Reproduced from Garden OJ,* Intraoperative and Laparoscopic Ultrasonography, *Blackwell Scientific Publications, Edinburgh, 1995, with the kind permission of the publishers.*

operator to identify various anatomical landmarks was assessed for three consecutive groups comprising 20 consecutive patient examinations each.[52] The gall bladder and portal vein were easily identified in all cases. There was a marked improvement in the ability of the operating surgeon to identify the supra-pancreatic bile duct, intrapancreatic bile duct and pancreatic duct, these structures being observed in 100 per cent, 80 per cent and 85 per cent of examinations in the last group of 20 patients compared to 85 per cent, 35 per cent and 30 per cent respectively in the first group. This improvement in performance undoubtedly reflects refinements in LapUS equipment and the technique and experience of the operator during this period of evaluation.

With appropriate training, the skills required to perform LapUS examination of the biliary tree during laparoscopic cholecystectomy may be rapidly acquired. This technique has the potential to be more widely utilized to implement a policy of 'superselective' operative cholangiography in the detection of common bile duct stones. Further experience with both linear array and sectoral probes will be required before it can be established which type of LapUS probe is of greater value during cholecystectomy.

USA), and for which both end-viewing and side-viewing probes are provided (LaparoScan U750F and U750S) (Fig. 10.17). The small transducer 'footprint' permits easy access and precise apposition with the viscera. Rotation of the probe shaft through 90° varies the scanning plane between longitudinal and transverse orientations, and this effect may be achieved with the probe placed via the umbilical or epigastric ports. However, this versatility may be at the expense of ease of image interpretation when compared with the more stable rectilinear image yielded by the larger flat 'footprint' of a linear array probe (Fig. 10.18).

In a prospective study of 60 patients undergoing laparoscopic cholecystectomy, we evaluated several prototypes of the LaparoScan system in comparison with routine intraoperative cholangiography.[52] The sonographic features of common duct stones were identified in nine patients, with one 'false-positive' and one 'false-negative' examination. The LaparoScan correctly identified previously unsuspected common duct stones in three out of four patients. In an attempt to quantify the 'learning curve' associated with the adoption of this technique, the ability of the

THE PANCREAS

Diseases of the pancreas may be difficult to evaluate radiologically due to the retroperitoneal location of the organ and its complex relationships with the adjacent vascular and ductal structures. Despite significant refinements in the various imaging techniques in recent years, the assessment of both inflammatory and neoplastic disorders of the pancreas remains challenging and controversial. Ultimately, it is the evaluation of the pancreas during laparotomy that often determines the operative approach, and even at this late stage surgical decision-making may still be a difficult process requiring an often demanding and hazardous retroperitoneal dissection. The practice of 'open and close' laparotomy following surgical biopsy in patients with pancreatic cancer was not an uncommon event in the past, although this fortunately appears to have diminished in frequency in recent years.[60] The relative shortcomings of various imaging techniques in satisfying the requirements of pancreatic surgeons has led to the development of

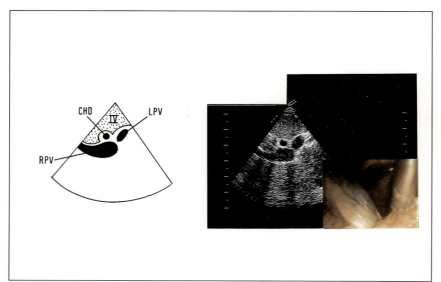

a

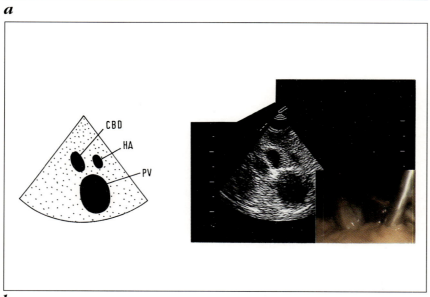

b

Figure 10.18 *All sonograms were obtained with the probe introduced via the subxiphoid port: (a) High transverse cut demonstrating the bifurcation of the portal vein behind hepatic segment IV, with a 5-mm common hepatic duct (CHD) lying anteriorly. LPV, left portal vein; RPV, right portal vein. (b) Typical 'Mickey Mouse' appearance of middle common bile duct (CBD), common hepatic artery proper (HA) and portal vein (PV).*

invasive ultrasound in an attempt to better evaluate pancreatic disease: hence the development of endoscopic ultrasonography (as described elsewhere) and techniques whereby small ultrasound probes may be inserted into the pancreatic and bile ducts either endoscopically or intraoperatively. Some surgeons have taken the opportunity to insert miniaturized ultrasound transducers designed for intravascular use into the superior mesenteric and portal vein during laparotomy in order to define its relationship with the adjacent pancreatic tumour

(H. van Urk, personal communication), although attempts to locally stage pancreatic cancer using intravascular ultrasound via the inferior vena cava have proved disappointing.[61]

The indications for IOUS of the pancreas include: (1) the operative assessment of acute or chronic pancreatitis and their sequelae; (2) the operative localization of neuroendocrine tumours of the pancreas, and (3) the operative assessment of resectability of pancreatic tumours, primarily in patients with carcinoma of the head of the pancreas

27. Jeffers L, Spieglman G, Reddy R et al, Laparoscopically directed fine needle aspiration for the diagnosis of hepatocellular carcinoma: a safe and accurate technique, *Gastrointest Endosc* (1988) **34**:235–7.

28. John TG, Greig JD, Crosbie JL et al, Superior staging of liver tumors with laparoscopy and laparoscopic ultrasound, *Ann Surg* (1994) in press.

29. Bleiberg H, Rozencweig M, Mathieu M et al, The use of peritoneoscopy in the detection of liver metastases, *Cancer* (1978) **41**:863–7.

30. Ohta Y, Yamazaki M, Torii M et al, A device of ultrasonic laparoscope, *Gastroenterol Endosc* (1981) **23**:1385–91.

31. Hirata K, Mima S, Fukuda M, High resolution ultrasonography in cancer diagnosis – advances and indications of intraluminal sonography, *Gan To Kagaku Ryoho* (1986) **13**:1661–7.

32. Oda M, Development of ultrasonic laparoscope, *Gastroenterol Endosc* (1982) **24**:884–93.

33. Frank K, Bliesze H, Bönhof JA et al, Laparoscopic sonography: a new approach to intra-abdominal disease, *J Clin Ultrasound* (1985) **13**:60–5.

34. Fukuda M, Mima S, Tanabe T et al, Endoscopic sonography of the liver – diagnostic application of the echolaparoscope to localize intrahepatic lesions, *Scand J Gastroenterol* (1984) **19** (Suppl. 102):24–8.

35. Fukuda M, Hirata K, Mima S, Preliminary evaluation of sonolaparoscopy in the diagnosis of liver diseases, *Endoscopy* (1992) **24**:701–8.

36. Bönhof JA, Linhart P, Bettendorf U, Holper H, Liver biopsy guided by laparoscopic sonography. A case report demonstrating a new technique, *Endoscopy* (1984) **16**:237–9.

37. Ido K, Kawamoto C, Ohtani M et al, Tumor biopsy under the peritoneoscopic ultrasonogram guidance, *Gastroenterol Endosc* (1989) **31**:1528–32.

38. Fornari F, Civardi G, Cavanna L et al, Laparoscopic ultrasonography in the study of liver diseases: preliminary results, *Surg Endosc* (1989) **3**:33–7.

39. Cuesta MA, Meijer S, Borgstein PJ et al, Laparoscopic ultrasonography for hepatobiliary and pancreatic malignancy, *Br J Surg* (1993) **80**:1571–74.

40. Mårvik R, Myrvold HE, Johnsen G, Røysland P, Laparoscopic ultrasonography and treatment of hepatic cysts, *Surg Laparosc Endosc* (1993) **3**:172–4.

41. Miles WFA, Paterson-Brown S, Garden OJ, Laparoscopic contact hepatic ultrasonography, *Br J Surg* (1992) **79**:419–20.

42. Knight PR, Newell JA, Operative use of ultrasonics in cholelithiasis, *Lancet* (1963) **i**:1023–5.

43. Eiseman B, Greenlaw RH, Gallagher JQ, Localization of common bile duct stones by ultrasound, *Arch Surg* (1965) **91**:195–9.

44. Sigel B, Coelho JCU, Nyhus LM et al, Comparison of cholangiography and ultrasonography in the operative screening of the common bile duct, *World J Surg* (1982) **6**:440–4.

45. Sigel B, Machi J, Beitler JC et al, Comparative accuracy of operative ultrasonography in detecting common duct calculi, *Surgery* (1983) **94**:715–20.

46. Sigel B, Coelho JCU, Spigos DG et al, Real-time ultrasonography during biliary surgery, *Radiology* (1980) **137**:531–3.

47. Lane RJ, Coupland GAE, Ultrasonic indications to explore the common bile duct, *Surgery* (1982) **91**:268–74.

48. Lane RJ, Glazer G, Intra-operative B-mode ultrasound scanning of the extra-hepatic biliary system and pancreas, *Lancet* (1980) **ii**:334–7.

49. Jakimowicz JJ, Rutten H, Jürgens PJ, Carol EJ, Comparison of operative ultrasonography and radiography in screening of the common bile duct for calculi, *World J Surg* (1987) **11**:628–34.

50. Ascher SM, Evans SRT, Goldberg JA et al, Intraoperative bile duct sonography during laparoscopic cholecystectomy: experience with a 12.5-MHz catheter-based US probe, *Radiology* (1992) **185**:493–6.

51. Röthlin M, Schlumpf R, Largiadèr F, Die technik der intraoperativen sonographie bei der laparoskopischen cholecystektomie, *Der Chirurg* (1991) **62**:899–901.

52. John TG, Banting SW, Pye S et al, Preliminary experience with intracorporeal laparoscopic ultrasonography using a sector scanning probe: a prospective comparison with intraoperative cholangiography in the detection of choledocholithiasis, *Surg Endosc* (1994) **8**:in press

53. Goletti O, Buccianti P, Decanini L et al, Intraoperative sonography of biliary tree during laparoscopic cholecystectomy, *Surg Laparosc Endosc* (1994) **4**:9–12.

54. Yamashita Y, Kurohiji T, Hayashi J et al, Intraoperative ultrasonography during laparoscopic cholecystectomy, *Surg Laparosc Endosc* (1993) **3**:167–71.

55. Yamamoto M, Stiegmann GV, Durham J et al, Laparoscopy-guided intracorporeal ultrasound accurately delineates hepatobiliary anatomy,. *Surg Endosc* (1993) **7**:325–30.

56. McIntyre RC, Van Stiegman G, Intraoperative, endoscopic, and laparoscopic ultrasound. In: Hunter JG, Sackier JM, eds, *Minimally Invasive Surgery*. (McGraw-Hill: New York, 1993) 15–21.

57. Machi J, Sigel B, Zaren HA et al, Technique of ultrasound examination during laparoscopic cholecystectomy, *Surg Endosc* (1993) **7**:544–9.

58. Jakimowicz JJ, Intraoperative ultrasonography during minimal access surgery, *J R Coll Surg Edinb* (1993) **38**:231–8.

59. Greig JD, John TG, Mahadaven M, Garden OJ, Laparoscopic ultrasonography in the evaluation of the biliary tree during laparoscopic cholecystectomy, *Br J Surg* (1994) **81**:1202–6.

60. Watanapa P, Williamson RCN, Surgical palliation for pancreatic cancer: developments during the past two decades, *Br J Surg* (1992) **79**:8–20.

61. Lehner K, Gerhardt P, Blasini R, Intravascular ultrasonography in tumour staging, *Endoscopy* (1992) **24** (Suppl. 1):376–8.

62. Sigel B, Machi J, Kikuchi T et al, The use of ultrasound during surgery for complications of pancreatitis, *World J Surg* (1987) **11**:659–63.

63. Zeiger MA, Shawker TH, Norton JA, Use of intraoperative ultrasonography to localize islet cell tumors, *World J Surg* (1993) **17**:448–54.

64. van Heerden JA, Grant CS, Czako PF et al, Occult functioning insulinomas: which localizing studies are indicated? *Surgery* (1992) **112**:1010–15.

65. Rothmund M, Localization of endocrine pancreatic tumours, *Br J Surg* (1994) **81**:164–6.

66. Plainfosse MC, Bouillot JL, Rivaton F et al, The use of operative sonography in carcinoma of the pancreas,. *World J Surg* (1987) **11**:654–8.

67. Serio G, Fugazzola C, Iacono C et al, Intraoperative ultrasonography in pancreatic cancer, *Int J Pancreatol* (1992) **11**:31–41.

68. Warshaw AL, Tepper JE, Shipley WU, Laparoscopy in the staging and planning of therapy for pancreatic cancer, *Am J Surg* (1986) **151**:76–80.

69. Warshaw AL, Gu ZY, Wittenberg J, Waltman AC,. Preoperative staging and asessment of resectability of pancreatic cancer, *Arch Surg* (1990) **125**:230–3.

70. Cuschieri A, Laparoscopy for pancreatic cancer: does it benefit the patient? *Eur J Surg Oncol* (1988) **14**:41–4.

71. Murugiah M, Paterson-Brown S, Windsor JA et al, Early experience of laparoscopic ultrasonography in the management of pancreatic carcinoma, *Surg Endosc* (1993) **7**:177–81.

72. John TG, Greig JD, Carter DC, Garden OJ, Carcinoma of the pancreatic head and periampullary region: tumor staging with laparoscopy and laparoscopic ultrasonography, *Ann Surg* (1995) **220**: in press.

73. John TG, Garden OJ, Laparoscopic ultrasound: extending the scope of diagnostic laparoscopy, *Br J Surg* (1994) **81**:5–6.

74. John TG, Garden OJ, Assessment of pancreatic cancer. In: Cuesta M, Nagy AG, eds, *Minimally Invasive Surgery in Gastrointestinal Cancer* (Churchill Livingstone: London, 1993) 95–111.

75. Okita K, Kodama T, Oda M, Takemoto T, Laparoscopic ultrasonography. Diagnosis of liver and pancreatic cancer, *Scand J Gastroenterol* (1984) **19** (Suppl. 94):91–100.

76. Pietrabissa A, Shimi SM, Vander Velpen G, Cuschieri A, Localisation of insulinoma by laparoscopic infragastric inspection of the pancreas and contact ultrasonography, *Surg Oncol* (1993) **2**:83–6.

77. Tio TL, Tytgat GNJ, Cikot RJLM et al, Ampullopancreatic carcinoma; preoperative TNM classification with endosonography, *Radiology* (1990) **175**:455–61.

78. Rösch T, Braig C, Gain T et al, Staging of pancreatic and ampullary carcinoma by endoscopic ultrasonography. Comparison with conventional sonography, computed tomography, and angiography, *Gastroenterology* (1992) **102**:188–99

79. Grimm H, Maydeo A, Soehendra N, Endoluminal ultrasound for the diagnosis and staging of pancreatic cancer, *Baillière's Clin Gastroenterol* (1990) **4**:869–88.

80. Leen E, Goldberg JA, Robertson J et al, Early detection of occult colorectal hepatic metastases using duplex colour Doppler sonography, *Br J Surg* (1993) **80**:1249–51.

81. Bismuth H, Kuntslinger F, Castaing D, Ultrasound and liver transplantation. In: Bismuth H, Kuntslinger F, Castaing D, eds, *A Text and Atlas of Liver Ultrasound* (Chapman and Hall: London, 1991) 126–35.

82. Lane RJ, Ackroyd N, Appleberg M, Graham J, The application of operative ultrasound following carotid endarterectomy, *World J Surg* (1987) **11**:593–7.

83. Steger AC, Lees WR, Shorvon P et al, Multiple-fibre low-power interstitial laser hyperthermia: studies in the normal liver, *Br J Surg* (1992) **79**:139–45.

84. Ravikumar TS, Kane R, Cady B et al, Hepatic cryosurgery with intraoperative ultrasound monitoring for metastatic colon carcinoma, *Arch Surg* (1987) **122**:403–9.

Chapter 11 Intravascular Ultrasound

Wui K Chong

Advances in transducer technology have resulted in the development of miniature probes that can be mounted on the end of a catheter. As with endoscopic ultrasound, arteries and veins can be visualized from within. Close proximity to the region of interest enables high-frequency transducers to be used, hence allowing greater resolution.

The earliest intravascular ultrasound (IVUS) system was a single-crystal 20-MHz forward-mounted transducer on an 8-Fr catheter.[1] The single crystal, acting as transmitter and receiver, was a pulsed Doppler device which measured velocities up to 10 mm from the catheter tip. Marcus et al[2] developed a 3-Fr Doppler catheter which was wire-guided and had a flexible tip. The transducer was a single-element piezoelectric crystal which was side-mounted and angled backwards at 45°. In vitro studies with this catheter showed a strong correlation between Doppler measurements of velocity and measured flow rates.

Development of imaging catheters had to wait for the development of miniature transducers (under 1 mm). Transducers this size have to operate at a high frequency (above 10 MHz) in order to focus the ultrasound beam adequately.[3] IVUS probes can be mechanical or multiple-element (electronic). Multiple-element systems use multiple transducers controlled by an integrated circuit at the catheter tip fired in sequence or phased array; hence they require more crystal elements than mechanical transducers, and the technical problem of fitting sufficient miniature transducers on a catheter tip is much greater. Multiple transducers also require multiple wires travelling the length of the catheter, which results in the generation of a lot of noise. The first catheter ultrasound imaging system, designed for intracardiac imaging, was a phased array system.[4] Electronic systems have no moving parts, so problems due to rotating cables and motors are avoided. However, electronic systems are intrinsically more complex than mechanical ones and it is doubtful whether they can be as cost-effective.

In a mechanical system a single miniaturized transducer lies on the end of rotating or push–pull metal cable. A major technical problem has been the need to maintain consistent rotation of the transducer at the end of a flexed or convoluted catheter. Mechanical IVUS catheters tend to be much stiffer and less maneuverable than electronic ones. IVUS catheters in clinical use are designed to be disposable because resterilization is difficult.

The greatest experience has been with mechanically rotated transducers, and several brands are commercially available. The catheter system illustrated is manufactured by Diasonics and Meditech/Boston Scientific Corporation. The IVUS probe consists of a mechanically rotated single-element transducer situated on the end of a flexible braided metal cable (Fig. 11.1). The probe rotates at 15 rev/s, with a pulse repetition frequency of 30 kHz. This fits inside a 6.6-Fr, 95-cm-long polyethylene catheter with a sonolucent window at its tip. Deaerated water is injected into the end of the catheter to provide an acoustic coupling medium. The ultrasound beam is directed radially with a forward angulation of 10° to reduce echoes from the catheter wall. It generates a real-time 360° cross-sectional image of arterial wall and lumen. The probe scans at 12–30 MHz and has a depth of field of 0.7–4.5 mm. Earlier models were blunt-tipped, while current models have a floppy tip and take a 0.025-inch guide wire on a monorail system (Fig. 11.2; see also Fig. 11.17). The system is designed for once-only use. Insertion of the catheter is best done through a sheath, and the 6.6-Fr wire-guided version fits within an 8-Fr sheath. The wire is advanced under fluoroscopic guidance through an area of interest identified on angiography; the catheter is then advanced over the wire until the transducer has passed through the area. For optimal imaging the catheter should be coaxial and the transducer centrally placed within the lumen. Apart from a few cases of transient coronary artery spasm, there have been no reported complications from IVUS.

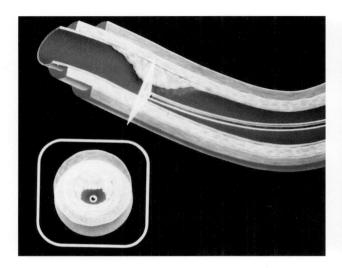

Figure 11.1 *The Boston Scientific IVUS catheter. The ultrasound beam emerges at an angle of 10° to the perpendicular, generating a cross-sectional image of vessel lumen and wall. (Courtesy Boston Scientific Corporation, Watertown, MA.)*

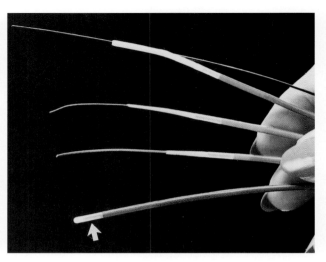

Figure 11.2 *Wire-guided (top 3) and blunt-tipped (bottom) IVUS catheters. The transducer lies behind a sonolucent window (arrow). Distilled water is injected through the tip of the catheter for acoustic coupling.*

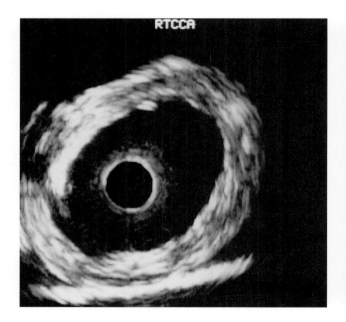

Figure 11.3 *Normal carotid artery. The wall is uniformly echogenic.*

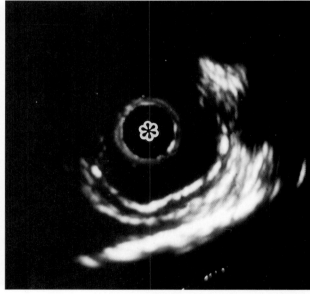

Figure 11.4 *In vitro image of superficial femoral artery showing normal three-layered appearance. The artery has been bisected. ∗, transducer.*

Images are recorded on multi-format camera or videotape. The images can be digitized from the videotape using a commercially available frame grabber for three-dimensional reconstruction. Luminal size, wall thickness and cross-sectional area can be directly measured at any point within the vessel.

Catheters are also commercially available in 9-, 4.5- and 3.5-Fr; the latter can access arteries as small as 1 mm in diameter. Devices that operate at frequencies up to 40 MHz (for coronary use) are being investigated. One electronic system is commercially available (Endosonics, Rancho Cordova, CA). This has 64 transducer elements arranged radially around the catheter tip. The catheters are available in 7.8-, 5- and 3.5-Fr sizes. At this time the image quality of mechanical systems is superior to phased array systems. The combined IVUS–angioplasty catheter is a new development which allows real-time ultrasound visualization of the effect of balloon inflation[5] on plaque and arterial wall.

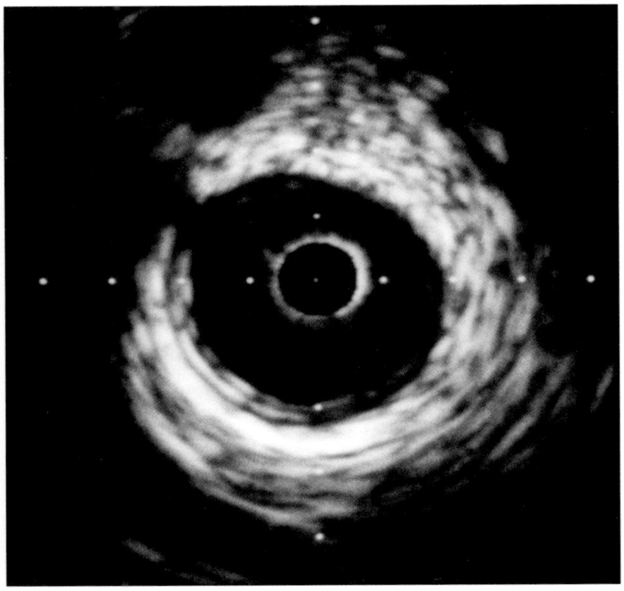

Figure 11.5 *Coronary artery showing layered appearance. 3.5-Fr/30-MHz catheter. (Courtesy of Boston Scientific Corporation, Watertown, MA.)*

NORMAL APPEARANCE OF ARTERIES

In vitro work with cadaver arteries has shown that the arterial wall has different ultrasonic characteristics depending on its composition.[6] The walls of arteries in which the media has a high elastin content (e.g. the carotid) will appear either uniformly echogenic or the media will appear more echogenic than the adventitia (Fig. 11.3). Muscular arteries such as the superficial femoral artery have a layered appearance: an inner hyperechoic layer, a middle hypoechoic layer and an outer hyperechoic layer (Fig. 11.4). These do not correspond directly to the three histological layers. Sonographic–pathological correlation suggests that the inner hyperechoic layer is caused by echoes arising from the interface between blood and intima, the intima itself and the intima–media interface. The middle layer arises from the central part of the media and appears hypoechoic due to its smooth muscle content. The outer layer is generated by the media–adventitia interface and the adventitia itself.

The normal coronary artery in young people is homogeneous without layering.[7] A layered appearance is seen in middle age and is associated with intimal thickening (Fig. 11.5).

PLAQUE CHARACTERIZATION

The earliest plaque deposits appear as thickening and increased echogenicity of the intima on ultrasound (Fig. 11.6). Histologically, these lesions consist of lipid-containing fibrocytes and smooth muscle. Larger deposits of plaque appear as heterogeneous areas within the intima. The echogenicity of these areas can range from very bright to almost anechoic, depending on their composition. Extracellular lipid appears hypoechoic on IVUS. As plaque grows the cellular matrix breaks down, leaving lipid and cholesterol deposits mingled with cellular debris. This appears heterogeneous on US; the lipid appears predominantly hypoechoic, while the cellular material appears as hyperechoic specks (Fig. 11.7).

Plaque composed primarily of fibrous tissue is moderately echogenic without acoustic shadowing (Fig. 11.8). Calcified plaque is strongly echogenic with acoustic shadowing (Figs. 11.9 and 11.10). Thrombus appears moderately echogenic and can usually be distinguished from plaque (Fig. 11.11).

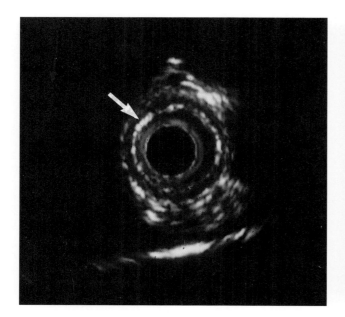

Figure 11.6 *Early plaque (arrow) shown as thickening of the innermost layer.*

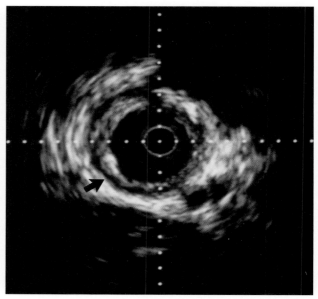

Figure 11.7 *Left superficial femoral artery. Circumferential plaque of mixed composition. The hypoechoic layer (arrow) representing the media marks the outer limit of the plaque. (Courtesy Boston Scientific Corporation, Watertown, MA.)*

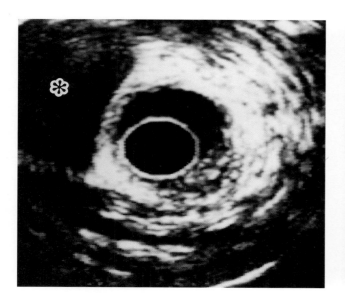

Figure 11.8 *Superficial femoral artery with fibrous plaque from 4 o'clock to 6 o'clock. ✽ , superficial femoral vein.*

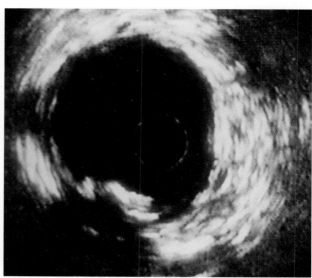

Figure 11.9 *Calcified plaque at 7 o'clock showing acoustic shadowing.*

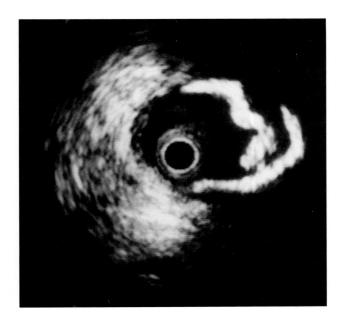

Figure 11.10 *Heavily calcified irregular plaque in the aorta from 12 o'clock to 6 o'clock which conceals the arterial wall behind it.*

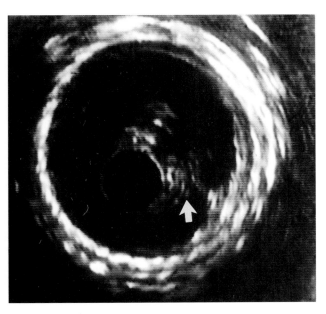

Figure 11.11 *Ribbed appearance of aortic dacron graft. Intraluminal thrombus (arrow) is present. (Courtesy of Dr Clare Allen.)*

IVUS is more sensitive than radiography to the presence of plaque: development of atheroma in coronary artery bypass grafts has been detected earlier with IVUS than with angiography.[8]

ASSESSMENT OF LUMINAL AREA

With the development of a variety of devices for restoring the lumen of occluded or stenosed arteries, the importance of knowing the normal dimensions of the arterial lumen is greater than ever. Knowledge of the volume and characteristics of the obstructing plaque is also useful. Angiography has until now been the gold standard for the assessment of arterial disease. However, the angiogram is a two-dimensional depiction of the vessel lumen, and the inaccuracy of angiographic assessment of luminal size is well recognized. Calculation of cross-sectional area from geometric measurements of the stricture assume that the luminal cross-section is circular or elliptical. Even with biplanar angiography, if the lumen is eccentric or has protruberant filling defects assessment of luminal cross-sectional area by angiography is inaccurate. Radiographic magnification and vessel tortuosity are other potential sources of error. Pathological–angiographic correlation has shown that inaccuracy of angiography in grading stenosis is greatest in mild or moderate disease. Even identifying which parts of the artery are free of disease may be difficult on angiography: segments of artery that appear normal on the angiogram may have diffuse atheroma. Conversely, an atheroma-free island lying within a diffusely atheromatous vessel may be mistaken for an aneurysm.

For the angiographer, identification of normal vessel is important for two reasons: it is necessary for calculation of the percentage stenosis, and knowledge of the normal vessel diameter determines the size of the angioplasty balloon. A diffusely diseased

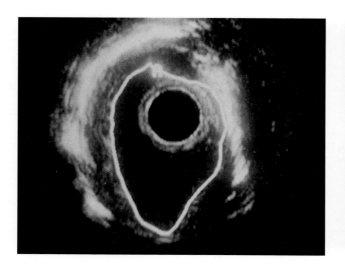

Figure 11.12 *The luminal cross-sectional area can be measured by tracing its outline.*

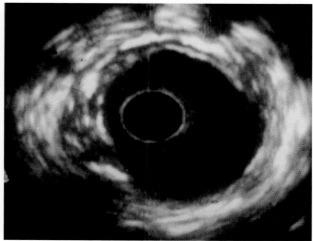

Figure 11.13 *Crescentic plaque from 7 o'clock to 12 o'clock. An area of calcification is seen at 7 o'clock. Between 11 o'clock and 2 o'clock the three-layered structure is preserved. Deep to the plaque the hypoechoic layer representing the media thins out and the thickness of the plaque cannot be determined with certainty.*

arterial wall can be mistaken for normal on the angiogram and can lead to an inadequate dilatation of a stenosis. In the coronary circulation IVUS has demonstrated significant amounts of atheroma in vessels that are angiographically normal, notably the left main coronary artery.[9] Vessels appear to respond to the development of plaque by expanding outward, preserving the arterial lumen. After angioplasty, in vessels in which there has been apparently successful restoration of the lumen on angiography, IVUS has shown a considerable amount of residual plaque.[10]

IVUS can potentially detect disease earlier than angiography. Luminal diameter and volume load can be quantified more precisely because the luminal diameter on IVUS is measured electronically. The cross-sectional area is obtained by tracing the outline of the lumen on the sonographic image (Fig. 11.12). This is intrinsically more accurate than deriving the area from angiographic measurements of diameter. IVUS measurements of cross-sectional area correlate well with histology and are unaffected by luminal eccentricity. In addition, unlike angiography, IVUS can identify the normal vessel wall. A baseline for angioplasty can therefore be obtained and the degree of stenosis measured more accurately. Thus IVUS is

likely to become the future gold standard for assessment of luminal stenosis.

Angiography provides indirect and limited information about the nature of the obstructing lesion. Calcification has to be very marked before it is visible radiographically. Plaque which is not calcified appears similar irrespective of its composition while the presence of thrombus or intimal hyperplasia can only be inferred.

IVUS can detect thrombus and, to a degree, characterize plaque as soft (lipid), hard (fibrous) or calcified. IVUS is much more sensitive to the presence of calcification than angiography.[11] Its ability to demonstrate changes in plaque following angioplasty suggests it may have a useful role in detecting post-angioplasty complications, possibly predicting the likelihood of restenosis or occlusion.

The 'normal' arterial wall can sometimes be assessed on IVUS even in the presence of overlying plaque. Where the hypoechoic middle layer is visible, it serves as a marker of the location of the media, and the amount of plaque within the lumen can be estimated. Unfortunately the middle layer is often not visible in severely atheromatous arteries. As plaque develops and thickens, thinning and atrophy of the middle layer occurs. With its disappearance, it is

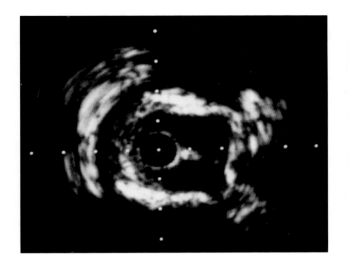

Figure 11.14 *Coronary artery after angioplasty. The lumen is rectangular due to remodelling. Extensive shadowing 11 o'clock to 2 o'clock and 5 o'clock to 8 o'clock due to calcific plaque. 3.5-Fr/30-MHz catheter. (Courtesy Boston Scientific Corporation, Watertown, MA.)*

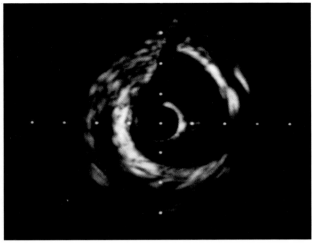

Figure 11.15 *Post-angioplasty of coronary artery showing distortion of lumen. Small side branch seen at 12 o'clock. 3.5-Fr/30-MHz catheter. (Courtesy Boston Scientific Corporation, Watertown, MA.)*

often difficult to see where plaque ends and wall begins (Fig. 11.13). The other factor which limits the use of IVUS is the presence of heavily calcified plaques. By attenuating the ultrasound beam behind the plaque, they prevent the assessment of plaque thickness (Fig. 11.9). The ability of IVUS to detect plaque load is therefore limited. Where plaque thickness or volume can be assessed, this information is clinically useful if atherectomy is contemplated; the risks of cutting into normal vessel wall and causing perforation would be reduced.

ASSESSMENT OF THE POST-ANGIOPLASTY ARTERY

IVUS is providing new insights into the mechanism of angioplasty. Analysis of iliac arteries with IVUS before and after angioplasty has shown that most of the increase in luminal cross-sectional area is due to cracking or compression of plaque. Remodelling of plaque and circumferential redistribution was seen (Figs. 11.14 and 11.15). Stretching of arterial wall was only a minor contributing factor to the increase in luminal size.[12] IVUS has revealed that there can be considerable residual obstruction after stenting even though the angiogram shows a significant improvement in lumen size.[13]

After recanalization of total occlusions, subintimal passage resulting in dissection is a common complication. The occurrence of arterial dissection appears to be related to plaque composition and occurs more frequently in plaques containing calcium.[14]

BALLOON ANGIOPLASTY

Histological examination of arteries after balloon angioplasty reveals cracking and fracture of plaque (Figs. 11.16 and 11.17), with calcified plaques more likely to fracture than non-calcified ones. This is not visible on angiography. IVUS demonstrated cracks in 78 per cent of plaques which had undergone balloon angioplasty.[15]

Dissections occur adjacent to areas of calcification and are larger in calcified than non-calcified vessels following balloon angioplasty (Fig. 11.18). The presence of calcification probably promotes dissection by increasing shear stresses within plaque.[16] IVUS is more sensitive than angiography

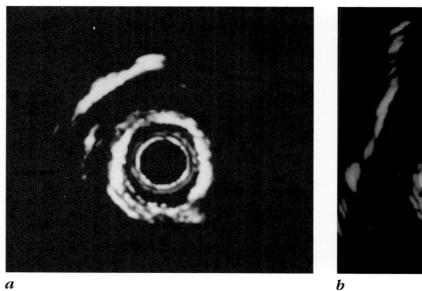
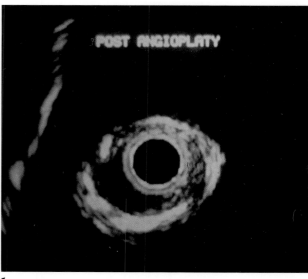

a *b*

Figure 11.16 *(a) Heavily calcified superficial femoral artery plaque with no through transmission. (b) Plaque fragmentation after balloon angioplasty is seen.*

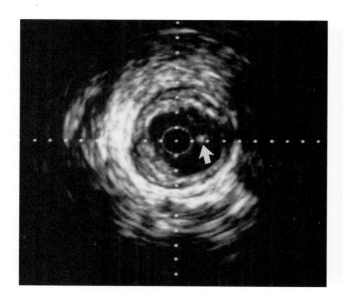
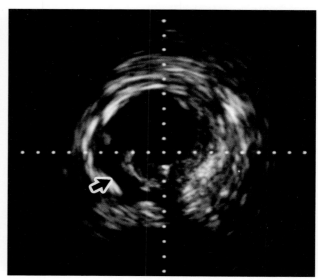

Figure 11.17 *Left superficial femoral artery post-angioplasty. Circumferential soft and fibrous plaque with crack from 12 o'clock to 2 o'clock. 4.8-Fr/20-MHz catheter on a monorail guide wire (arrow). (Courtesy Boston Scientific Corporation, Watertown, MA.)*

Figure 11.18 *Post-angioplasty dissection (arrow) in right iliac artery. (Courtesy Boston Scientific Corporation, Watertown, MA.)*

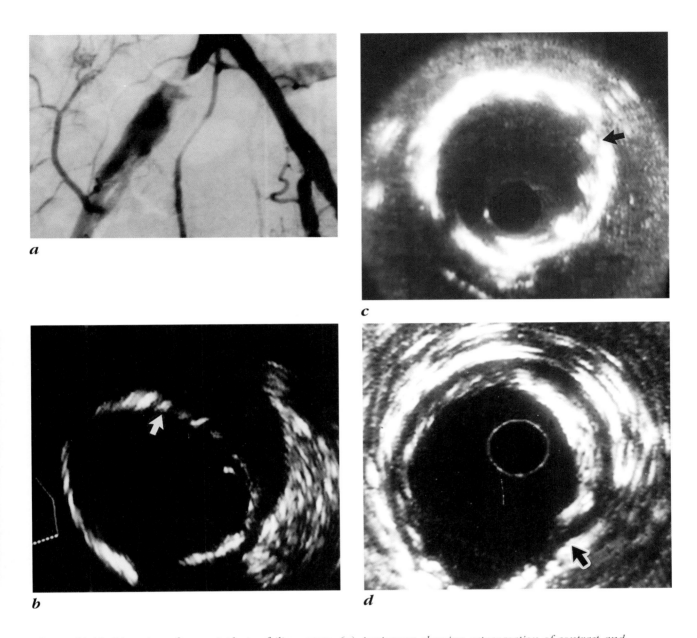

Figure 11.19 *Dissection after angioplasty of iliac artery. (a) Angiogram showing extravasation of contrast and narrowing of the right iliac artery. The intimal flap is not visible. (b) The dissection flap (arrow) separates the true and false lumens. (c) After the dissection is treated with a metal stent, the position of the struts (arrow) can be seen. (d) After stenting, the false lumen is markedly reduced in size. IVUS shows the communication between the true and false lumens (arrow). (Courtesy of Dr Clare Allen.)*

for detecting post-angioplasty dissection, which can be treated with endoluminal stent insertion (Fig. 11.19). The IVUS appearances of arteries which have undergone laser-assisted balloon angioplasty do not appear different to arteries which have undergone balloon angioplasty.

ATHERECTOMY

Arteries that have been subjected to rotational atherectomy have a smooth, circular appearance on IVUS, with less plaque disruption, even in heavily calcified vessels.[17] Lumen area was increased and plaque area

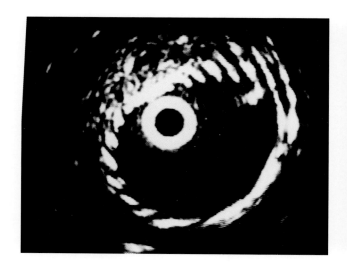

Figure 11.20 *Metal Wallstent (Schneider, Minneapolis, MN) in a transjugular intrahepatic portosystemic shunt.*

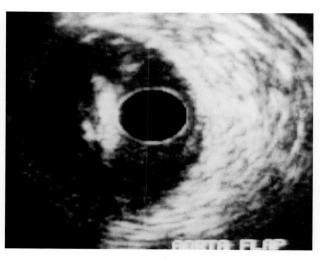

Figure 11.21 *Aortic dissection, showing flap adjacent to the catheter.*

decreased. Plaque reduction was greater with hypo-echoic than echogenic plaque. Restenosis after atherectomy was associated with a three-layered appearance. The incidence of restenosis was higher with hypo-echoic than with echogenic plaque.[18] As with balloon angioplasty, IVUS has shown that angiography underestimates the amount of residual plaque.[19]

STENTING

Metal stents are well visualized with IVUS, appearing as intensely echogenic lines or dots with acoustic shadowing (Figs. 11.19 and 11.20). IVUS can show the degree of apposition of the stent to the arterial wall, and indicate underexpansion or overexpansion. A smooth vessel wall is also seen after stenting. The presence of dissection, thrombus, intimal hyperplasia or recoil after stent insertion can be demonstrated.[20] Comparing IVUS before and after stent insertion shows that the stent tends to compress rather than crack the atheroma. Dissection caused by balloon angioplasty can be treated by stenting, and stent positioning is aided by IVUS.

IVUS is therefore likely to play an increasingly important role in monitoring and detecting complications of the various devices now available for vessel recanalization.[21] In the future the ability of IVUS to detect calcification in a lesion may favor selection of stenting or atherectomy instead of balloon angioplasty.

Spontaneous aortic dissections are well visualized on IVUS (Fig. 11.21). Although the diagnosis can be made with computed tomography (CT), IVUS is particularly useful in identifying the point of entry and re-entry (Fig. 11.19d). In the pulmonary arteries diminished pulsatility is visible on IVUS in patients with pulmonary hypertension and cardiomyopathy.[22,23]

DOPPLER VELOCITY CATHETERS AND VASOMOTOR RESPONSE

Blood velocity can be measured with ultrasound catheters using the Doppler principle. A single piezo-electric crystal operating at 12–20 MHz is mounted on the end or side of a 3-Fr catheter. Both end- and side-mounted catheters can make accurate and reproducible velocity measurements and have been used mainly in the coronary arteries for calculation of coronary flow reserve.

Vasodilatation mediated through vascular endothelium occurs in response to sympathetic stimulation. There is progressive reduction in the endothelial vasoactive response in the early stages of atherosclerosis which is ultimately lost as disease progresses. Administration of a vasodilator like papaverine, nitroglycerin or adenosine causes an increase in coronary blood flow in normals. The coronary flow reserve can be calculated by the ratio of the peak flow velocity to the baseline flow velocity. A reserve of less than 3.5 is considered abnormal. Coronary flow reserve has been used to assess the hemodynamic significance of stenoses and is also reduced in vasculitis, hypertension and patients with cardiac ischemia with normal coronary arteries (syndrome X).

The ability of IVUS to provide real-time cross-sectional images of vessel lumen has given investigators a new tool to study the vasomotor response of the coronary arteries in vivo. The physiological change in serial cross-sectional area of the coronary artery in response to vasoconstrictors or vasodilators like nitroglycerine can be directly measured.[24] Normal coronary arteries dilate in response to sympathetic stimulation, but vasoconstriction is seen in patients with atherosclerosis. Pinto et al[25] used IVUS in the coronary arteries of cardiac transplants to show that in rejection there was significantly less increase in luminal area, indicating a reduced vasodilator response. The ratio between end-diastolic and end-systolic lumen area is a measure of vessel distensibility. Hodgson[26] found that the distensibility index was approximately 13 per cent in normal vessels but only 5 per cent in atheromatous vessels. The distensibility index was inversely related to wall thickness.

Doppler catheters can only provide velocity information from the proximal coronary arteries. Recently, ultrasound guide wires which can be passed through stenoses and can take balloon catheters and other interventional devices have become available. The doppler Flowire (Cardiometrics; Mountain View, CA) is a 175-cm-long 0.018-inch guide wire with a 12-MHz transducer at its tip, allowing for the first time velocity measurements beyond a stenosis and from the distal coronary arteries, and permitting monitoring of flow during intervention. Studies with the Flowire have shown a diastolic/systolic flow ratio of >1.5 between the proximal and distal coronary arteries in normal vessels. In atherosclerotic arteries, there is a reduction in diastolic flow velocity, with relatively preserved systolic velocity proximally. Distal to the obstruction, significantly lower diastolic and systolic velocities are observed.[27] A high proximal/distal velocity ratio is seen across a severe stenosis which is reduced after angioplasty. This may be a useful measure of stenosis severity as well as adequacy of angioplasty. Anderson et al[28] used the Doppler guide wire to monitor coronary flow velocity during and after angioplasty. Following each inflation of the balloon, an increase in velocity was seen. Elastic recoil following angioplasty caused a gradual reduction in velocity over 30 min. Spasm of the coronary artery and resolution after treatment with nitroglycerin

was found. Cyclic flow variations were associated with angiographic evidence of thrombus. They are caused by platelet accumulation on the damaged endothelium at the site of angioplasty. As the platelet aggregation enlarges, velocity declines. A pressure gradient builds up across the platelet mass, which eventually dislodges and breaks off, with an abrupt increase in velocity. In several cases, administration of monoclonal antiplatelet antibody resulted in resolution of the thrombus on angiography and attenuation of the cyclic flow pattern. The Doppler wire can accommodate most IVUS catheters. Isner et al[29] found that the Flowire could be made to serve as a guide wire for an IVUS catheter and used the combination to assess stenoses and monitor angioplasty. The Doppler wire and IVUS were complementary, one providing physiological and the other anatomical data. In ambiguous cases, information from one could corroborate data from the other.[29]

VEINS

On intravascular ultrasound, the normal venous wall appears as a thin homogeneously echogenic structure (Fig. 11.22). IVUS can identify valves and

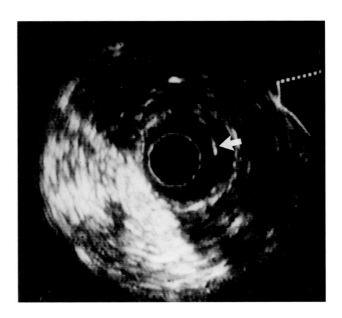

Figure 11.22 *Femoral vein. Valve cusps (arrow) are shown. (Courtesy of Dr Clare Allen.)*

thrombus within veins. The most likely use for IVUS is for assessing the IVC and iliac veins. These vessels are difficult to evaluate with percutaneous ultrasound while contrast dilution and flow artifacts often cause poor visualization on pedal venography. McCowan et al[30] found IVUS to be superior to cavography and percutaneous ultrasound in detecting thrombus in the inferior vena cava after filter insertion. IVUS was better than cavography in defining the cross-sectional area of the lumen, while cavography was superior in determining the craniocaudad extent of thrombus.

IVUS imaging of stenosed saphenous vein coronary bypass grafts has shown that the atheroma is usually poorly echogenic and calcification is unusual.[31] IVUS is more sensitive than angiography in detecting atheroma.[32] After intervention, angiography shows the improvement in luminal diameter, but, as with arteries, the difference between balloon angioplasty, which results in fissuring and cracking of plaque, and the smooth effaced appearance of the arterial wall after stenting and atherectomy can be clearly seen on IVUS. Intimal hyperplasia and fibrosis in the wall of the vein can be differentiated from atheroma.

THREE-DIMENSIONAL RECONSTRUCTION

Three-dimensional reconstruction of IVUS images can be performed by using the same algorithms as are used for CT and magnetic resonance (MR) reconstruction. Multiple cross-sectional images are acquired by advancing or withdrawing the catheter through a segment of vessel. The data are digitized, and then processed and manipulated using a workstation. The system we devised for this purpose is based on multiple transputers, rated at 100 MIPS (millions of instructions per second) and programmed in a parallel processing language (OCCAM) modified to handle ultrasound data.[33] This was coupled to the IVUS system through a motion sensor to detect the linear position of the probe within the vessel. One hundred to two hundred axial images 1 mm apart were acquired in a typical run, acquisition taking about 10 s. The axial images were preprocessed for edge detection, smoothing and region-of-interest selection. The data sets recorded could be reformatted along any selected section through the vessel, providing orthogonal sagittal reconstructions (Fig. 11.23). The data can also be examined

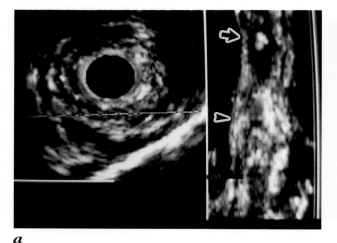
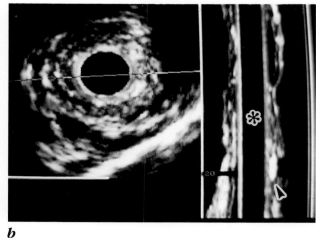

a   *b*

Figure 11.23 *Sagittal reconstruction of the superficial femoral artery. (a) The standard axial view is shown on the left, with the cut line passing through the vessel wall. On the right, sagittal reconstruction through this line shows a calcified plaque at the top (arrow) with fibrous plaque below (arrowhead). (b) Reconstructing through a cut line bisecting the vessel shows the transducer in the center (*). Calcified plaque with acoustic shadowing (arrowhead) is seen on one wall, with normal three-layered appearance on the opposite side.*

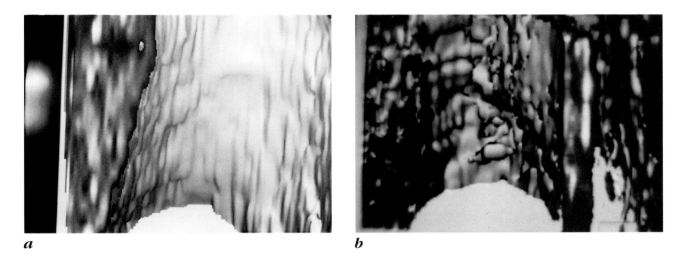

Figure 11.24 *Surface-contoured depth-shaded reconstruction accentuating the difference between (a) light and (b) heavy plaque.*

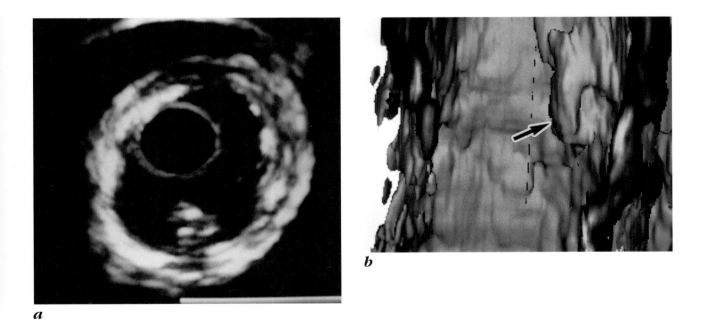

Figure 11.25 *(a) Heterogeneous plaque with flecks of calcification protrudes into the lumen. (b) Depth-shaded reconstruction showing the contour of the plaque (arrow).*

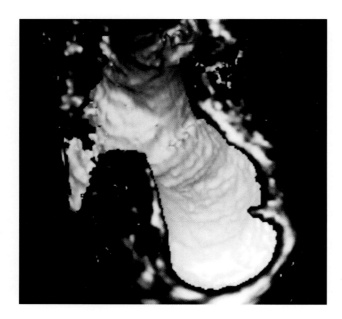

Figure 11.26 *Surface-contoured depth-shaded reconstruction of aortic bifurcation. Speckle reduction processing has been applied to create a smoother image.*

for surface characteristics. Depth-shaded surface views were created by selecting an echo-level threshold and generating corresponding surfaces viewed from within the vessel (Figs. 11.24 and 11.25). The sagittal and three-dimensional depth-shaded contour reconstructions provide views of the distribution of plaque along the long axis which are easier to correlate with angiograms. An in vitro study IVUS–pathological correlation[34] has shown that three-dimensional reconstruction facilitates the evaluation of the length and depth of post-angioplasty dissection. Volume estimation of plaque and lumen is possible from the data. The depth-shaded images provide better perception of shape and surface features and these can be improved further by speckle reduction processing (Fig. 11.26).

LIMITATIONS OF INTRAVASCULAR ULTRASOUND

IVUS is an invasive procedure and involves the same risks as intravascular catheterization. Mechanical

systems tend to rotate unevenly or stop rotating if the catheters take a tortuous or angulated course. Uneven rotation leads to a distorted image. The wire-guided mechanical catheter operates on a monorail system which works less well than a catheter with a central lumen.

Currently, IVUS catheters are expensive and are designed to be disposed of after single use. Expense is a major reason why their use has been limited. Whether IVUS is going to be cost-effective in a clinical setting has yet to be determined.

If the angle of incidence of the ultrasound beam is not perpendicular to the arterial wall, the quality of the image is degraded and artifacts simulating dissections appear.[35] For optimum imaging the IVUS catheter should lie coaxially within the vessel. Maintaining the catheter in such a position in vivo in a tortuous or large vessel such as the aorta can be difficult. An additional problem with large vessels is the limited range of the probe: with 20-MHz probes the effective range is 2 cm. The inability with current IVUS devices to image forward of the catheter is a disadvantage because a stenosis that cannot be traversed by the catheter cannot be imaged.

FUTURE DEVELOPMENTS AND APPLICATIONS FOR IVUS

Combination catheters with ultrasound/atherectomy, ultrasound/laser catheters and imaging/Doppler capabilities are currently under development. Also being developed are angioscopes with ultrasound capabilities. IVUS guidance will lead to more appropriate use of atherectomy and stent placement. If further miniaturization of transducers can be achieved, ultrasound guide wires with imaging capabilities that can be passed through conventional catheters will become feasible. Forward-viewing transducers would permit visualization of occluded vessels. Multifrequency ultrasound catheters will be able to image large and small vessels. Advances in image processing will lead to on-line, real-time, three-dimensional imaging and atheroma quantification.[36] IVUS measurement of vessel distensibility and lumen size in response to vasomotor drugs may provide important insights into flow reserve and the hemodynamic effects of atheroma. Early work using the Doppler guide wire suggests that it is useful for determining the severity of a stenosis and for monitoring improvement in flow after angioplasty.

There is angiographic evidence that coronary artery lumen can increase after therapy with antilipid agents. Because it is better able to quantify plaque volume and luminal cross-sectional area, IVUS may be useful for monitoring effectiveness of therapy.

Intravascular ultrasound is safe and technically straightforward. It allows the angiographer to quantify lumen size and plaque volume much more accurately and to determine the character of plaque. It can demonstrate complications resulting from angioplasty, such as thrombus and dissection. The Doppler guide wire is an important advance that provides hemodynamic information beyond a stenosis. IVUS will probably play an increasing role in vascular imaging.

FURTHER READING

Pandian, NG, Intravascular and intracardiac ultrasound imaging, An old concept, now on the road to reality, *Circulation* (1989) 80:1091–4.

Tobis JB, Yock PG (eds) *Intravascular Ultrasound Imaging* (Churchill Livingstone: New York, 1992).

Bom N, Roelandt JR, *Intravascular Ultrasound: Techniques, Developments, Clinical Perspectives* (Kluwer: Norwell, 1989).

REFERENCES

1. Hartley CJ, Cole JS, A single-crystal ultrasonic catheter-tip velocity probe, *Med Instrum* (1973) **8**:241–3.

2. Marcus M, Wright C, Doty D et al, Measurements of coronary velocity and reactive hyperemia in the coronary circulation of humans, *Circ Res* (1981) **49**:877–91.

3. Meyer CR, Fitting DW, Chiang EH et al, High resolution intravascular imaging via ultrasonic catheters: proof of concept, *Proc IEEE* (1988) **76**:1074–8.

4. Bom N, Lancee CT, van Egmon FC, An ultrasonic intracardiac scanner, *Ultrasonics* (1972) **10**:72.

5. Violaris AG, Linnemeier TJ, Campbell S et al, Intravascular ultrasound imaging combined with coronary angioplasty, *Lancet* (1992) **339**:1571–2.

6. Gussenhoven EJ, Essed CE, Lancee CT, Arterial wall characteristics determined by intravascular ultrasound imaging: an in-vitro study, *J Am Coll Cardiol* (1989) **14**:947–52

7. Fitzgerald PJ, St Goar FG, Connolly AJ et al, Intravascular ultrasound imaging of coronary arteries. Is three layers the norm? *Circulation* (1992) **86**:154–8

8. Schroeder JS, Gao SZ, Hunt SA et al, Accelerated graft coronary artery disease: diagnosis and prevention, *J Heart Lung Transplant* (1992) **11**:S258–65.

9. Hermiller JB, Buller CE, Tenaglia AN et al, Unrecognised left main coronary artery disease in patients undergoing interventional procedures, *Am J Cardiol* (1993) **71**:173–6

10. Ehrlich S, Honye J, Mahon D et al, Unrecognised stenosis by angiography documented by intravascular ultrasound, *Cathet Cardiovasc Diagnosis* (1991) **3**:198–201.

11. Potkin BN, Keren G, Mintz GS et al, Arterial responses to balloon coronary angioplasty: an intravascular ultrasound study, *J Am Coll Cardiol* (1992) **20**:942–51.

12. Losardo DW, Rosenfield K, Pieczek A et al, How does angioplasty work? Serial analysis of human iliac arteries using intravascular ultrasound, *Circulation* (1992) **86**:1845–58.

13. Laskey WK, Brady ST, Kussmaul WG et al, Intravascular ultrasonographic assessment of the results of coronary artery stenting, *Am Heart J* (1993) **125**:1576–83.

14. Potkin BN Keren G, Mintz GA et al, Arterial responses to balloon coronary angioplasty: an intravascular ultrasound study, *J Am Coll Cardiol* (1992) **10**:942–51.

15. Isner JM, Rosenfield K, Losordo DW et al, Percutaneous intravascular ultrasound as adjunct to catheter-based interventions: preliminary experience in patients with peripheral vascular disease, *Radiology* (1990) **175**:61–70.

16. Fitzgerald PJ, Ports TA, Yock PG, Contribution of localised calcium deposits to dissection after angioplasty, *Circulation* (1992) **86**:64–70.

17. Mintz GS, Potkin BN, Keren G et al, Intravascular ultrasound evaluation of the effect of rotational atherectomy in obstructive atherosclerotic coronary disease, *Circulation* (1992) **86**:1383–93.

18. Suarez de Lezo J, Romero M, Medina A et al, Intracoronary ultrasound assessment of directional coronary atherectomy: immediate and follow-up findings, *J Am Coll Cardiol* (1993) **21**:298–307.

19. White NW, Webb JG, Rowe MH et al, Atherectomy guidance using intravascular ultrasound: quantitation of plaque burden, *Circulation* (1989) **80**:II–374 (abst).

20. Katzen BT, Current status of intravascular sonography, *Radiol Clin North Am* (1992) **30**:895–905.

21. Yock PG, Fitzgerald PJ, Linker DT, Angelsen BAJ, Intravascular ultrasound guidance for catheter based coronary interventions, *J Am Coll Cardiol* (1991) **17**:39B–45B.

22. Porter T, Taylor D, Pandian N et al, Characterization of pulmonary arterial stiffness by simultaneous intravascular ultrasound and hemodynamic studies in patients with congestive heart failure, *Circulation* (1991) **84**:II–1 (abst).

23. Porter T, Taylor D, Mohanty PK et al, Direct in vivo evaluation of pulmonary artery pathology by catheter-based intravascular ultrasound imaging, *Circulation* (1991) **84**:II–702.

24. Dupuoy, P, Geschwind HJ, Pelle G, et al, Assessment of coronary vasomotion by intracoronary ultrasound, *Am Heart J* (1993) **126**:76–85

25. Pinto FJ, St Goar FG, Fischell TA et al, Nitroglycerin-induced coronary vasodilation in cardiac transplant recipients. Evaluation with in vivo intracoronary ultrasound, *Circulation* (1992) **85**:69–77.

26. Hodgson JM, Coronary imaging and angioplasty with an electronic array catheter system. In: Tobis JB, Yock PG, eds, *Intravascular Ultrasound Imaging* (Churchill Livingstone: New York, 1992) 161–70.

27. Ofili EO, Labovitz AJ, Kern MJ, Coronary flow velocity dynamics in normal and diseased arteries, *Am J Cardiol* (1993) **71**:3D–9D.

28. Anderson HV, Kirkeeide RL, Stuart Y et al, Coronary artery flow monitoring following coronary interventions, *Am J Cardiol* (1993) **71**:62D–69D.

29. Isner JF, Kaufman J, Rosenfield K et al, Combined physiologic and anatomic assessment of percutaneous revascularisation using a doppler guide wire and ultrasound catheter, *Am J Cardiol* (1993) **71**:70D–86D.

30. McCowan TC, Ferris EJ, Carver DK, Inferior vena caval filter thrombi: evaluation with intravascular US, *Radiology* (1990) **177**: 783–8.

31. Keren G, Douek P, Oblon C et al, Atherosclerotic saphenous vein grafts treated with different interventional procedures assessed by intravascular ultrasound, *Am Heart J* (1992) **124**:198–206.

32. Nase-Hueppmeier S, Uebis R, Doerr R, Hanrath P, Intravascular ultrasound to assess aorto-coronary venous bypass grafts in vivo, *Am J Cardiol* (1992) **70**:455–8.

33. Chong WK, Lawrence R, Gardener J, Lees WR, The appearance of normal and abnormal arterial morphology on Intravascular ultrasound, *Clin Radiol* (1993) **48**:301–7.

34. Coy KM, Park JC, Fishbein MC et al, In vitro validation of three-dimensional intravascular ultrasound for the evaluation of arterial injury after balloon angioplasty, *J Am Coll Cardiol* (1992) **20**:692–700.

35. Di Mario C, Madretsma S, Linker D et al, The angle of incidence of the ultrasonic beam: a critical factor for the image quality in intravascular ultrasonography, *Am Heart J* (1993) **125**:442–8.

36. Pandian NG, Hsu TL, Intravascular ultrasound and intracardiac echocardiography: concepts for the future, *Am J Cardiol* (1992) **69**:6H–17H.

Chapter 12 Nonvascular Applications of Catheter-Based Ultrasound Transducers

Ji-Bin Liu
Barry B Goldberg

Since the 1980s, new electronic and acoustic technology has permitted the development of miniaturized intraluminal ultrasound systems to evaluate a variety of vascular and nonvascular lumina throughout the body. Successful acquisition of intraluminal ultrasound involves a combination of both ultrasound transducer and catheter technologies. During the last 5 years, miniature catheter-based ultrasound transducers have become commercially available and have been used in a variety of studies, in both animals and humans, to establish their efficacy within blood vessels and nonvascular lumina.[1-7] This chapter will discuss the nonvascular applications of these catheter-based miniature ultrasound transducers.

It should be pointed out that the utility of placing transducers within lumina has been established through the use of transvaginal and transrectal ultrasound probes and transducers incorporated into flexible gastroscopes. They can be inserted through the vagina to image the uterus and ovaries, through the rectum to display the prostate, and through the esophagus into the stomach, and even into the duodenum, to produce cross-sectional ultrasound images not only of the walls of the gastrointestinal tract but also of the areas beyond. Transvaginal and transrectal ultrasound techniques have become the routine clinical procedures for the evaluation of various pelvic abnormalities.[8,9] Endoscopic ultrasound has proved useful in the identification of submucosal masses and in the differentiation of the cause of extrinsic mass effect on the gastrointestinal tract.[10,11] In addition, when malignancy is present, this technique can help to determine tumor extension and the involvement of adjacent lymph nodes. Abnormalities in adjacent organs, such as the pancreas, liver and gall bladder, have also been evaluated using this method.[12] Thus, there already is a basis on which to predict the success of utilization of much smaller transducer-containing catheters in various regions of the body.

TECHNICAL CONSIDERATIONS

There are three types of miniature catheter-based ultrasound transducers which were originally designed for intravascular ultrasound applications. The first is a mechanical rotating transducer with a central drive shaft connected to a motor on the ultrasound unit that turns the transducer, located at the tip of the shaft, to produce a 360° real-time cross-sectional image. The second is a fixed transducer with a rotating mirror attached to a central wire that is turned by a motor, resulting in the movement of the mirror producing a real-time cross-sectional image. The third is an electronic phased array employing multiple crystals distributed around the transducer tip, resulting in a cross-sectional two-dimensional image.

While there are several endoluminal ultrasound instruments, as well as a variety of miniature ultrasound catheters available, for our research we have used the IVUS ultrasound system (Diasonics, Milpitas, CA) in association with the Sonicath catheter-based transducers (Medi-Tech/Boston Scientific, Watertown, MA). The single-element transducer is mounted on the end of a wire (core), which is connected to a motor on the ultrasound system. The core can be inserted into the flexible catheter, and the motor rotated to produce a 360° real-time cross-sectional image. Sterile water (0.5–1.0 ml) is introduced between the core and the catheter to eliminate air, which could interfere with transmission of the ultrasound beam. The transducer sends and

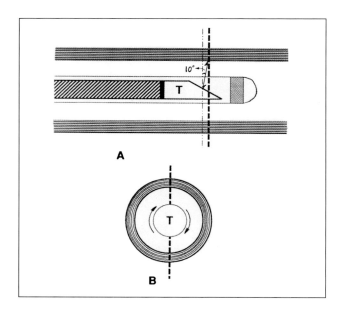

Figure 12.1 *Diagrammatic representation of an endoluminal transducer (T) sending and receiving the ultrasound signal at an angle 10° off from perpendicular to the long axis of the catheter: (A) longitudinal view; (B) cross-sectional view corresponding with the scanning plane.*

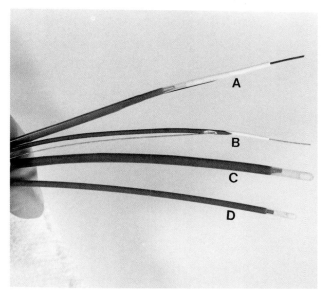

Figure 12.2 *Variety of transducer-containing catheters: (A) 6.2-Fr over a guide wire; (B) 4.8-Fr over a guide wire; (C) 9-Fr blunt tip; (D) 6-Fr blunt tip.*

receives the ultrasound signal at an angle 10° from perpendicular to the long axis of the catheter (Fig. 12.1). A variety of catheters are available, including 4.8-, 6.2- and 9-Fr (70–126 cm in length), containing either a 20- or 12.5-MHz transducer. They are either blunt tipped or over guide wires which are useful in advancing into smaller lumina (Fig. 12.2). The catheters and inner-core transducers can be sterilized using standard gas sterilization techniques. For the procedure in humans, the catheter was used only once but the transducer could be reused. The operating frequency of the 20-MHz transducer results in an axial resolution of 0.1 mm and a penetration of about 2.0 cm. Real-time images were recorded on videotape for later evaluation.

GENITOURINARY TRACT

Since the ultrasound transducer-containing catheters are no more than 2–3 mm in diameter they can be easily passed into the urethra without the need for dilatation. When they are positioned within the urethra it is possible to demonstrate areas of abnormality such as plaque or fibrosis. Endoluminal urethral ultrasound in conjunction with transrectal ultrasound has been utilized to guide Teflon injection into the external urinary sphincter in men with urinary incontinence after radical prostatectomy. This technique allows the urologist to inject Teflon precisely to the region of the sphincter and to measure the exact depth and volume of the injected material.

Transurethral ultrasound has also been used to assess the deployment of the intraprostatic and intrasphincter urethral stent placement. It can precisely identify the proximal and distal margins of the stent deployment and measure the stent diameter. Follow-up endoluminal ultrasound can be used to determine if there is any breakage in the stent wires, alteration in the stent diameter, abscess or calculi formation and/or neoepithelium growth through the stent openings (Fig. 12.3). Thus, these miniature catheter-based transducers have been able to provide important information to

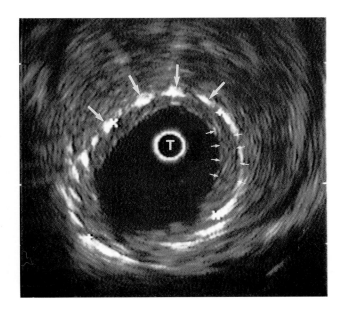

Figure 12.3 *Cross-sectional ultrasound image of a urethral stent (large arrows) covered by neoepithelium (small arrows) in a patient with a neurogenic bladder. The stent diameter can be precisely measured. T, ultrasound transducer.*

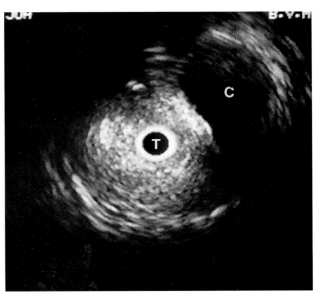

Figure 12.4 *The endoluminal transducer (T) located within the urethra delineates a cystic lesion (C) consistent with the diagnosis of a urethral diverticulum.*

the urologist for the long-term follow-up of intra-urethral stents. In addition, endourethral ultrasound is ideal for the delineation of urethral diverticula, which can be difficult to visualize using either cystoscopy or urethrography (Fig. 12.4).

Although rigid transurethral ultrasound transducers have been used to assess the urinary bladder, these small, flexible transducer-containing catheters can also be used to evaluate the urinary bladder.[13] It is possible to visualize all the layers of the bladder wall, including the hyperechoic mucosa, hypoechoic muscular media and hyperechoic adventitia. Small tumors can be clearly identified and their degree of invasion evaluated (Fig. 12.5).

Endoluminal ultrasound evaluation of the ureter is easily performed during uroendoscopic procedures. The flexible 6.2-Fr catheter is stabilized by its passage through the channel of an endoscope and a guide wire is used to stabilize the probe as it is directed into the ureter, thus minimizing the risk of perforation. It can also be placed through a nephroscope into the renal pelvis and ureter. These ultrasound catheters have been used to evaluate the ureters in over 100 patients undergoing endoscopic procedures with no complications. The use of this high-frequency catheter-based ultrasound transducer enabled the ureteral wall to be imaged. Extramural structures adjacent to the ureter, such as blood vessels, lymph nodes and muscles, could also be delineated. These transducer-containing catheters have proven useful for detecting stones embedded in the submucosa in both the ureter and renal pelvis (Fig. 12.6). Stones which can be seen on X-ray but not detected endoscopically can be located and their exact size and depth beneath the mucosal surface clearly documented and measured. The information provided by this approach has proven of value in assisting the urologist in making surgical decisions concerning stone removal.

Endoluminal ultrasound localization of blood vessels outside the ureter has also proven to be clinically useful. The size of the vessel and its exact location can be accurately delineated (Fig. 12.7). This information has proven helpful prior to endopyelotomy to define the location and size of the crossing vessel. Differentiation between pulsatile arteries and

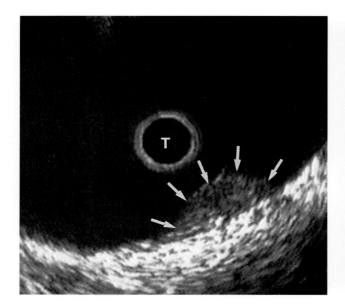

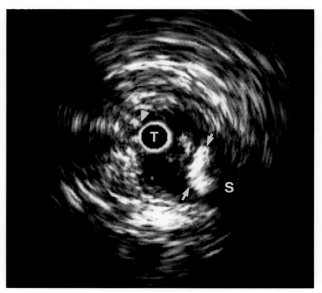

Figure 12.5 *Urinary bladder tumor (arrows) is seen arising from the posterior wall with no evidence of invasion. T, transducer. (Reproduced with permission from Goldberg BB, Liu JB, Scand J Urol Nephrol (1991) 137:147–54.)*

Figure 12.6 *Endoluminal ultrasound transducer (T) within the ureter demonstrates thickened mucosa in which is embedded a stone (arrows) which is producing distal acoustic shadowing (S). Note reflection from guide wire (arrowhead) located between the transducer and mucosal surface.*

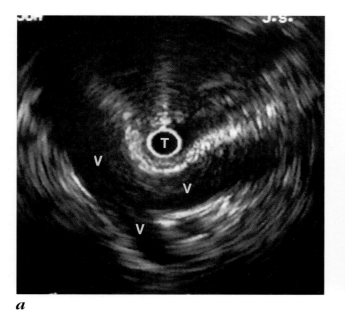

a

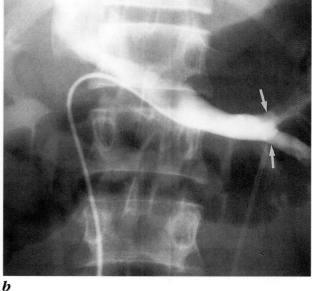

b

Figure 12.7 *(a) Endoluminal ultrasound transducer located at the site of ureteral narrowing demonstrates the presence of a crossing vessel (V), which was the cause of the resulting hydronephrosis. (b) There was excellent correlation with a subsequent angiogram (arrows). T, transducer.*

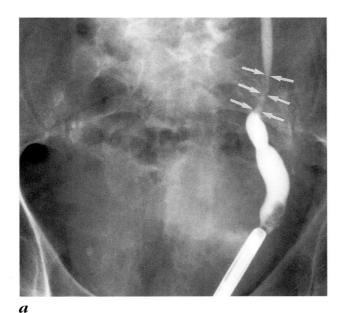

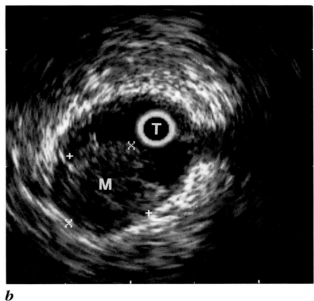

a   *b*

Figure 12.8 *(a) A retrograde contrast urogram shows an area of ureteral narrowing (arrows). (b) Endoluminal ultrasound transducer (T) located within the ureter at that level demonstrates the presence of a solid mass (M) consistent with the diagnosis of ureteral tumor, which was subsequently biopsied and proven to be transitional cell carcinoma.*

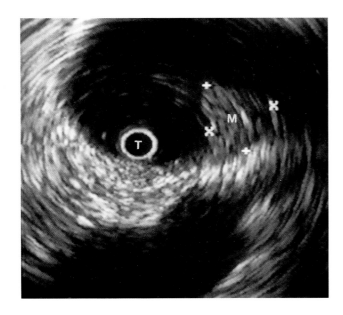

Figure 12.9 *Endoluminal ultrasound transducer (T) located within the renal pelvis demonstrates a solid mass (M) measuring 0.6 × 0.5 cm. This was proven to be a transitional cell carcinoma by biopsy.*

nonpulsatile veins can be easily identified. Endoluminal ultrasound has also been successful in demonstrating ureters invaginating into the renal pelvis. Thus, this technique has proven to be of considerable value in determining the cause of ureteropelvic junction obstruction, particularly when treatment by endopyelotomy is contemplated.[14]

High-resolution endoluminal ultrasound has been able to detect the presence and extent of ureteral and renal pelvis neoplasms, providing information not available with such other imaging techniques such as conventional ultrasound, computed tomography (CT), magnetic resonance imaging (MRI) and intravenous urography (Figs. 12.8 and 12.9). Even ureteroscopy cannot provide this information, since it can only visualize lesions that involve the luminal surface. This technique has also been able to differentiate between areas of focal thickening or extrinsic mass. However, complete staging of ureteral and renal pelvic malignancies has been limited by the lack of significant penetration due to the high frequency of the transducer.

Orientation during endoluminal sonography may be difficult. However, some landmarks can be identified, such as the level of the urinary bladder, the ureteral orifice, the iliac vessels, the psoas muscle and the renal pelvis. In order to know the exact anteroposterior and lateral position of these transducer-containing catheters within the urinary tract, it has been necessary to use several different techniques. Within the ureter and renal pelvis, the reflection from the adjacent guide wire visualized as a bright reflector with distal acoustic shadowing is used to determine the orientation. The guide wire is then imaged fluoroscopically and localized to the medial or lateral aspect of the ultrasound probe. With this information the relationship of the bright reflection (guide wire) on the ultrasound image to its true anatomical location can then be determined and the ultrasound image appropriately orientated. This is important when documenting the exact location of stones embedded within the mucosa of the ureter or renal parenchyma as well as the orientation of crossing vessels relative to the ureter or renal pelvis prior to any intraluminal surgical procedures.

High-resolution endoluminal sonography has proven useful in the evaluation of the urinary tract. In most cases, significant additional information was provided to the urologist, aiding in appropriate treatment decisions. When used as an adjunct to endoscopy this approach has been able to obtain more information than other conventional external imaging modalities. Thus, endoluminal ultrasound has the potential to become an important new tool for the evaluation of a variety of urologic abnormalities.

GASTROINTESTINAL TRACT

Placement of an endoluminal ultrasound transducer into the gastrointestinal tract was first reported in 1956 by Wild and Reid.[15] They used an ultrasound transducer in the rectum to evaluate the wall of the bowel in an attempt to identify malignant tumors. In the early 1980s the concept of combining a flexible endoscope with an ultrasound transducer to image the gastrointestinal tract was developed and results were published by Fukuda et al[16] and DiMagno et al[17] with the use of 7.5- to 12.5-MHz transducers. Using these transducers it was possible to image both the mural structures of the gastrointestinal tract and structures adjacent to the gastrointestinal tract wall.[10,11] This approach proved useful in the preoperative diagnosis and staging of esophageal and gastric cancers.[18,19]

These miniature catheter-based ultrasound transducers differ from the routinely used endoscopic ultrasound transducers in a number of aspects. First, the ultrasound catheter is much smaller than the dedicated endoscopic transducers. These 6.2-Fr catheters are so small that they fit easily through a nasogastric tube or the biopsy channel of conventional endoscopes and insert into the bile and pancreatic ducts through the surgically created openings. In addition, the small size of these catheters allows them to be inserted through strictured areas that dedicated endoscopic ultrasound probes cannot be placed through. The second major difference is that the frequency of 20 MHz is much higher than the frequency currently used clinically, which ranges from 7.5 to 12 MHz. This higher frequency increases the axial resolution of the image so that mural gastrointestinal structures can be seen with much greater resolution. However, the penetration of the ultrasound waves is limited by the higher frequency. The third major difference is that these transducers are not surrounded by a water-filled balloon as are the transducers embedded in the dedicated endosonoscopes. Because of the smaller size and the lack of compression there is much less distortion of small mural structures such as esophageal and gastric varices. The disadvantage is that there may be loss of acoustic coupling in organs filled with air, such as the stomach and the small intestine.

UPPER GASTROINTESTINAL TRACT

Although five layers had been previously described in the human gastrointestinal tract,[20] it is usually only possible to see three sonographic layers in the human esophagus using standard endoscopic ultrasound technology. This is probably because of compression by the water-filled balloon on the esophageal wall. The three layers which are normally seen in the esophagus are the first hyperechoic layer, which corresponds to the balloon and mucosa–submucosa interface together with the submucosa–muscularis propria interface, the second hypoechoic layer, which corresponds to the muscularis propria, and the third hyperechoic layer, which represents the interface between the muscularis propria and the surrounding tissue.[21]

In order to better understand and evaluate the human esophagus a number of human autopsies were done in which the esophagus was evaluated using 20-MHz ultrasound transducers. The histological

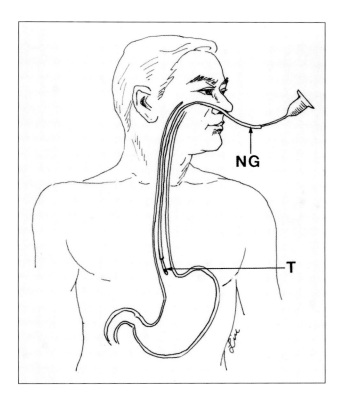

Figure 12.10 *Schematic diagram shows the catheter-based transducer (T) passed transnasally through a nasogastric tube (NG) into the esophagus.*

observations on cross-section were compared with the cross-sectional endoluminal sonography at the corresponding levels. Analysis of images obtained in the in vitro fluid-filled esophagus revealed seven reproducible and distinct alternating hyper- and hypoechoic layers in the esophageal wall. Each of these seven layers corresponded to distinct histological structures. The first hyperechoic layer corresponded to the mucosa, the second thin hypoechoic layer appeared as the muscularis mucosae, the third very bright hyperechoic layer corresponded to the submucosa, the fourth hypoechoic layer to the circular smooth muscle, the fifth thin hyperechoic layer to the intermuscular connective tissue, the sixth hypoechoic layer to the longitudinal smooth muscle, and the seventh hyperechoic layer to the adventitia (Fig. 12.11). The difference between the non-fluid-filled and the fluid-filled esophagus is that the first layer in the non-fluid-filled esophagus appears as a mixed echoic layer corresponding to the squamous epithelium, lamina propria and muscularis mucosae. This is probably due to the first three histological layers

(squamous epithelium, lamina propria and muscularis mucosae) being folded and contracted around the transducer. Therefore, the sound waves pass through redundant layers of tissue and the summation effect is a relatively hypoechoic or mixed echogenic pattern. When filled with fluid the first three histological layers are no longer redundant, so that the sound waves pass through each layer in an orderly sequence. Additionally, the near field of the ultrasound image has lower resolution than the mid field of the ultrasound image. Therefore, when fluid within the lumen pushes the mucosal layer away from the transducer there is better resolution of the mucosal layer, which can then be separated into two distinct echo structures.

After completion of in vitro experiments, these transducers were tested in normal human volunteers to see if these findings could be reproduced in vivo. The method used to introduce the 6.2-Fr ultrasound catheters into the human stomach and esophagus was to first place a 16-Fr nasogastric tube transnasally through the esophagus into the stomach. The ultrasound catheter was then inserted through the nasogastric tube into the stomach (Fig. 12.10). By manipulating the nasogastric tube and the ultrasound catheter it was possible to image the entire esophagus and most of the stomach as well as the duodenum.

In normal volunteer studies all the layers seen in the autopsy esophageal specimens were also seen in the in vivo human esophagus. When the esophagus was at rest, six layers were seen similar to the non-fluid-filled autopsy esophageal specimens. In the esophagus, during the swallowing of a 5–10-ml water bolus, seven layers were seen, similar to the fluid-filled autopsy esophageal specimen.

By using a digital computer analysis system (MicroSonic software), repetitive measurements could be made of the circular smooth muscle, longitudinal smooth muscle and total muscle thickness in each individual volunteer subject (Fig. 12.12). It was found that each muscle layer was significantly thicker at the lower esophageal sphincter (LES) when compared to the same structure 5–10 cm above the LES (Table 12.1) (Fig. 12.13). To our knowledge, this is the first in vivo demonstration of muscular thickening at the LES compared with at the esophageal body.[22]

The stomach and duodenum can also be imaged using the 20-MHz catheter-based transducer. In the stomach, five layers are visualized, similar to the five layers which are seen with the lower frequency endoscopic ultrasound (Fig. 12.14). The stomach is imaged by having the subject drink 200–400 ml of water. The transducer is then placed within the water to promote acoustic coupling. By manipulating the

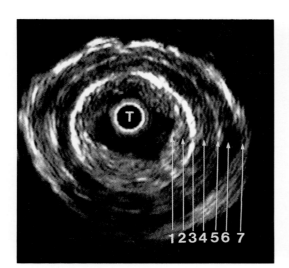

a

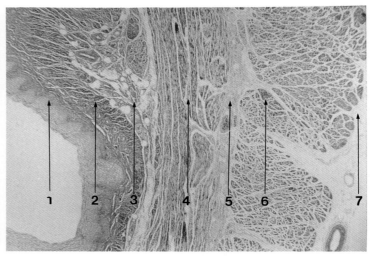

b

Figure 12.11 *(a) A 20-MHz ultrasound transducer (T) located within a saline-filled human esophageal specimen delineates seven layers of the esophageal wall. (b) Close correlation is seen between this cross-sectional histological slice and the ultrasound imaging. 1, mucosa; 2, muscularis mucosae; 3, submucosa; 4, circular smooth muscle; 5, intermuscular connective tissue; 6, longitudinal smooth muscle; 7, adventitia. (Reproduced with permission from Miller LS, Liu JB, Klenn PJ et al, Gastroenterology (1993) 105:31–90.)*

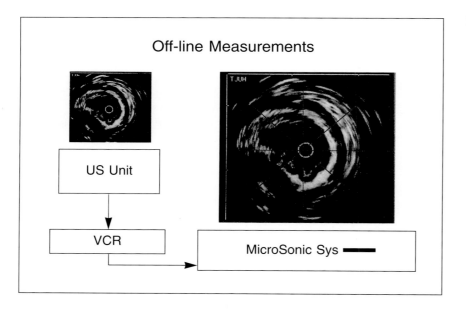

Figure 12.12 *Demonstration of the off-line measurement system.*

Table 12.1 Mean muscle thickness at the lower esophageal sphincter and 5–10 cm above the lower esophageal sphincter (N = 17). (Reproduced with permission from Liu JB, Miller LS, Goldberg BB et al, Radiology (1992) 184:721–7.)

	Circular smooth muscle	Longitudinal smooth muscle	Total width of muscle
Lower esophageal sphincter	0.134 cm ± 0.034 cm	0.079 cm ± 0.013 cm	0.236 cm ± 0.046 cm
5–10 cm above LES	0.072 cm ± 0.026 cm	0.051 cm ± 0.011 cm	0.130 cm ± 0.039 cm

transducer and repositioning the subject, most of the stomach can be imaged. The pyloric area of the stomach can be entered and imaged with the ultrasound catheter. In this area the pyloric sphincter appears as a markedly thickened muscle layer. In addition, the ultrasound catheter can often be inserted into the proximal duodenum and the image of the duodenum can be obtained (Fig. 12.15).

Once the normal sonographic anatomy of the esophagus was defined in vivo using the 20-MHz transducer, it was possible to look for abnormalities in patients with various esophageal disorders. In patients with achalasia of the esophagus, the endoluminal ultrasound images demonstrated increased thickness of the two muscular layers in the region of the LES (Fig. 12.16). The thickness of the circular smooth muscle, longitudinal smooth muscle and total muscle were significantly greater in achalasia patients than in the control group with the *P*<0.001 (Table 12.2).[22]

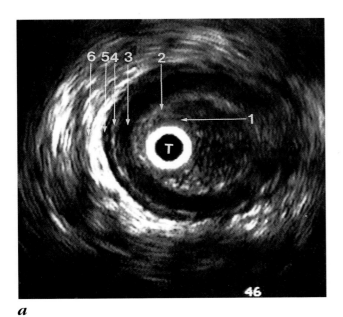
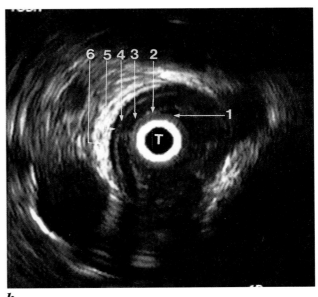

a *b*

Figure 12.13 *The catheter-based transducer (T) positioned (a) within the LES region, and (b) 6 cm above the LES in a normal volunteer delineates the various normal layers of the esophageal wall. Note that the thickness of the muscular layers in the LES region are greater than those in the body of the esophagus. 1, mucosa; 2, submucosa; 3, circular smooth muscle; 4, intermuscular connective tissue; 5, longitudinal smooth muscle; 6, adventitia.*

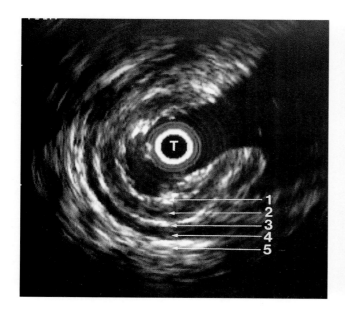

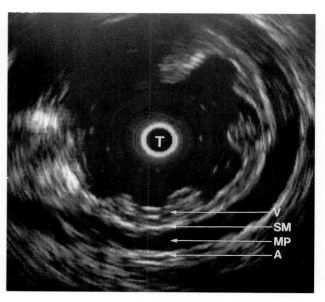

Figure 12.14 *Endoluminal ultrasound image obtained from the body of the stomach demonstrates the normal five layers of the gastric wall, which are: 1, the hyperechoic mucosa; 2, hypoechoic deep mucosa and muscularis mucosae; 3, hyperechoic submucosa; 4, hypoechoic muscularis propria; 5, hyperechoic serosa. T, transducer.*

Figure 12.15 *A cross-sectional image obtained from within the duodenum delineates multiple layers, these are villi (V), submucosa (SM), muscularis propria (MP), and adventitia (A). T, transducer.*

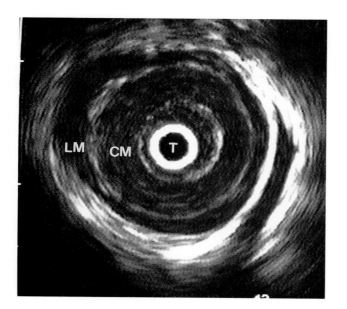

Figure 12.16 *In a patient with achalasia, endoluminal ultrasound demonstrates an increased thickness of the two muscular layers in the LES region. Note that the circular muscle layer (CM) is much thicker than the longitudinal muscle layer (LM). T, transducer.*

Table 12.2 Muscle thickness measurements at the LES in achalasia patients (N = 8). (Reproduced with permission from Liu JB, Miller LS, Goldberg BB et al, Radiology (1992) 184:721–7.)

	Maximum (cm)	Minimum (cm)	Mean ± SD (cm)
CSM	0.600	0.187	0.339 ± 0.161
LSM	0.145	0.092	0.119 ± 0.020
TM	0.783	0.333	0.496 ± 0.180

SD, standard deviation; LES, lower esophageal sphincter; CSM, circular smooth muscle; LSM, longitudinal smooth muscle; TM, total muscle.

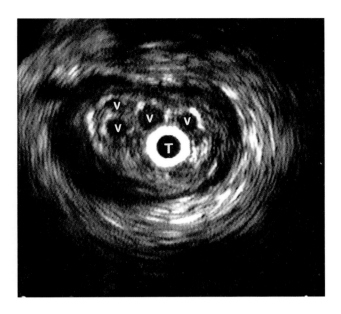

Figure 12.17 *In a patient with portal hypertension, anechoic round areas (V) representing varices can be seen in the submucosa of the distal esophagus. T, transducer.*

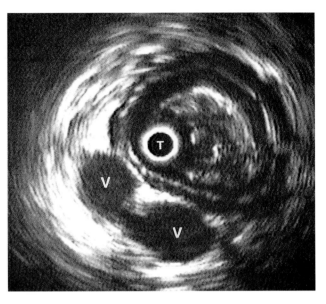

Figure 12.18 *Periesophageal varices (V) can be seen adjacent to the esophageal wall in a patient with portal hypertension. T, transducer.*

Endoluminal ultrasound was also used in the evaluation of esophageal and gastric varices. With the 20-MHz transducer-containing catheters, esophageal and gastric varices, as well as periesophageal and perigastric varices, can be clearly imaged (Figs. 12.17–12.19). Because of the higher resolution and lack of compression of the varices by the catheter-based transducer, submucosal varices in the esophagus are well delineated and their size can be precisely measured. We believe high-resolution endoluminal sonography to be the more precise and reproducible way of evaluating the presence and size of esophageal varices. We found that video-endoscopy, compared to endoluminal sonography, for the detection of gastric varices had a sensitivity of 48 percent and a specificity of 50 percent and for the detection of esophageal varices had a sensitivity of 94 percent and a specificity of 17 percent. We feel that this inability to define the presence or absence of gastric varices is due to the endoscopist's inability to discriminate between varices and normal gastric folds.[23]

There are three reasons why high-resolution endoluminal sonography appears to be better than conventional endoscopic ultrasound in quantitating

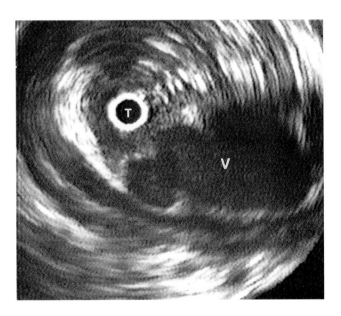

Figure 12.19 *Endoluminal ultrasound image demonstrates submucosal gastric varices (V) in the fundus of the stomach. T, transducer.*

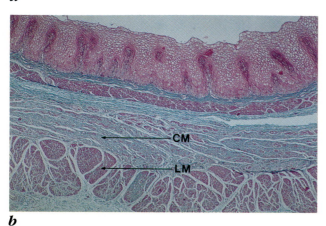

a

b

Figure 12.20 *(a) A cross-sectional ultrasound image was obtained from the distal esophagus of an autopsy specimen with sclerodermatous involvement. It can be seen that there is a hyperechoic abnormality (fibrosis) completely obliterating the circular smooth muscle (CM) and partially obliterating the longitudinal smooth muscle (LM). T, transducer. (b) This esophageal histological section with Masson's stain was taken from the same level as in (a). There is marked fibrosis (blue) obliterating the circular smooth muscle (CM). However, the longitudinal smooth muscle remains relatively well-preserved (LM). (Reproduced with permission from Miller LS, Liu JB, Klenn PJ et al, Gastroenterology (1993) **105**:31–9.)*

the size of esophageal varices: (1) The higher frequency (20 MHz) ultrasound imaging allows for improved resolution of submucosal structures; (2) the catheter-based transducer itself is so small that it does not distort the size or shape of the varix; and (3) there is no water-filled balloon around the transducer to distort the anatomy of the esophagus and varix. In addition, high-resolution endoluminal sonography gives additional valuable information that cannot be obtained endoscopically, including the exact size of the varices and the wall thickness of the varix, the presence or absence of perigastric and periesophageal varices and the presence or absence of perforating veins.

There are many potential clinical applications using high-resolution endoluminal sonography in the setting of portal hypertension. We have already used high-resolution endoluminal sonography clinically to determine the size of esophageal varices before and after transjugular intrahepatic portosystemic shunts (TIPS), to follow patients during sclerotherapy in order to determine the patency of the varices, and to image the stomach for the presence or absence of gastric varices when there was a question about their endoscopic visualization. In addition, this imaging modality may be used in the future to assess the effects of various therapeutic drug regimens on the size of esophageal varices as well as to predict the incidence of bleeding and rebleeding in patients with portal hypertension based on the exact measured size of the varices.

Scleroderma is a generalized connective tissue disorder characterized by fibrosis and microvascular obliteration in the skin, gastrointestinal tract, lung, heart and kidneys. The esophagus is the most frequent gastrointestinal tract organ affected in scleroderma. A study evaluating esophageal involvement by scleroderma was undertaken using high-frequency endoluminal sonography.[24] Three parts of this study were carried out. First, esophageal autopsy specimens were compared histologically and sonographically both from patients with scleroderma and from those with diseases unrelated to the esophagus. Second, the esophagi of normal controls and scleroderma patients were evaluated in vivo using this technology to determine whether or not there were sonographic abnormalities consistent with the sonographic abnormalities seen on the autopsy specimens. In the first part of the study, a hyperechoic abnormality was seen in the normally hypoechoic muscularis propria in patients with scleroderma which was not detected in patients who died of non-esophageal-related diseases. This hyperechoic abnormality correlated with the presence

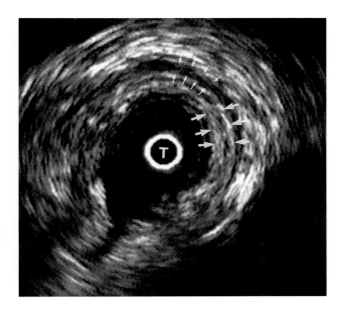

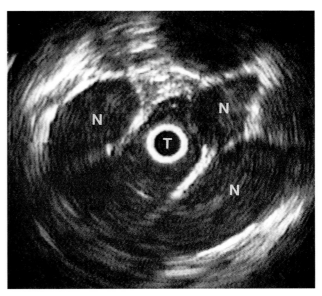

Figure 12.21 *In a patient with scleroderma, endoluminal ultrasound shows a diffusely increased echogenicity in the distal esophageal wall (large arrows). The normal delineation of the various wall structures has disappeared and the esophageal lumen remains slightly dilated in the resting state. Note that the normally hypoechoic longitudinal muscle (small arrows) was not completely replaced by fibrosis. T, transducer.*

Figure 12.22 *A cross-sectional ultrasound image obtained from a patient with scleroderma demonstrates enlarged lymph nodes (N) adjacent to the esophagus. T, transducer.*

of fibrosis on histological sections from these autopsy specimens (Fig. 12.20). In the second part of the study similar hyperechoic abnormalities (fibrosis) were seen in most of the patients evaluated with scleroderma while no hyperechoic abnormalities were seen in any of the normal volunteer subjects. It was found that there was a significant difference between the presence of these hyperechoic abnormalities in scleroderma patients and the absence of these hyperechoic abnormalities in the normal control population (P <0.001) (Fig. 12.21). The distal esophageal lumen was slightly dilated at rest in 82 percent of patients with scleroderma (Fig. 12.21). In contrast to the muscular contraction seen in the normal subjects, these patients showed weak or absent muscular contraction in response to a swallowed water bolus. In addition, one-third of the patients with scleroderma were found to have prominent periesophageal lymph nodes (Fig. 12.22). Comparison of chest CT images to endoluminal sonography for the detection of lymph nodes in

the periesophageal area demonstrated that endoluminal ultrasound was more sensitive.

Since high-resolution endoluminal sonography reflects the degree of histological fibrosis in the distal esophagus, we anticipate that this technology will be utilized clinically in longitudinal studies to follow the progression of fibrosis in the esophagus. Furthermore, it may be useful in the evaluation of various therapeutic drug regimens which may modify the progression of fibrosis in the distal esophagus in scleroderma patients.

Due to the high-resolution of endoluminal ultrasound, imaging of the gastrointestinal tract for submucosal lesions, particularly within the esophagus, is exquisitely sensitive. As with the lower frequency endoscopic ultrasound transducers, various submucosal lesions have characteristic echogenicities and echotextures and arise from characteristic areas of the gastrointestinal tract wall. The major advantage of the high-frequency endoluminal ultrasound technology is

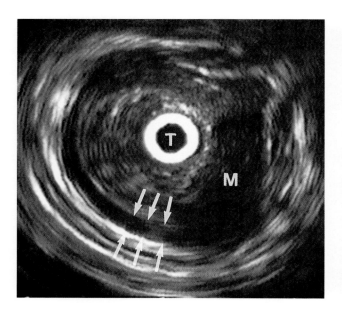

Figure 12.23 *Cross-sectional endoluminal ultrasound image demonstrates a hypoechoic mass (M) arising from the muscularis propria, which was a leiomyoma. Arrows denote adjacent normal region. T, transducer.*

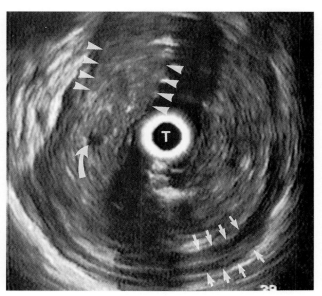

Figure 12.24 *In a patient with ulcerative esophagitis, the cross-sectional endoluminal ultrasound image demonstrates thickening of the submucosa (arrowheads) in the lower portion of the esophagus. A dilated vessel (curved arrow) can be seen within the submucosa. Note that the two muscular layers (arrows) are not involved. T, transducer.*

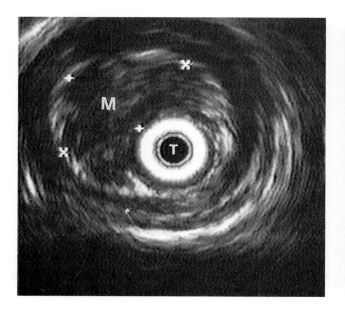

Figure 12.25 *A cross-sectional endoluminal ultrasound image delineates a 0.6 × 1.1 cm hypoechoic mass (M) located in the mid-esophageal wall. There is no evidence of the lesion penetrating the submucosa or extending into the muscular layers. Biopsy of the region confirmed the presence of an esophageal carcinoma. T, transducer.*

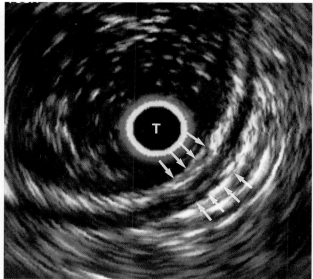

Figure 12.26 *A cross-sectional ultrasound image obtained from the colon via a sigmoidoscope demonstrates the normal multiple layers of the colon wall (arrows). T, transducer.*

that very small lesions can be imaged with high resolution and without compression artifact. Leiomyomas appear as hypoechoic masses contiguous with the muscularis propria. They have a smooth outer margin (Fig. 12.23). Lipomas appear hyperechoic and arise from the submucosa. A number of patients with acute esophagitis documented by endoscopy have been imaged with this technique. Imaging of patients with esophagitis revealed specific abnormalities, including diffuse thickening in the submucosa associated with small dilated vessels imaged within this region (Fig. 12.24).

High-frequency endoluminal sonography is useful in detecting esophageal and gastric malignancies, which may be either hypo- or hyperechoic (Fig. 12.25). Small masses can be detected and staged with great accuracy because the high resolution of the transducer provides high delineation of the area of interest. However, the low penetration (2 cm) limits the direct application of these ultrasound transducers in larger malignancies, since advanced extension far beyond the wall of the esophagus and lymph nodes will be out of the range of the penetration of the ultrasound beam. A major advantage of the 6.2-Fr ultrasound catheters is that they are able to traverse almost any stricture due to either esophageal carcinoma or radiation fibrosis and, therefore, can image the area of narrowing as well as the area below the tumor.

LOWER GASTROINTESTINAL TRACT

Use of high-resolution endoluminal sonography in the gastrointestinal tract has not been limited to the esophagus, stomach and duodenum. We have also imaged the colon, rectum and anal canal. Preliminary work has shown the feasibility of using these miniature transducers in association with endoscopes in the evaluation of the colon (Fig. 12.26). These miniature transducers can be passed through biopsy channels in a sigmoidoscope and then used to visualize areas of interest. Thus, with this approach the presence of a tumor, either superficial or within the wall of the colon, can be evaluated. The ability to image beneath the surface mucosa provides information about the extent of tumor invasion. There is the potential to use this approach to evaluate inflammatory bowel diseases, or, with even longer catheters, to evaluate abnormalities of the small bowel.

The anal canal and rectum were also evaluated by using a 9-Fr catheter containing a 12.5-MHz transducer. In the anal canal the hypoechoic mucosa, hyperechoic submucosa and hypoechoic internal

anal sphincter (IAS), as well as a part of the external anal sphincter (EAS), were identified (Fig. 12.27). The images obtained from the anal canal in 20 subjects were digitally stored on a MicroSonic computer system and measurements were made at eight octants for the IAS and first band of the EAS. The mean width of the IAS was 3.5 ± 0.5 mm, ranging from 1.6 mm to 3.2 mm. The mean width of the first band of the EAS was 2.3 ± 0.5 mm, ranging from 1.6 mm to 3.2 mm.[25] In addition, this imaging approach can be used for the evaluation of the rectal tumors (Fig. 12.28) and holds promise for the staging of early malignant lesions of the anal canal and rectum.

In summary, high-resolution endoluminal sonography is a promising new ultrasound imaging approach for the investigation of the gastrointestinal tract. The major advantages of this technique are increased resolution and the ability to image mural structures without distortion of those structures. Its current major limitation appears to be lack of penetration for staging of gastrointestinal malignancies and for evaluation of structures not within the immediate vicinity of the lumen. We believe that this technology will progress so that catheters of varying sizes and transducers of various frequencies will become available for a variety of lesions in the gastrointestinal tract.

BILIARY SYSTEM

It has been possible to pass these miniature transducer-containing catheters through previously established percutaneous openings into the biliary system to demonstrate the presence and extent of cholangiocarcinoma and to evaluate the effectiveness of the biliary stents (Fig. 12.29).[26–28] Adjacent lymph nodes and blood vessels could also be visualized. In addition, it was possible to insert these catheters at the time of surgery directly via an opening in the duodenum into the biliary system to image the bile duct walls as well as to visualize beyond the lumen into the surrounding tissues. Normal structures, depending on their proximity to the bile ducts, such as adjacent vessels, the liver and the head of the pancreas, could be also imaged.

The most common abnormality demonstrated by this approach is the delineation of wall thickening and mass effect due to either primary cholangiocarcinoma or extrinsic tumors involving adjacent structures. Limited penetration of the ultrasound makes

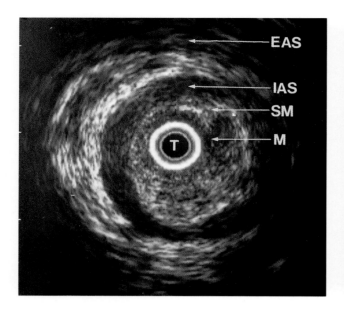

Figure 12.27 *Catheter-based transducer (T) within the anal canal demonstrates the hypoechoic mucosa (M), hyperechoic submucosa (SM), hypoechoic internal anal sphincter (IAS), and hypoechoic external sphincter (EAS).*

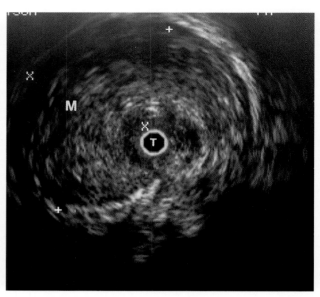

Figure 12.28 *A cross-sectional ultrasound image delineates a hypoechoic mass (M) arising from the distal rectal wall. This proved to be a rectal carcinoma. T, transducer.*

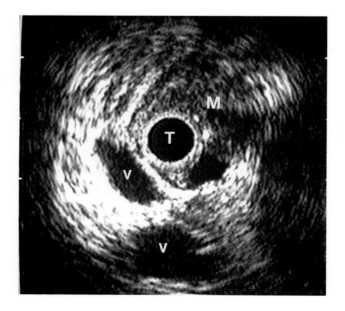

Figure 12.29 *In a patient with known cholangiocarcinoma, the endoluminal ultrasound image demonstrates a hypoechoic mass (M) arising from the distal common bile duct. V, vessel; T, transducer.*

this approach difficult for the staging of malignancies. However, it can show the mass, thickening and irregularity produced by tumor surrounding the bile duct and give some idea of the extent of the involvement of the biliary system through which the transducer could be passed. Endoluminal ultrasound thus often provides more information than was obtainable with just the injection of iodinated contrast into the biliary system. While the contrast showed stricture and irregularity of the bile ducts, the extent and distribution of tumor within the bile duct walls and surrounding tissues and lymph node could not be demonstrated. The results of treatment, either radiation or chemotherapy, resulting in decrease of tumor mass, could also be evaluated using these miniature transducers.

These catheter-based transducers have been utilized to visualize the pancreas at the time of surgery. They can be inserted either through the ampulla of Vater by opening the duodenum or by direct insertion into the surgically exposed pancreatic duct. With either of these approaches it is possible to visualize almost the entire pancreas from the ampulla of Vater to its tail. The normal uniform echotexture

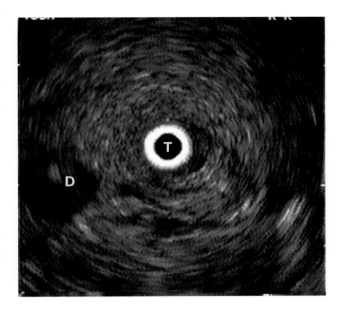

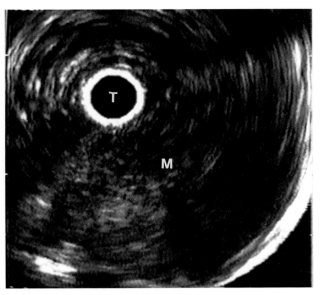

Figure 12.30 *The ultrasound catheter (T) has been inserted into the pancreatic duct through a small surgically created opening. A cross-sectional ultrasound image of the head of the pancreas shows its uniform echotexture. The echo-free area represents a portion of the common bile duct (D). (Reproduced with permission from Goldberg BB, Liu JB, Ultrasound Quarterly (1992) 9:245–70.)*

Figure 12.31 *In a patient with a suspected pancreatic tumor, the endoluminal ultrasound image demonstrates a complex mass (M). Pathological finding was a microcystic adenocarcinoma.*

of the pancreas surrounding the duct can be identified. Within the head of the pancreas, blood vessels and the bile duct can be imaged (Fig. 12.30). This approach has proven useful to the surgeon as an aid in determining the extent of a primary tumor that is to be resected (Fig. 12.31). In addition, this approach can be used to establish that there are no other smaller satellite tumors within other portions of the pancreas not seen by standard, noninvasive imaging, or by palpation or standard intraoperative ultrasound.

In addition to the evaluation of tumors, it has been possible to demonstrate the presence of calcifications in patients with chronic pancreatitis. Also, pancreatic duct stones have been identified. This technique has been an aid to surgeons in the removal of stones, by helping to establish their location as well as confirming that the removal was successful. In the future, it should be possible to pass these miniature transducers via a flexible endoscope through the duodenum, then past the ampulla of Vater into the bile and pancreatic ducts, as is done with an endoscopic retrograde cholangiopancreagram (ERCP). Preliminary work in animals has shown the feasibility of using longer transducer-containing catheters that can be

inserted through standard biopsy channels of endoscopes into the biliary system.

TRACHEOBRONCHIAL TREE

Flexible fiberoptic bronchoscopy, introduced in the late 1960s to directly visualize the tracheobronchial tree, is a well-established technology.[29,30] With this instrumentation it is possible to detect abnormalities of the tracheobronchial tree, including intra- and extraluminal masses, acute and chronic inflammation, and lymphadenopathy. Bronchoscopic signs of disease, including mural deformity and fixation as well as endoluminal obstruction, are used to determine the site for biopsy in order to obtain tissue either directly from the suspected primary pathology or from involved lymph nodes. In spite of radiographic guidance and visible deformity, the precise location of extraluminal masses or lymph nodes viewed through the bronchoscope may not be obvious. It is usually not possible to identify hilar

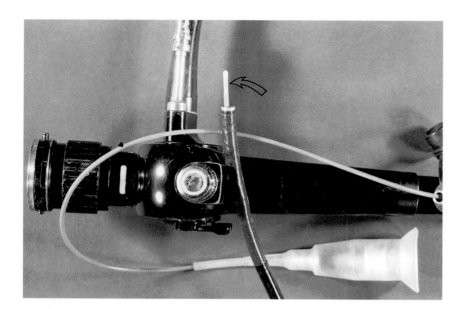

Figure 12.32 *The catheter-based transducer (arrow) has been passed through the biopsy channel of the fiberoptic bronchoscope.*

pulmonary and mediastinal blood vessels. If the lesion is peripheral it may not be clear even with fluoroscopy whether a biopsy is obtained from the abnormality itself or from nearby non-representative tissue.[31] Because of these limitations of the bronchoscopic technique miniature catheter-based transducers have been used in conjunction with flexible bronchoscopy to image beyond the luminal surface, providing information about the exact location of masses, lymph nodes and such normal structures as blood vessels (Fig. 12.32).[32]

In the trachea and major bronchi it was not possible to obtain a 360° cross-sectional image because the lumen diameters were much larger than the catheter-based transducers. Thus, only that portion of the transducer which was in contact with the mucosal surface yielded an ultrasound image. To evaluate masses in the periphery of the lung, the ultrasound catheter can be advanced beyond the distal end of the bronchoscope. It was usually possible to obtain a 360° cross-sectional image at the level of the 4th to 6th bronchi.

The masses were usually of decreased echogenicity compared to the surrounding tissue, or complex, exhibiting both hyper- and hypoechogenic reflections. Peripherally located masses often had sharply defined borders due to the strong reflective interfaces produced between the aerated lung and the lesion.

In addition to the simple identification of the mass in question, dimensions of the lesion could also be delineated up to 2 cm from the bronchial wall. This limitation was not serious since the dimensions of the tumor were usually appreciated from inspection of the previously obtained chest X-ray or CT. More importantly, the location of the tumor in relation to the bronchus in which the transducer was located could be determined. Although the tracheal and bronchial walls were normally hyperechogenic, when the tumor invaded the bronchial wall this pattern disappeared and the bronchial wall tended to blend in with the adjacent hypoechogenic tumor.

As the transducer was moved along the surface of the bronchus or trachea, the extent of the tumor and its depth could be demonstrated. This was most dramatically seen with peripheral tumors, where the relatively small bronchus usually permitted complete contact with the transducer, resulting in a 360° cross-sectional ultrasound image (Fig. 12.33). These peripheral tumors were usually beyond the reach of the bronchoscope and, thus, additional information not previously available by standard bronchoscopy was provided by these miniature transducers.

Lymph nodes were characterized as discrete well-marginated hypoechogenic structures, usually with an ovoid or round configuration (Fig. 12.34). With endoluminal ultrasound, the distance of lymph nodes

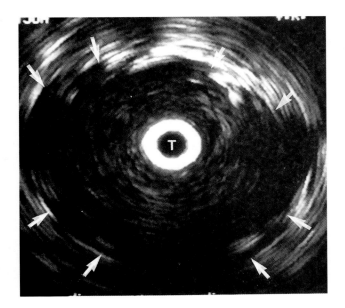

Figure 12.33 *Catheter-based ultrasound transducer (T) located within a distal small bronchus demonstrates a hypoechoic mass (arrows). Transbronchoscopic biopsy showed a poorly differentiated non-small cell carcinoma.*

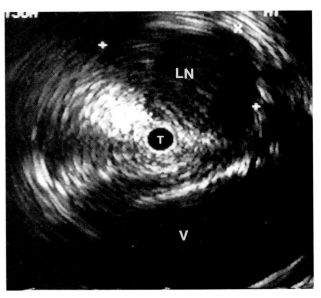

Figure 12.34 *Endoluminal ultrasound image demonstrated an enlarged lymph node (LN) adjacent to a pulsatile blood vessel (V). The ultrasound information was used to avoid puncturing this vessel during the biopsy procedure.*

from the tracheal or bronchial wall can be measured, and biopsies can be carried out under ultrasound localization. Blood vessels were demonstrated as either anechoic tubular or oval structures. Arteries demonstrated pulsatility. However, veins were free of pulsations unless transmitted from adjacent vascular or cardiac structures. The veins usually contained slowly moving echoes due to reflections related to red blood cell rouleau formation. The diameter of the blood vessels could be measured and their position relative to the bronchus, tumor or lymph nodes could be demonstrated (Fig. 12.34). With this information it was possible to avoid puncturing blood vessels by choosing a site for transbronchial biopsy away from these vital structures.

Endoluminal ultrasound has the advantage over fluoroscopy in locating the lesion in relationship to the bronchus in which the biopsy forceps or needle is placed. Unlike fluoroscopy, ultrasound can show whether the lesion lies beyond the mucosa or demonstrates mucosal invasion. It can also evaluate the depth of the mass and the presence or absence of lymph nodes adjacent to the bronchial wall. In addition, ultrasound catheters have the capability of distinguishing blood vessels from nonvascular masses. This may reduce the incidence of hemorrhage.

The limitations of the procedure could be avoided by improvements in the ultrasound catheter and bronchoscopic technology. For example, the addition of an inflatable balloon to the transducer-containing catheter that could be dilated so as to maintain contact of the transducer to the wall in the larger bronchi would be helpful.[33] Future bronchoscopes may, in fact, have built-in ultrasound transducers similar to gastroscopic endoscopes. This, however, would not solve the problem of peripheral tumors in which a separate ultrasound catheter would be preferable.

The preliminary results suggest that this new ultrasound procedure will become an important diagnostic tool during bronchoscopy due to its ability to locate structures beyond the lumen of the tracheobronchial tree.

GYNECOLOGY

These miniature catheter-based transducers have been passed through the cervical os into the endometrial canal without the need for dilatation, unless there was a stricture present. It has been possible to image the endometrium and adjacent myometrium. Initial results have shown it to be useful in helping to differentiate many causes of uterine bleeding.[34] Endoluminal ultrasound images have demonstrated submucosal myomas, endometrial polyps and synechia, as well as endometrial and cervical carcinoma. In addition, the cervical nabothian cysts have been identified. This technique was performed in a number of cases both before and during surgery. Subsequent cross-sectional anatomical slices allowed us to correlate the ultrasound findings with the pathology results. Close correlation of those results confirmed our ability to delineate a variety of gynecological abnormalities. For instance, with myomas a

typical hypoechoic appearance was seen. Their relationship to the endometrium could be shown (Fig. 12.35). A hyperechogenic endometrial polyp could also be imaged. It was possible to demonstrate the presence of both endometrial and cervical cancer (Fig. 12.36).

Transabdominal and endovaginal ultrasound are still the primary tools for the evaluation of a variety of gynecological abnormalities. The concept is that when these established approaches are unsuccessful, then endoluminal ultrasound should be considered. The higher frequency transducers (12.5 or 20 MHz) should enable us to image smaller abnormalities. These catheters have also been inserted into the endometrial canal to image embryos.[35]

Preliminary work has been carried out in utilizing these ultrasound catheters in the evaluation of the fallopian tube. The catheter has been directed through a hysteroscope into the fallopian tube. With this approach it may be possible to detect some causes for infertility such as masses blocking the

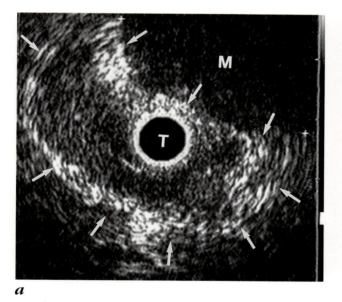

a

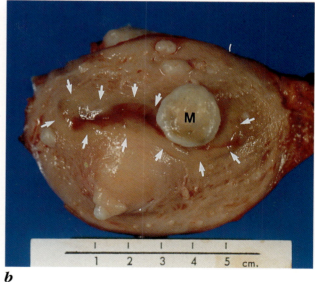

b

Figure 12.35 *(a) Endoluminal ultrasound transducer (T) within the endometrial canal demonstrates the presence of a hypoechoic mass (M) impinging on a portion of the hyperechoic endometrium (arrows). It measured 1.8 cm (+). (b) Subsequent hysterectomy confirmed the presence of a submucosal myoma (M) impinging on the hyperplastic endometrium (arrows). (Reproduced with permission from Goldberg BB, Liu JB, Merton DA et al,* J Ultrasound Med *(1991)* **10***:583–90.)*

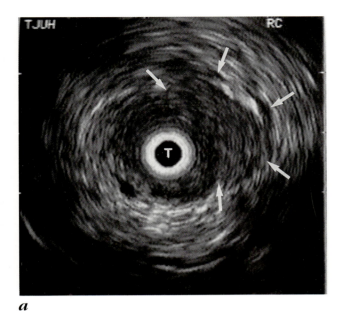
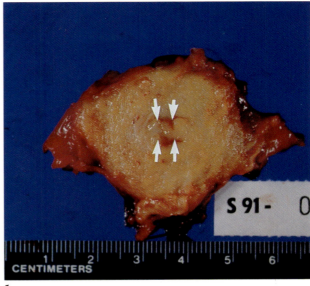

a   *b*

Figure 12.36 *(a) Endoluminal catheter-based transducer (T) located within the endometrial canal demonstrates the presence of an irregular solid mass (arrows) extending from the endometrium into a portion of the myometrium. (b) This was confirmed pathologically to be a grade 1 endometrial carcinoma with minimal invasion of the adjacent myometrium (arrows). (Reproduced with permission from Goldberg BB, Liu JB, Merton DA et al, J Ultrasound Med (1991)* **10**:*583–90.)*

canal. External approaches with insertion of these catheters through a laparoscope are also under investigation. This approach could prove helpful in the detection of small ovarian or tube abnormalities, including early ectopic pregnancies. In our initial studies, these miniature transducers have shown great promise as an aid to the gynecologist during laparoscopic procedures.

REFERENCES

1. Goldberg BB, Liu JB, Merton DA et al, Endoluminal US: experiments with nonvascular uses in animals, *Radiology* (1990) **175**:39–43.

2. Dake MD, Intravascular ultrasound, *Current Opin Radiol* (1991) **3**:181–7.

3. Meyer CR, Chiang EH, Fechner KP et al, Feasibility of high-resolution, intravascular ultrasonic imaging catheters, *Radiology* (1988) **168**:113–16.

4. Pandian NG, Kreis A, Brockway B et al, Ultrasound angioscopy: real-time, two-dimensional, intraluminal ultrasound imaging of blood vessels, *Am J Cardiol* (1988) **62**:493–4.

5. Nishimura RA, Welch TJ, Stanson AW et al, Intravascular US of the distal aorta and iliac vessels: initial feasibility studies, *Radiology* (1990) **176**:523–5.

6. Yock PG, Linker DT, White NW et al, Clinical applications of intravascular ultrasound imaging in atherectomy, *Int J Cardiac Imaging* (1989) **4**:117–25.

7. Isner JM, Rosenfield K, Losordo DW et al, Percutaneous intravascular US as adjunct to catheter-based interventions:

preliminary experience in patients with peripheral vascular disease, *Radiology* (1990) **175**:61–70.

8. Mendelson EB, Bohm-Velez M, Joseph N et al, Gynecologic imaging: comparison of transabdominal and transvaginal sonography, *Radiology* (1988) **166**:321.

9. Rifkin MD, Kurtz AB, Goldberg BB, Sonographically guided transperineal prostatic biopsy: preliminary experience with a longitudinal linear-array transducer, *AJR* (1983) **139**:745–7.

10. Heyder N, Endoscopic ultrasonography of tumours of the oesophagus and the stomach, *Surg Endosc* (1987) **1**:17–23.

11. Gordon SJ, Rifkin MD, Goldberg BB, Endosonographic evaluation of mural abnormalities of the upper gastrointestinal tract, *Gastrointest Endosc* (1986) **32**:193–8.

12. Boyce GA, Sivak MV, Endoscopic ultrasonography in the diagnosis of pancreatic tumors, *Gastrointest Endosc* (1990) **36**:S28–32.

13. Holm HH, Northeved AA, A transurethral ultrasonic scanner, *J Urol* (1974) **111**:238–48.

14. Goldberg BB, Bagley D, Liu JB et al, Endoluminal sonography of the urinary tract: preliminary observations, *AJR* (1991) **156**:99–103.

15. Wild JJ, Reid JM, Diagnostic use of ultrasound, *Br J Phys Med* (1956) **19**:248–57.

16. Fukuda M, Hirata K, Saito K et. al, On the diagnostic use of echoendoscope in abdominal disease. I. Diagnostic experiences with a new type of echoendoscope on gastric diseases, *Proc Jap J Med Ultrasound* (1980) **37**:409–10.

17. DiMagno EP, Regan PT, Wilson DA et al, Ultrasonic endoscope, *Lancet* (1980) March:**1**:629–31.

18. Botet JF, Lightdale CJ, Zauber AG et al, Preoperative staging of esophageal cancer: comparison of endoscopic US and dynamic CT, *Radiology* (1991) **181**:419–25.

19. Botet JF, Lightdale CJ, Zauber AG et al, Preoperative staging of gastric cancer: comparison of endoscopic US and dynamic CT, *Radiology* (1991) **181**:426–32.

20. Kimmey MB, Martin RW, Hagitt RC et al, Histologic correlates of gastrointestinal ultrasound images, *Gastroenterology* (1989) **96**:433–41.

21. Caletti G, Ferrari A, Brocchi E et al, Normal EUS anatomy: the gut wall. In: *Endoscopic Ultrasonography: A Tutorial.* (Course Syllabus for Symposium sponsored by the Cleveland Clinic Foundation, March 21–22, 1992) 35–42.

22. Liu JB, Miller LS, Goldberg BB et al, Transnasal US of the esophagus: preliminary morphologic and function studies, *Radiology* (1992) **184**:721–7.

23. Liu JB, Miller LS, Feld RI et al, Gastric and esophageal varices: 20 MHz transnasal endoluminal US, *Radiology* (1993) **187**:363–6.

24. Miller LS, Liu JB, Klenn PJ et al, Endoluminal ultrasonography of the distal esophagus in systemic sclerosis, *Gastroenterology* (1993) **105**:31–9.

25. Alexander AA, Miller LS, Liu JB et al, High frequency endoluminal ultrasound evaluation of anal canal, *J Ultrasound Med* (1992) **11**:S54.

26. Engstrom CF, Wiechel KL, Endoluminal ultrasound of the bile ducts, *Surg Endosc* (1990) **4**:187–90.

27. Shapiro MJ, Bonn J, Sullivan KL et al, Endoluminal biliary ultrasound: initial clinical experience, *SCVIR* (1991) **2(1)**:11–12.

28. vanSonnenberg E, D'Agostino HB, Sanchez RL et al, Percutaneous intraluminal US in the gallbladder and bile ducts, *Radiology* (1992) **182**:693–6.

29. Ikeda S, Flexible broncho-fiberoscopy, *Ann Otolaryngol, Rhinol, Laryngol* (1970) **79**:916–23.

30. Shure D, Fiberoptic bronchoscopy—diagnstic applications, *Clin Chest Med* (1987) **8**:1–13.

31. Shure D, Fedullo PF, Transbronchial needle aspiration of peripheral masses, *Am Rev Respir Dis* (1983) **128**:1090–2.

32. Goldberg BB, Steiner RM, Liu JB et al, US-assisted bronchoscope with use of miniature transducer-containing catheters, *Radiology* (1994) **190**:233–7.

33. Hurter TH, Hanrath P, Endobronchial sonography: feasibility and preliminary results, *Thorax* (1992) **47**:565–7.

34. Goldberg BB, Liu JB, Kuhlman K et al, Endoluminal gynecologic ultrasound: preliminary results, *J Ultrasound Med* (1991) **10**:583–90.

35. Ragavendra N, McMahon JT, Perrella RR et al, Endoluminal catheter-assisted transcervical US of the human embryo, *Radiology* (1991) **181**:779–83.

Chapter 13 Miniature Endoscopic Ultrasound

Andreas Müller
Adrian RW Hatfield

Gastrointestinal endoscopy is a major diagnostic and therapeutic tool for disease of the gastrointestinal tract; however, the view obtained is limited to the surface. Endoscopy may suggest the presence of a mass within or outside the gastrointestinal wall, but it cannot further determine the location or extent of an extraluminal mass. As there is no extracoporeal imaging method with sufficient resolution to examine the gastrointestinal wall, endoscopic ultrasound (EUS) was developed. After over a decade of clinical experience, EUS has proved to be a valuable addition to endoscopic techniques, enabling further assessment of lesions to be made. The limiting factors are the cost of the equipment and that an additional endoscopic examination is required which causes discomfort to the patient and makes the method more expensive. EUS is difficult to operate and further problems may be encountered as the diameter of the probe, which is larger than a conventional endoscope, can prevent its easy passage through tight strictures. Endoscopic imaging is limited, as the view is reduced by the water-filled balloon which is necessary as an interface between the tranducer and the gut wall preventing disturbance from air.

In the late 1980s, the first miniature endoscopic ultrasound (MEUS) prototypes, which could be introduced through the instrument channel of a conventional endoscope, were developed. These probes were initially used intravascularly.[1] However, the potential for extending the technique to clinical gastroenterology was soon recognized.

INSTRUMENT TECHNOLOGY

The transducer of the miniprobe is mounted at the tip of a catheter which is approximately 200 cm in length, whereas in the conventional EUS the transducer is mounted at the tip of a specially designed endoscope. This allows the probe to pass through the endoscopic biopsy channel and protrude beyond the end of the endoscope for endoluminal scanning. The plastic housing around the transducer is filled with physiological solution to allow penetration of the ultrasound beams.

Two imaging systems exist. The first generates a linear, two-dimensional image. The second produces a cross-sectional, two-dimensional image that gives a tomographic slice through the region imaged. Both techniques have their advantages and disadvantages. As in conventional EUS, MEUS usually uses the cross-sectional imaging. It produces better understanding of the three-dimensional structure.

MEUS prototypes operate at a higher frequency than conventional EUS (12–30 MHz compared to 7–12 MHz). In doing so, high resolution is achieved but the penetration distance into the tissue is reduced. This means that currently available MEUS prototypes are only able to produce useful images approximately 2–3 cm circumferentially from the transducer.

Several probes long enough to protrude from the end of a standard endoscope are already commercially available (Table 13.1 and Fig. 13.1). They all use mechanical systems with one or two rotating crystals or a rotating reflector.

Shorter probes are also available but their application is limited to percutaneous or transnasal use. Prototypes have been developed that use an electronic system with multiple piezoelectric crystals at the tip of the cannula. Microprocessors intensify and digitalize the signals, which are sent, as in the mechanical MEUS systems, to an external processor and a monitor. This may improve picture quality. Some probes have the advantages of a guide wire system (Boston Scientific, Cardiovascular Imaging Systems) or a balloon catheter that can be filled with water and through which the transducer can be passed (Olympus UM-2/3 R). The balloon is used as an interface between transducer and gastroduodenal wall to avoid the disturbance from air. One prototype from Fujinon (SP-501) is interchangeable between linear and rotating scanning.

Table 13.1 Commercially available miniature endoscopic ultrasound probes that can be introduced through a conventional endoscope.

	Ultrasonic probe UM-2/3R (Olympus)	*Sonoprobe SP 101 (Fujinon)*	*EndoSound (Microvasive[a])*	*Insight III (CVIS[b])*	*SSD 550 (Aloka)*
Diameter	2.4 mm	2.6 mm	4.8–6.2 Fr	4.3 Fr	2.0–2.4 mm
Ultrasound image	Radial	Linear	Radial	Radial	Radial
Ultrasound-frequency (MHz)	12–20	15–20	12.5–20	30	15–20

[a] Microvasive, Boston Scientific Corporation.
[b] Cardiovascular Imaging Systems.

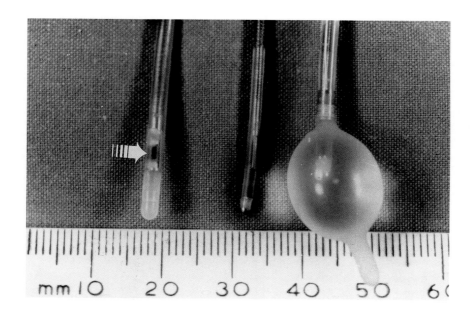

Figure 13.1 *Distal ends of Ultrasonic probe catheters (Olympus), from left to right: UM-3R (arrow points to the transducer), prototype probe with 1.6-mm diameter, UM-2R inside a balloon catheter. (Probes kindly provided by KeyMed, England.)*

CLINICAL INDICATIONS AND EXPERIENCE

MEUS probes were developed principally because of the limitations of conventional EUS. Narrow tumour stenoses, especially in oesophageal carcinoma, prevent passage of the conventional EUS probe and therefore cannot be assessed. The smaller diameter of the miniprobes allows cannulation of the biliary tree and the main pancreatic duct. Operation of a MEUS probe is easier and quicker than that of the conventional EUS. Most importantly, MEUS can be performed at the same time as the standard endoscopy, saving the patient the discomfort of an additional examination. Therefore, MEUS is not only a supplementary method to EUS, but has the potential for replacing conventional EUS in certain clinical situations. Initial clinical experience with the newer MEUS probes has revealed that fine anatomical structures can be imaged well. Comparative studies of EUS versus MEUS are awaited with interest.

In the *oesophagus*, initial experience with the probes reveals similiar staging results as those obtained with EUS. T1–3 stages can be easily determined by MEUS because the oesophageal wall layers lie close to the transducer and the high-frequency

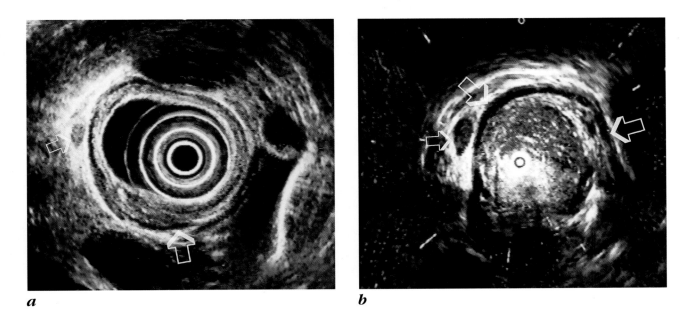

a *b*

Figure 13.2 *Ultrasound pictures of a T1 oesophageal cancer. (a) Produced with an EUM-20 (Olympus).Transducer is in the centre of the picture. The tumour is confined to the mucosa and submucosa. Muscularis propria (hypoechogenic, large arrow) is difficult to define. Note adjacent lymph node (small arrow). (b) Produced with Ultrasonic probe UM-3R (Olympus, probe kindly provided by KeyMed, England). Ttransducer is in the centre of the picture with surrounding tumour tissue. Note well-demarcated muscularis propria (large arrows) and lymph node (small arrow).*

probes produce high-resolution images (Fig. 13.2). However, the quality of the picture is often good only in the sector where the transducer has direct contact with the gastrointestinal wall.

The small probes pass easily through oesophageal strictures but low penetration into more advanced tumours means that staging is limited. Whether MEUS will replace EUS in staging tumours will be assessed by controlled trials. However, it is highly likely that MEUS will also find a place as a clinical investigation tool in oesophageal cancer patients undergoing laser therapy, photodynamic therapy and radiotherapy. Miniprobes provide the opportunity to assess such lesions at the time of a therapeutic procedure, and the resolution of MEUS pictures may allow tumour growth to be followed.

Liu et al[2] introduced miniprobes transnasally via a nasogastric tube blindly into the oesophagus to evaluate oesophageal wall structure.They were able to gather important data in patients with oesophageal abnormalities including achalasia, scleroderma, carcinoma and oesophagitis and were able to measure the size of oesophageal varices precisely and reproducibly.[3] Therefore, MEUS may be used in the future to assess the effect of various therapeutic drugs and procedures in patients with oesophageal varices.

Taniguchi et al[4] have developed a miniature ultrasound device that attaches to the gastrointestinal mucosa by suction. Animal studies have evaluated the motility of the muscle layers of the gut using this device. Such studies may herald the application of this technology to gastrointestinal motility disorders in humans.

In the *stomach*, the different wall layers can be clearly identified by MEUS (Fig. 13.3) and the extent of a pathological finding can be visualized quickly during the initial endoscopy. Takemoto et al[5] showed the usefulness of MEUS before and after endoscopic mucosectomy in early gastric cancer. Even though the MEUS enables high resolution imaging, initial clinical experience revealed that, like conventional EUS, MEUS cannot replace histology but can perform well in staging tumours. Additionally, MEUS has

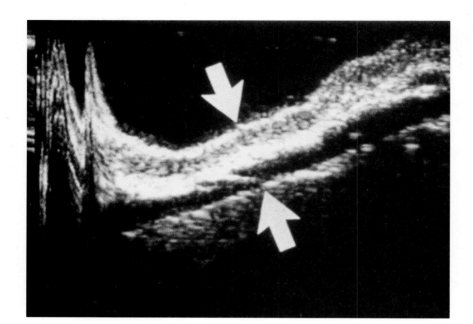

Figure 13.3 *Layers of normal stomach wall demonstrated by Sonoprobe SP 101 (Fujinon). Upper arrow pointed at the mucosa, lower arrow at the serosa. (Photograph kindly provided by Fujinon (Europe).)*

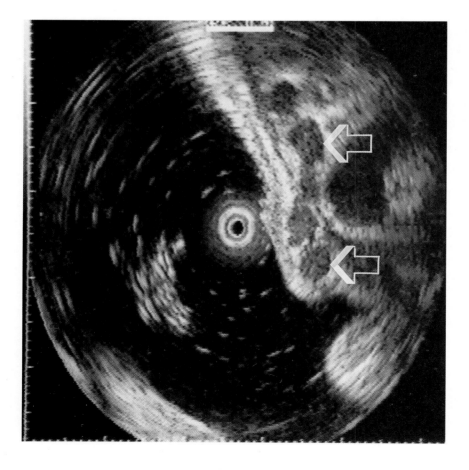

Figure 13.4 *Partially thrombosed varices (marked by arrows) in the stomach wall. Ultrasound pictures taken with the Aloka miniprobe SD 550; (Photograph kindly provided by Dr N. Frank, Stiftsklinik Augustinum, Munich, Germany.)*

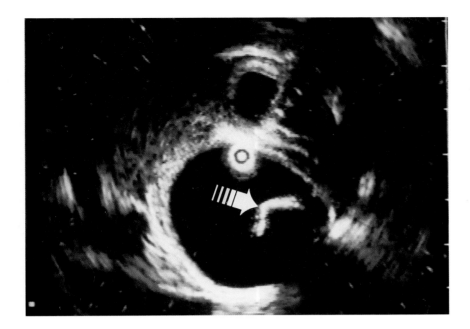

Figure 13.5 *Stone (arrow) inside a dilated common bile duct. Transducer of Ultrasonic probe UM-3R (Olympus, probes kindly provided by KeyMed, England) in the centre of the picture.*

proved to be a more sensitive modality in detecting gastric varices than endoscopy[2] (Fig. 13.4).

The newer MEUS probes have a small-diameter transducer that allows endoscopic intubation of the *biliary tree* and *pancreatic duct*. This may be performed without a previous sphincterotomy in approximately 75 per cent of patients.[6] The localization of the transducer is performed under fluoroscopic control. Use of a guide wire helps cannulation of the pancreatic duct to display the body and tail of the pancreas and facilitates passage of the probe through biliary strictures.

With MEUS the fine structure of the ampulla of Vater can be demonstrated with greater clarity than with any other imaging method in vivo. The sphincter is slightly hyperechogenic in comparison with the surrounding pancreatic tissue. It seems that there is a large interindividual variation in the size of the sphincter and distribution of local blood vessels (Müller et al, unpublished data). There may be a role for pre-sphincterotomy MEUS to estimate the optimal size of sphincterotomy and to reduce the complications from haemorrhage and perforation.

With the high-frequency probes it is possible to variably demonstrate three layers in the common bile duct wall.[7,8] Two layers are hyperechogenic and these are separated by a hypoechogenic layer. This probably represents the anatomical structure of the common bile duct wall: the epithelium is the innermost layer surrounded by elastic tissue with some muscle fibres (corresponding to the echo-poor layer). Around this is the adventitia.

It is also possible to use MEUS via a percutaneous transhepatic biliary tract established for cholangioscopy.[9]

Some common bile duct stones are difficult to reveal on ERCP X-ray films. With a pre-sphincterotomy MEUS small stones can be easily visualized. MEUS could therefore become the new gold standard for detecting common bile duct stones, particularly in patients with dilated bile ducts (Fig. 13.5).

Characteristically, cholangiocarcinomas cause strictures of the biliary tree. Typically, hilar cholangiocarcinomas are small. The extent and exact location may be difficult to determine at operation, and therefore preoperative staging is important. Other imaging methods for these lesions are unsatisfactory. Conventional ultrasound and computed tomography (CT) scanning are widely used but often fail to show a clear distinction between tumour and normal liver tissue. EUS may give better imaging results but has a tendency to overstage T2 cholangiocarcinomas, possibly due to compression of blood vessels, simulating penetration by tumour on ultrasound

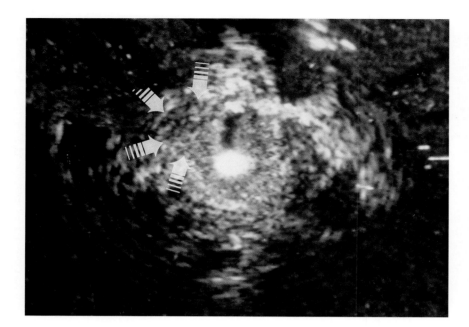

Figure 13.6 *Cholangiocarcinoma of the common hepatic duct causing stricture. Tumour tissue around the transducer. Transmural infiltration marked by arrows. (Olympus Ultrasonic probe UM-2R, probes kindly provided by KeyMed, England.)*

examination.[10] It is hoped that, with high resolution from MEUS probes scanning radially, the transmural extent (T stage) of cholangiocarcinomas[11] (Fig. 13.6) will be able to be assessed with greater accuracy. The assessment of the longitudinal spread must be done with the aid of fluoroscopy. Before passing a MEUS probe through a stricture, prior dilatation may be necessary and a guide wire probe could have a great advantage in this setting.

It is likely that MEUS will prove to be a valuable imaging method in cholangiocarcinoma in addition to endoscopic retrograde cholangiopancreagram (ERCP), EUS, abdominal ultrasound and CT, but further evaluation is needed.

Conventional EUS is the method of choice for staging pancreatic cancer and is superior to the combination of CT and ERCP.[12] In pancreatic cancer MEUS may be especially useful in diagnosing intra-ductal tumours, in which other imaging methods often fail. In these lesions MEUS has already been proven to offer valuable diagnostic information in addition to ERCP.[13] The high-resolution imaging of the ductal and paraductal tissue may be used to differentiate between the different forms of pancre-atic lesions. However, depth of penetration with the high-frequency probes is as yet too low to assess

invasion into the adjacent structures. There are no studies comparing conventional EUS to MEUS in this situation. However, limited experience with MEUS seems to suggest that the echo patterns in normal pancreas, chronic pancreatitis and cancer differ.[13] Therefore MEUS should be evaluated in combination with ERCP and EUS in determining main pancreatic duct strictures.

In the *colon* and *rectum* measurement of extent and staging of tumours can be done quickly at the time of standard endoscopy. However, again, there are no controlled studies comparing MEUS with conventional EUS.

The application of miniprobes in laparascopic procedures and in extragastrointestinal investigations such as imaging bronchial tumours is yet to be assessed.

To date, no reports of cholangitis, pancreatitis or perforation during or after examinations with MEUS have been published.

Most of the currently available probes are rather fragile. This becomes a problem when they are used during ERCP. Extra stresses are placed on the probe as it is necessary to bend it during cannulation of the common bile or pancreatic duct. On occasions this may result in breakage.

CONCLUSIONS

Conventional EUS has developed dramatically since its introduction into gastroenterology using an endoscopic probe in 1976[14] and is in clinical use at many gastroenterology centres throughout the world.

In this paradoxical age where advancing medical technology must be tempered by a need to decrease medical expenditure, before introducing a new procedure into general use it must be either superior to existing techniques or offer useful additional information. It must also be cost-effective and easy to use. EUS has not been able to satisfy all these points and has several disadvantages in comparison with other imaging techniques. It is difficult to operate and therefore needs a very experienced endoscopist and ultrasonographer. EUS causes discomfort for the patient as it cannot be performed at the same time as standard endoscopy and therefore means an additional examination for the patient. The EUS endoscope has a large diameter and it is often impossible to pass the instrument through a tumour stricture, making staging impossible. In summary, EUS has certain disadvantages compared to existing techniques such as ultrasound and CT.

By comparison, MEUS is easier to operate, and saves examination time and the need for a separate examination by conventional EUS. The first MEUS prototype probes produced low image quality. The newer probes have been improved and high-resolution imaging is now possible. There is little doubt as to the potential future for this new method in clinical gastroenterology. Controlled studies will be necessary to prove that the information gained from MEUS images is comparable to that from conventional EUS, and the probes have to be further improved technically. Interchangeable probes may increase depth of penetration by using lower frequency. Resolution of imaging must be improved further and the durability of the probes must be prolonged to lower the costs. Guide wires must be available for probes designed for the biliary tree and pancreatic duct. Finally, anatomical orientation with EUS would be facilitated by adding Doppler ultrasound, and this might also improve the assessment of tumour involvement to include adjacent blood vessels.

ACKNOWLEDGEMENT

This study was supported by the Sassella Foundation, Zürich, Switzerland.

REFERENCES

1. Bon N, Hoff T, Lancee C et al, Early and late intraluminal ultrasound devices, *Int J Cardiac Imag* (1989) **4**:79–88

2. Liu J, Miller L, Feld R et al, Gastric and esophageal varices: 20-MHz transnasal endoluminal US, *Radiology* (1993) **187**:363–6.

3. Miller L, Liu J, Klenn P et al, Endoluminal ultrasonography of the distal esophagus in systemic sclerosis, *Gastroenterology* (1993) **105**:31–9.

4. Taniguchi D, Martin R, Trowers E et al, Changes in esophageal wall layers during motility: measurements with a new miniature ultrasound suction device, *Gastrointest Endosc* (1993) **39**:146–52.

5. Takamoto T, Yanai H, Tada M et al, Application of ultrasonic probes prior to endoscopic resection of early gastric cancer, *Endoscopy* (1992) **24**(Suppl.1):329–33

6. Müller A, Hatfield A, Fairclough P et al, The use of high frequency ultrasound miniprobes in the biliary tree and pancreatic duct, *Gastroenterology* (1994) **106**:A351 (abstract).

7. Jaffe P, Hawes R, Sherman S et al, Intrabiliary and intrapancreatic ductal catheter ultrasonography: A prospective look at the indications, applications, and complications, *Endoscopy* (1994) abstract, in press.

8. Furukawa T, Naitoh Y, Tsukamoto Y et al, New techniques using intraductal ultrasonography for the diagnosis of diseases of the pancreatobiliary system, *J Ultrasound Med* (1992) **11**:607–12.

9. Engström C, Wiechel K, Endoluminal ultrasound of the bile ducts, *Surg Endoscopy* (1990) **4**:187–90.

10. Tio T, Cheng J, Wijers O et al, Endosonographic TNM staging of extrahepatic bile duct cancer: comparison with pathological staging, *Gastroenterology* (1991) **100**:1351–61.

11. Yasuda K, Mukai H, Nakajima et al, Clinical application of ultrasonic probes in the biliary and pancreatic duct, *Endoscopy* (1992) **24**(Suppl. 1):370–5.

12. Rösch T, Braig C, Gain T et al, Staging of pancreatic and ampullary carcinoma by endoscopic ultrasonography, *Gastroenterology* (1992) **102**:188–99.

13. Furukawa T, Tsukamoto Y, Naitoh Y et al, Evaluation of intraductal ultrasonography in the diagnosis of pancreatic cancer, *Endoscopy* (1993) **25**:577–81.

14. Lutz H, Rösch W, Transgastroscopic ultrasonography, *Endoscopy* (1976) **8**:203–5.

Chapter 14 **Contrast-Enhanced Ultrasonography**

William R Lees

The search for agents capable of altering the echogenicity of hollow viscera, blood vessels and tissue has continued for 30 years, but it is only recently that safe and practical echo-enhancers have approached commercial and clinical reality.

ENHANCING THE HOLLOW VISCUS

Saline and water infusions have long been used as negative contrast agents to distend and outline the stomach and duodenum and, in more recent years, to outline the lower gastrointestinal tract, the vagina, endometrial cavity and fallopian tubes (Figs. 14.1 and 14.2).

ULTRASOUND CONTRAST-ENHANCED HYSTEROSALPINGOGRAPHY

Ultrasound contrast-enhanced hysterosalpingography (HSG) uses intrauterine contrast media to increase the diagnostic value of plain transvaginal ultrasound. The endocervix is cannulated with a small balloon-tipped catheter as with the X-ray technique, and saline or positive contrast (Echovist (Schering, Berlin) or Albunex (Nycomed, Oslo)) is injected under moderate pressure to distend the cavity and traverse the tubes. Ultrasound saline HSG is superior for delineating the endometrial cavity, demonstrating endometrial polyps and for showing the relationship of fibroids to the cavity (Figs. 14.3–14.5). We have recently compared this to magnetic resonance imaging (MRI) for planning transendometrial resection of fibroids. MRI showed better the total number, size and distribution of fibroids, but the long scanning times preclude adequate distension of the cavity and, therefore, the ultrasound technique is better for submucosal fibroids,

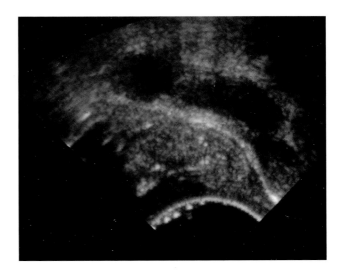

Figure 14.1 *Rectal water infusion using contrast to show the full extent of a villous adenoma.*

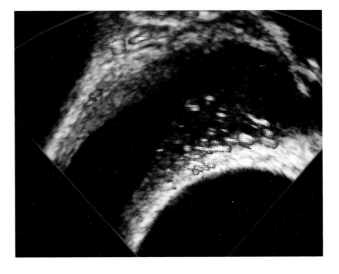

Figure 14.2 *Vaginal water infusion using a Foley catheter to demonstrate wall thickening in association with a vaginal sarcoma. The echoes within the mass are vessels visualized by colour flow imaging.*

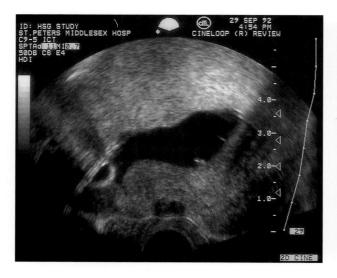

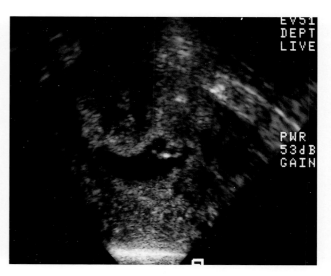

Figure 14.3 *Saline HSG–normal distension of the cavity. The saline was infused via a balloon-tipped catheter to include the endocervix.*

Figure 14.4 *Submucosal fibroid indenting an otherwise normal endometrial cavity.*

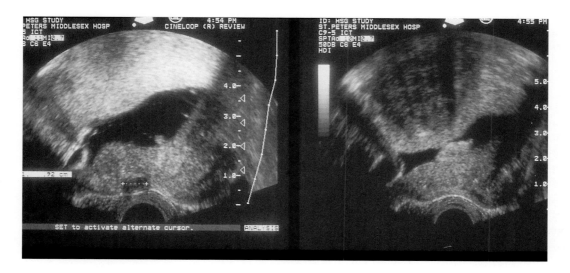

Figure 14.5 *Small endometrial polyps visualized by saline HSG.*

which are more suitable for hysteroscopic resection than myometrial fibroids (Figs. 14.6a, b).

Tubal patency can be demonstrated by observing the flow of saline into the peritoneal recesses of the pelvic cavity, but a positive contrast agent is significantly more sensitive. The intense B-mode enhancement produced by Echovist will outline the lumen of the tubes even though their diameter is well under a millimeter. Individual bubbles and bubble trains can be tracked in their passage down the tubes, but the flow is better seen with duplex or colour Doppler. Degenhardt has reported a sensitivity of 100 per cent in determining tubal patency under general anaesthesia compared with a standard laparoscopic technique.[1] As an outpatient

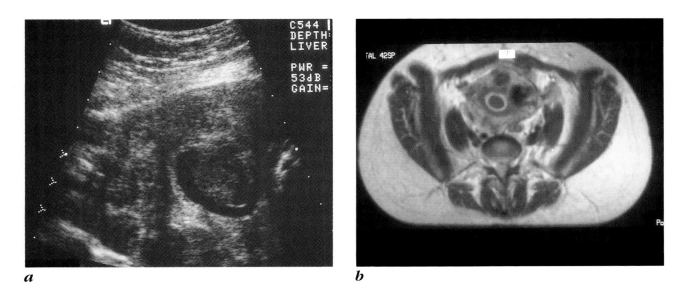

Figure 14.6 *(a) A large submucosal polyp outlined by saline. (b) MRI scan showing the low-signal polyp surrounded by the high-signal intensity of the endometrium.*

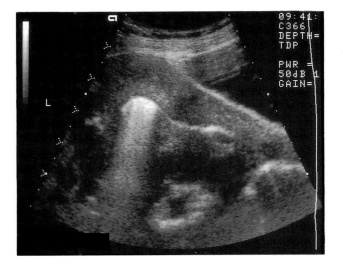

Figure 14.7 *A positive contrast study (Echovist). The posterior wall of the uterus is obscured by the intense reverberation effect produced by the microbubbles.*

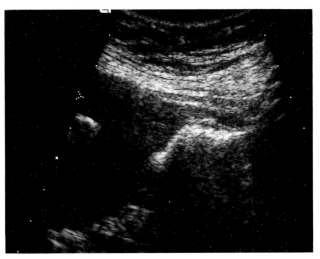

Figure 14.8 *HyCoSy study. Scan shows filling of the fallopian tube with free spill into the peritoneal cavity.*

procedure without anaesthesia, pain and tubal spasm may produce a false positive rate for tubal blockage of approximately 5 per cent, comparable to X-ray HSG. In our own series, we had two unusual false negatives where the tubes were correctly shown to be patent but adhesions from previous pelvic inflammatory disease (PID) did not allow free peritoneal spill. This was better seen on fluoroscopy (Figs. 14.7, 14.8). It seems clear that this simple office-based or out-patient procedure will confirm tubal patency in most infertile patients and displace X-ray HSG. Usually it is obvious that pain or spasm are limiting tubal flow. These cases and those of true blockage can be assessed further radiographically or by laparoscopy under general anaesthesia.[2]

INTRAVASCULAR ECHO-ENHANCERS

The use of saline and indocyanine green as an intravascular agent for use in echocardiology dates back to Gramiak's work in 1968.[3] Such simple infusions have a very brief echo-enhancing effect and the recent focus has been to develop stable bubble based agents to enhance the blood pool.[4]

These are of three main types:

1. Crystalline galactose carrying and stabilizing an air bubble of 2–8 μm diameter. The first commercially developed agent from Schering is Echovist which is now licensed for right heart cardiac studies and ultrasound HSG (HyCoSy). This agent has been further developed by the addition of a small quantity of palmitic acid, which has the effect of stabilizing the bubble sufficiently to allow passage through the pulmonary circulation with persistence in the systemic circulation for 2–4 min (Fig. 14.9). An increase of B-mode or Doppler sensitivity of 10–15 dB is gained but with current equipment only the Doppler enhancement is useful. The agent is currently undergoing Phase 3 clinical trials.[5]

2. Polymer microspheres encapsulating air or nitrogen. The earliest of these was Albunex from Nycomed which has limited transpulmonary properties and is mainly for right heart use. Other new biodegradable polymers have been developed with similar echo-enhancing properties, but with greater stability in the blood pool.[6–11]

3. Purely gaseous agents. Free gas bubbles are very efficient backscatters and may produce a signal two to three orders of magnitude greater than a bubble with a rigid shell. Simple gas bubbles are, however, very unstable and it is difficult to control the bubble size in suspension. Fluorocarbons have been developed as blood substitutes and have been shown to be remarkably safe and biological inert. Much effort has been expended in finding fluorocarbons which can form stable free bubbles of 2–4 μm diameter. One very promising agent is dodecafluoropentan (DDFP). This is a liquid at room temperature and undergoes a phase change at around body temperature. Initially, 0.3 μm droplets of the liquid form are suspended in an emulsion, stabilized by two surfactants. After intravenous injection the DDFP boils to form bubbles of 2–5 μm diameter. It readily clears the pulmonary vascular bed and persists in the blood pool for up to 30 min. The agent has a very high Q factor, improving its resonant properties compared to a

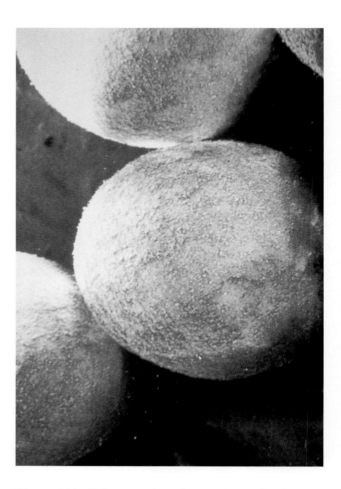

Figure 14.9 *Galactose microspheres prior to dissolution and injection.*

similar sized air bubble. As with other fluorocarbons, it is remarkably inert with a toxic dose over 600 times the clinical dose. This agent is currently undergoing Phase 2 clinical trials.[12,13]

TISSUE-ENHANCERS

Altering the grey scale properties of tissue has been achieved with perfluorocarbon compounds (e.g. perfluoroctylbromide, PFOB), but despite over 15 years experimentation these have not yet proved to be of practical use. Large doses of the agent are needed, typically 5 ml/kg, with the maximum contrast effect obtained 2 days after injection. The effect is to enhance the echogenicity of normal parenchyma and vascularized tumour parenchyma.[14–16] The agent is highly specific for liver and spleen. More recent studies have shown that PFOB alters the acoustic properties of tissues in a linear fashion over a wide range of concentrations, which opens up the possibility of quantitative analysis of liver and other tissue properties.[12] Iodipimide ethyl ester (IDE) can be formulated as dense small particles which are taken up by the Kupffer cells of the hepatic sinusoids within 10–20 min after injection. During uptake these act as scattering particles to increase the echogenicity of normal tissue. Tumours and other lesions lacking Kupffer cells do not significantly enhance.[17]

A recent development has been the 'Cavisome' (Schering, Berlin), which is a bubble agent stable enough to be taken up by the reticular endothelial system and the Kupffer cells of the liver where the resonant effects of the bubble can be used to enhance normal liver tissue.

HARMONIC IMAGING

The resonant properties of bubbles have recently been exploited in a novel way. A gas bubble or encapsulated microsphere will resonate in a highly non-linear fashion, with much of the energy in the returned echo concentrated in harmonics of the insonating frequency. Much of the energy of the backscattered signal is concentrated in or around the second harmonic. Many modern transducer/receiver systems have sufficient bandwidth to exploit this by insonating at the main resonant frequency of the bubble and filtering the returned signal to detect the second harmonic only. This enables complete separation of the signal derived from the contrast agent from the background tissue signal. This not only gives a pure contrast effect but, if used in Doppler mode, greatly suppresses the clutter signal which comes from tissue motion with echo amplitudes 30–35 dB greater than the Doppler signal.[18]

APPLICATIONS OF BLOOD POOL AGENTS

CONVENTIONAL VASCULAR DOPPLER

Useful enhancement of the Doppler signal will last for 2–4 min depending on the concentration of the agent used. A peak enhancement of up to 25 dB can be gained. This will improve the signal-to-noise ratio of the Doppler signal and also improve detection of both high- and low-flow velocities, which may otherwise fall below the threshold of detection of the Doppler apparatus. The obvious application is to increase the strength of signal in deep and difficult vessels such as the intracranial arteries and the renal arteries, but with higher frequency transducers such as those used for intra-cavity investigations it will enable detection of much smaller vessels and vessels flowing at a poor Doppler angle (Fig. 14.10). Also,

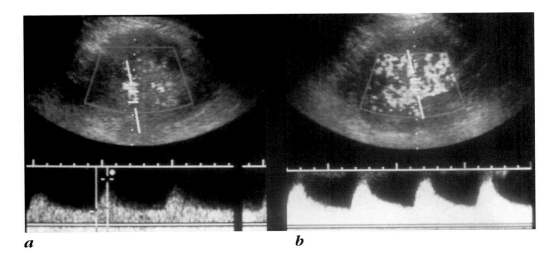

a *b*

Figure 14.10 *Enhancement of the blood pool by Levovist as seen on colour Doppler and spectral Doppler. (a) Pre-contrast; (b) post-contrast.*

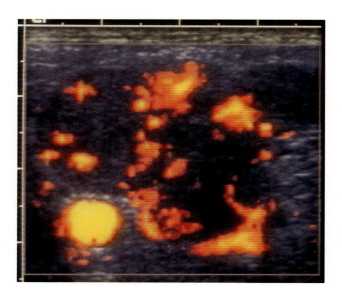

Figure 14.11 *Contrast-enhanced blood flow in a thyroid tumour (power Doppler).*

high-velocity, low-volume flows in arteriovenous shunts will be detected more reliably (Fig. 14.11). The technique has also been used with transoesophageal echocardiography to demonstrate viability of ischaemic myocardium.[19,20]

The technique is also suitable for quantitative studies. As long ago as 1978, Voci showed that classic dye dilution formulae could be modified for use with echo contrast to measure renal blood flow over a wide range of flow levels compared with direct measurement by an electromagnetic flow meter with a correlation coefficient of 0.92.[21] Schwartz has more recently produced experimental and animal models of volume blood flow determination using Levovist (Schering, Berlin). He compares three ultrasonic intensity methods i.e. radio frequency, video and Doppler, and shows that Doppler methods are best suited to estimation of volume flow.[22]

In solid organs such as the liver, breast, ovary and prostate much interest has centred on studies of tumour blood flow. The neovascular circulation of any tumour more than a few millimetres in diameter has typical properties. Vessels are chaotic in their size and spatial distribution and lack the regular branching pattern of a normal vascular bed. They show tangles, communications and high-velocity aterio-venous shunts. The abnormal vessels also lack mechanisms for controlling vasomotor tone and hence will have an intrinsically low impedance flow pattern in their feeding arteries. This may be to some extent

countered by a high interstitial tissue pressure in many tumours, and the duplex Doppler waveform may be mimicked by naturally low impedance circuits such as in the corpus luteum or in trophoblasts. Despite this, a combination of colour and duplex Doppler imaging can demonstrate most of these features, but both methods have until now been mainly limited by poor signal-to-noise ratios even in accessible organs such as the ovary or prostate.[23,24]

We have recently demonstrated the value of contrast-enhanced vascular studies of the prostate using a three-dimensional acquisition and reconstruction technique to build up maps of blood flow with solid tissue.[25] This method is designed to highlight abnormal vascular patterns and increases in regional blood flow. Colour blooming may overemphasize vessel size and it is clear that the ultrasound equipment manufacturers will modify their machines to use the extra signal available from echo contrast to improve the sensitivity, spatial, temporal or velocity resolution in the final display. Tumour blood flow maps require high sensitivity, high spatial resolution but low temporal and velocity resolution (Figs. 14.12a, b). This study was limited by contrast availability to only 20 patients with suspected prostate cancer. Two out of 12 cancers showed abnormal blood flow signals only after contrast administration. Accuracy for Doppler analysis alone was 100 per cent for the diagnosis of malignancy and was even 86 per cent when studying the distribution of cancer on a quadrant by quadrant basis.

We have also recently reported the application of power Doppler in diagnosis of prostate cancer using similar methods to the study described above in 40 patients.[25] This was less sensitive, although the relative angle independence and lack of aliasing produced significantly better three-dimensional maps. The combination of power Doppler with contrast enhancement promises to be much better than either alone. Second harmonic imaging promises even greater sensitivity with fewer artifacts.

It is tempting to relate the pixel density seen on Doppler imaging with volume blood flow, but this is not correct. Doppler pixel counts distinguish badly between arterial and venous flow, and only give an indication of the volume of blood flowing through tissue and not the volume flow or perfusion. Pathological and physiological studies of prostate cancers show that they are usually poorly vascularized and perfused compared to normal prostatic tissue, yet our own and other studies have shown that over 85 per cent show an increased colour Doppler signal.[25] The paradox can be explained if we accept an abnormal distribution of vessel size, with

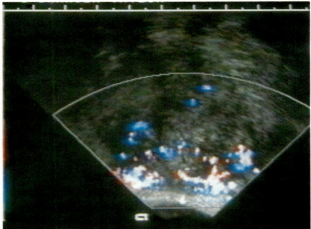

a

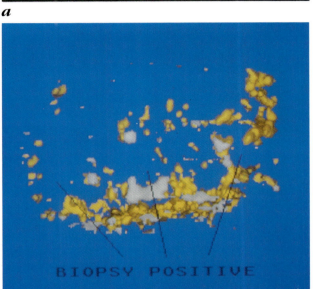

b

Figure 14.12 *(a) Contrast-enhanced Doppler study of blood flow in a prostate cancer. (b) Three-dimensional reconstruction of the blood flow signal within a prostate showing intense flow asymmetrically placed within the gland in the area of malignant infiltration.*

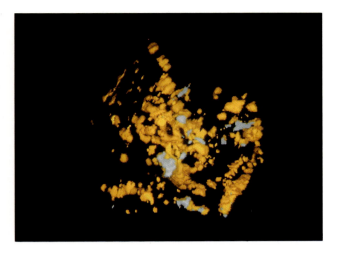

Figure 14.13 *Three-dimensional reconstruction of blood flow through a tumour showing chaotic distribution of vessels with numerous interconnections.*

different types.[26] It lends geometrical quantitation to the Doppler image (Fig. 14.13). Cosgrove et al (unpublished work) have made an interesting observation in their contrast-enhanced studies of blood flow in breast cancer, that is, cancers tended to show a more rapid maximum increase in colour Doppler signal strength than benign lesions. They hypothesize that this is due to early venous filling from arteriovenous shunts in the vascular halo around the lesion. They also showed a longer persistence of enhancement within the cancers, probably due to pooling in abnormal tumour vessels.

Contrast-enhanced Doppler imaging shows great promise not only for mapping the distribution of tumour vessels but also for studying the dynamics of contrast passage through normal and abnormal tissue. It is theoretically possible to use these techniques to study perfusion in tumour tissue which will undoubtedly be of use in monitoring response to treatment (Rubin J, personal communication).

more large vessels running through the tumour tissue which will be preferentially detected because of greater signal intensity with suppression of signal in smaller and more numerous normal vessels.

Three-dimensional acquisition, reconstruction and display of Doppler images is not difficult to achieve and is readily applied to invasive transducers of many

INTRA-ARTERIAL USE OF CONTRAST AGENTS

Many different agents have been injected into the hepatic artery during angiography to enhance the detection of liver lesions. Gaseous carbon dioxide will strongly enhance vascular lesions such as

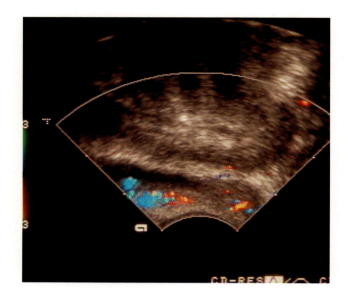

Figure 14.14 *A novel use for ultrasound contrast: the ultrasound sinogram. Contrast has been instilled into a perianal fistula and the track outlined in the rectal wall by contrast flow seen by colour Doppler imaging.*

hepatocellular carcinoma, as will blood pool agents such as Levovist.[27] Oily lipiodol is trapped in vascular lesions for many days after injection and can be seen as an area of increased echogenicity on ultrasound where it has been used to guide biopsy and also as a marker for intra-operative surgical use.[28]

Intravascular ultrasound has some limitations in respect of accurate measurement of the lumen of very small vessels such as the coronary arteries and after interventions such as angioplasty and atherectomy. These can be overcome by simultaneous use of an echogenic contrast agent. Adequate contrast opacification will also delineate the vessel wall surface to show cracks, ulcers and adherent clots (Fig. 14.14).[29]

BOUND AGENTS

Finally, an interesting new use of the principles of echo-enhancement is the production of enhancing polymers bound to needles and catheters to increase their visibility during invasive procedures such as biopsy (Acuson, Mountain View, CA).[30]

REFERENCES

1. Degenhardt F, hystero-contrast-sonography—a new alternative for the monitoring of fallopian tube patency, *Zentralbl Gynakol* (1991) **113**:799–801.

2. Balen FG, Allen CM, Siddle NC et al, Ultrasound contrast hysterosalpingography – evaluation as an out-patient procedure, *Br J Radiol* (1993) **66**:592–9.

3. Gramiak R, Shah PM, Kramer DH, Ultrasound cardiography: contrast studies in anatomy and function, *Radiology* (1969) **92**:939–48.

4. Butler BD, Production of microbubbles for use as echo contrast agents, *J Clin Ultrasound* (1986) **14**:408–12.

5. Schlief R, Schurman R, Niendorf HP, Basic properties and results of clinical trials of ultrasound contrast agents based on galactose, *Ann Acad Med Singapore* (1993) **22**:762–7.

6. Christiansen C, Kryvi H, Sontum PC et al, Physical and biochemical characterization of Albunex, a new ultrasound contrast agent consisting of air-filled albumin microspheres suspended in a solution of human albumin, *Biotechnol Appl Biochem* (1994) **19**:307–20.

7. Schneider M, Bussat P, Barrau MB et al, A new ultrasound contrast agent based on biodegradable polymeric microballoons, *Invest Radiol* (1991) **26**(Suppl 1):S190–1; discussion S198–202.

8. Carroll BA, Turner RJ, Tickner EG et al, Gelatin encapsulated nitrogen microbubbles as ultrasonic contrast agents, *Invest Radiol* (1980) **15**:260–6.

9. de Jong N, Hoff L, Ultrasound scattering properties of Albunex microspheres, *Ultrasonics* (1993) **31**:175–81.

10. Schneider M, Broillet A, Bussat P et al, The use of polymeric microballoons as ultrasound contrast agents for liver imaging, *Invest Radiol* (1994) **29**(Suppl 2): S149–51.

11. Wheatley MA, Schrope B, Shen P, Contrast agents for diagnostic ultrasound: development and evaluation of polymer-coated microbubbles, *Biomaterials* (1990) **11**:713–17.

12. Andre M, Nelson T, Mattrey R, Physical and acoustical properties of perfluoroctylbromide, an ultrasound contrast agent, *Invest Radiol* (1990) **25**:983–7.

13. Mattrey RF, Wrigley R, Steinbach GC et al, Gas emulsions as ultrasound contrast agents. Preliminary results in rabbits and dogs, *Invest Radiol* (1994) **29**(Suppl 2):S139–41.

14. Satterfield R, Tarter VM, Schumacher DJ et al, Comparison of different perfluorocarbons as ultrasound contrast agents, *Invest Radiol* (1993) **28**:325–31.

15. Long DM, Long DC, Mattrey RF et al. An overview of perfluoroctylbromide – application as a synthetic oxygen carrier and imaging agent for X-ray, ultrasound and nuclear magnetic resonance, *Biomater Artif Cells Artif Organs* (1988) **16**:411–20.

16. Mattrey RF, Leopold GR, vanSonnenberg E et al, Perfluorochemicals as liver and spleen seeking ultrasound contrast agents, *J Ultrasound Med* (1983) **2**:173–6.

17. Parker KJ, Baggs RB, Lerner RM et al, Ultrasound contrast for hepatic tumors using IDE particles, *Invest Radiol* (1990) **25**:1135–9.

18. Burns PN, Ultrasound contrast agents in radiological diagnosis, *Radiol Med (Torino)* (1994) **87**:71–82.

19. Vandenberg BF, Kerber RE, Skorton DJ, Detection of myocardial viability with ultrasound tissue characterization: myocardial contrast echocardiography and integrated backscatter imaging, *Am J Card Imaging* (1994) **8**:113–22.

20. Schrope B, Newhouse VL, Uhlendorf V, Simulated capillary blood flow measurement using a nonlinear ultrasonic contrast agent, *Ultrason Imaging* (1992) **14**:134–58.

21. Voci P, Heidenreich P, Aronson S et al. Quantification of renal blood flow by contrast ultrasonography: preliminary results, *Cardiologia* (1989) **34**:1001–6.

22. Schwarz KQ, Bezante GP, Chen X et al, Volumetric arterial flow quantification using echo contrast. An in vitro comparison of three ultrasonic intensity methods: radio frequency, video and Doppler, *Ultrasound Med Biol* (1993) **19**:447–60.

23. Goldberg BB, Hilpert PL, Burns PN et al, Hepatic tumours: signal enhancement at Doppler US after intravenous injection of a contrast agent, *Radiology* (1990) **177**:713–7.

24. Violante MR, Parker K, Lerner R, Particulate contrast agents for improved ultrasound detection of liver metastases, *Invest Radiol* (1990) **25**(Suppl 1):S165–6.

25. Lees WR, Balen F, Allen CM et al, Diagnostic value of 3D blood flow maps derived from Doppler data, *Radiology* (1994) **193**:335.

26. Kelly IG, Gardener J, Lees WR, Three dimensional foetal ultrasound, *Lancet* (1992) **339**:1062–4.

27. Veltri A, Capello S, Faissola B et al, Dynamic contrast-enhanced ultrasound with carbon dioxide microbubbles as adjunct to arteriography of liver tumours, *Cardiovasc Intervent Radiol* (1994) **17**:133–7.

28. Lau WY, Arnold M, Leung NW et al, Hepatic intra-arterial lipiodol ultrasound guided biopsy in the management of hepatocellular carcinoma, *Surg Oncol* (1993) **2**:119–24.

29. Hausmann D, Sudhir K, Mullen WL et al, Contrast enhanced intravascular ultrasound: validation of a new technique for delineation of the vessel wall boundary, *J Am Coll Cardiol* (1994) **23**:981–7.

30. Widder DJ, Simeone JF. Microbubbles as a contrast agent for neurosonography and ultrasound-guided catheter manipulation: in vitro studies, *AJR* (1986) **147**:347–52.

Chapter 15 **Future Directions for Invasive Ultrasound**

John E Gardener

Every new idea in science must pass through three phases. In Phase 1 everybody says the man is crazy and the idea is all wrong. In Phase 2 they say that the idea is correct but of no importance. In Phase 3 they say that it is correct and important, but we knew it all along.

S. Freud

INTRODUCTION

In this chapter we will examine a number of new technical developments in enough detail to allow the reader to form opinions as to their likely application to invasive procedures. An important focus will be on techniques related to imaging in three or more dimensions. These techniques require position-sensing, in some form, to locate the ultrasound echo samples in space. This position-sensing technology then integrates in other important ways, e.g. in guiding instruments for invasive procedures. We will look at some of the problems associated with acquisition of three-dimensional ultrasound and at what the different technical and clinical possibilities are. Several other new techniques which also may have importance for invasive ultrasound studies will also be examined.

Whilst this book is focused on invasive ultrasound and we are directing our attention in this direction, it is clear that the methods we describe have more general application. Some of the sample illustrations given are not specific to noninvasive techniques but are included in order to provide a full range of ideas for potential application to invasive procedures.

SCOPE FOR IMPROVEMENTS IN INVASIVE IMAGING

Invasive techniques principally provide for close access to the tissues of interest. There is minimal overlying tissue and problems of skin contact are removed. This means firstly that higher frequencies may be used, with the associated improved resolution. Minimal overlying tissue also means reduced artifact and distortion due to refraction, scattering and absorption. The images obtained are therefore usually of a higher quality than those obtained with conventional probes and there is considerable potential for processing and more sophisticated presentation.

More of a problem is that these transducers are usually less readily manipulated than conventional probes. For example, intravascular ultrasound (IVUS) probes take only transverse sections across the vessel. It is currently impractical to construct an IVUS probe scanning both transverse and longitudinal planes, either mechanically or as an array. This means that the views acquired will be much more restricted than with most conventional sonography.

Three-dimensional image acquisition produces a solid volume of tissue image recorded as a block. Since this solid set contains high-quality data, there is scope for specialized reconstruction and display processing for various purposes. Most importantly, image reconstruction and various types of display produced from these data can allow the limitations of the accessibility and manipulation of the viewing plane to be overcome.

THREE-DIMENSIONAL IMAGING

It has been clear for many years that there ought to be benefits from imaging with ultrasound in three dimensions.[1,2] The ultrasound beam even from a simple transducer is three-dimensional, as the anatomy to be interrogated usually is also. In the case when the anatomy is moving it might be of course be described as four-dimensional, which we will discuss later. The acquisition and storage of a three-dimensional volume allows the possibility of 'rescanning' this recorded data at a later stage, providing in principle all the information available at the scan. In this way ultrasound investigations could become to a significant extent 'scan and review' procedures, similar to computed tomography (CT) and magnetic resonance imaging (MRI), with expert scan interpretation or reinterpretation being made without the patient present. More importantly for immediate use in invasive ultrasound, this rescanning allows for display of views which would be inaccessible from conventional operation.

In CT and MRI, the use of three-dimensional representations has been increasing, to the extent that most new equipment now has some form of three-dimensional display facility. The most common applications for the three-dimensional facilities are in: surgery planning; assessment of complex anatomy and pathology; measurement in three dimensions; prosthesis manufacture; and better diagnosis.[3]

When we display a normal two-dimensional ultrasound cross-sectional view there are many elements of the image which will not be correctly recognized as components of a three-dimensional structure, or at least not perceived in their true spatial relationships. For invasive ultrasound in general the problems will be in assessing anatomy and in characterizing tissue structure and type. Both of these will benefit from the ability to image volumes of tissue. We will therefore begin by trying to clarify some basic principles of three-dimensional imaging, since it is important to recognize the problems associated with visualization of three (or more) dimensional structures.

WHAT IS A THREE-DIMENSIONAL IMAGE?

The term 'three-dimensional image' is used in a variety of different ways. In some clinical areas, such as those associated with laparoscopy, the term 'three-dimensional' implies a way of viewing surfaces stereoscopically. It is also applied widely to surface-rendered views produced by shading techniques on image workstations. Both these are limited to viewing of surfaces within the data.

We believe that the term three-dimensional image is most appropriately applied to the three-dimensional set of data. One then employs a variety of techniques in order to project representations of the three-dimensional image on a two-dimensional display. A large number of these projections is necessary in order to convey the full sense of the three-dimensional structure to the viewer, including the surface representations just mentioned, where appropriate. This is very much in agreement with the mathematical use of the term 'image', in that it is a representation in another form of the three-dimensional structure of the object. This usage can also be applied directly to an arbitrary number of dimensions.

DISPLAYING THREE-DIMENSIONAL INFORMATION

In almost all practical displays the user is presented with a two-dimensional view. This is not surprising, considering that the fundamental viewing instrument is the retina of the eye, which is two-dimensional. In using two eyes, one can form an impression of the relative position of two-dimensional surfaces in a three-dimensional space. The important limitation of this, of course, is that one cannot see behind the surface. With ultrasound imaging we are usually looking at a three-dimensional structure which contains a solid volume of echoes, and which therefore does not readily translate onto a two-dimensional projection. In routine clinical scanning, the operator forms a mental representation of the three-dimensional anatomical structure, while viewing a large series of two-dimensional slices interactively. In this case, the operator is using manual sense information about the physical location of the individual slices in building up three-dimensional subjective impressions.

The problem with conveying the full three-dimensional information on a two-dimensional screen is seen in Fig. 15.1. A solid volume of tissue is scanned to form a three-dimensional representation. The details of how this is done need not concern us at this stage. Following the paths of rays projected from the three-dimensional image onto the viewer's screen, we see that each point on the screen represents a ray projected through the data. All the data all along this ray could contribute in some way to the brightness and colour of the screen at this point. For example, we might choose the sum of all the points, the brightness of the nearest point, or any of a large number of other projections. Now for most displays there is a limit of at most 8 bits of intensity information which can be represented at any point on the screen. Suppose we have a modest array size of $128 \times 128 \times 128$ making up the three-dimensional image (data set); each ray must pass through at least 128 voxels. There is roughly 128 times too much information for the screen to display.

With simple bone images this is not a serious difficulty, since segmentation simplifies the picture – we

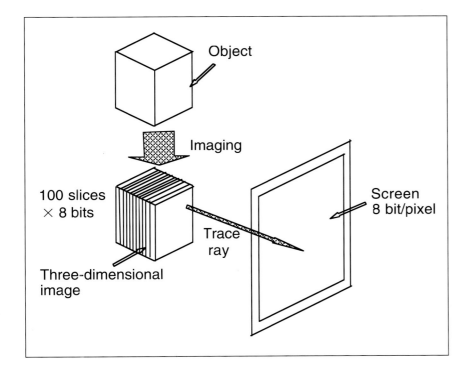

Figure 15.1 *The problem of displaying the information. Each screen display point (pixel) is generated by casting a ray through the three-dimensional image (data set), sampling typically at least 128 voxels, each of 8 bits. The display screen capacity of about 8 bits is very much less than this.*

are interested only in very restricted components, the bony surfaces. With any type of soft tissue imaging, however, this is clearly a serious problem. Obscuring the view of whatever we choose to see there will generally be a large amount of overlying structure competing for display on each pixel. It is easy to be tempted, by a clinical request for example, to produce an image to 'show all the internal three-dimensional structure'. One might then naively set about devising some clever scheme to represent a solid volume, with different tissues in different translucent colours and shades, overlooking the basic limitations of the two-dimensional display and the eye. Except in simple cases where the image is particularly simple, this cannot be done. If we were to find a way of simplifying the image by isolating particular elements, this would be no problem. However, this segmentation process is a major difficulty for ultrasound, presently largely unsolved.

What must be used instead is a selection of different types of representation, chosen to best display the particular required features, operated interactively by the viewer.

Surface Shading from Ray Tracing

Surface-shaded views such as that shown in Fig. 15.2 of a skull imaged by X-ray CT are most commonly referred to as true three-dimensional images: These are produced using segmentation by ray tracing to a simple fixed threshold, followed by artificial shading (rendering). This technique has sometimes been called 2½-dimensional imaging. The segmentation generates a surface, and where each tracing ray, projected from the viewing screen, meets the surface threshold, a shading colour is generated, determined by (1) the angle of incidence, (2) the depth, and (3) the surface character (which may be simply an adjustable parameter). In the presentation used on our own workstation software,[4] true surfaces found by thresholding are coloured using an amber scale; cut sections, either at the edge of the data or deliberately cut, are shown as grey scale in the format of the generating images. Thus the three-dimensional ultrasound images shown below usually present both natural surfaces and grey scale ultrasound cross-sections. Viewing these surface-shaded images rotating interactively on an image

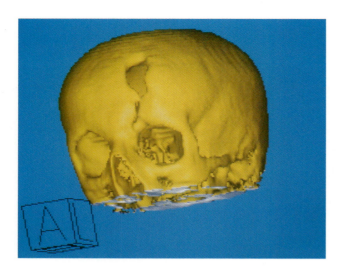

Figure 15.2 *A skull, taken from an X-ray CT study of a head, rendered as a three-dimensional surface image by ray tracing.*

workstation provides a very convincing impression of the three-dimensional structure of the surfaces.

This type of surface shading has been applied to ultrasound with good effect in cases where there are clearly defined boundaries, although the concept of applying a fixed threshold to an extended region of ultrasound image is not strictly correct. The signal level varies widely with position and orientation in most cases, so that there should be better ways of segmenting ultrasound data based on other than a fixed threshold.

Volume Rendering

Alternatively, if one wants to see the internal structure, a volume representation may be chosen. In this, one allows the ray to pass through the data and contributions from different depths are added together in some way and used to construct the image pixel on the screen. Examples include maximum intensity (MIP), minimum intensity and summed voxel projections, combined with positional or intensity weighting, used to produce pseudo-radiographic images, which give a translucent volume appearance under interactive rotation.

Multiplanar Reformatting (MPR)

This is probably the most useful means of displaying internal structure. Multiple cuts through the data along regular orthogonal planes select out particular features of anatomy in three simultaneous section images, referred to a surface view. Whilst these may not appear obviously three-dimensional, they are a valid and extremely useful way of interactively viewing a three-dimensional soft tissue image. Compare this with how one would physically examine the structure of a solid tissue specimen, say a kidney, by sectioning. Used interactively these views are equivalent to applying physical movement in examining real physical objects. There can sometimes be difficulty in retaining a perception of where the cut planes lie, in some implementations of the technique.

Rapid Sectioning

In some cases the ability to display two-dimensional sections, rapidly flipping back and forth through the image data set, provides a very useful way to perceive the internal structure, particularly if the motion required to generate the interactive selection is closely matched to the geometry of the selected planes. In this case why not simply eliminate the three-dimensional acquisition, using the transducer to show live images? This will work if this type of scanning is possible. Very often it is not, and the need to maintain careful contact, or to minimize, for example, intravascular damage, dictates a careful single-pass acquisition. It is the separation of the display function from the acquisition function which is important.

Modelling

In attempting to present images to a user it is important to consider what function is required. If the object is primary diagnosis then it is of course essential to preserve the maximum amount of information. If the user is planning some type of surgical procedure then it may be appropriate to reduce the information somewhat in order to present it in a more accessible way, e.g. by performing a volume segmentation or interpretation, and colouring the components as a diagram or 'model'. In diagnosis this pre-interpretation is not acceptable.

It is clear that we are using a number of different methods in order to convey the information from the original object which was scanned onto the screen. Nevertheless these images do give a considerable realism, particularly when the generated image can be rotated interactively on a workstation.

Extending to Multidimensional Studies

The term multidimensional imaging includes extensions of two-dimensional images into three spatial dimensions, together with spatio-temporal combinations: two and three spatial dimensions with time. The obvious application for spatio-temporal imaging is in the heart, where gating of the acquisition can provide a series of three-dimensional time samples spanning the heart cycle. This is discussed in a later section.

The term can also be used to describe techniques in which information from different modalities is combined to give a composite image or data set, requiring a more complex display of some form. The registration of image data sets from different modalities is a subject of much current interest. The two images clearly cannot be registered unless one of them is three-dimensional. A slice may be registered inside a three-dimensional image, but two slices will in general intersect only in a line. For complete fusion two three-dimensional images are merged, usually on the basis of registration of common landmarks, either natural or attached markers. This registration is a complex problem, a subject of much current research. In a typical usage, multi-modal imaging refers to a combination of anatomical and functional images, such as for example an MRI of the brain combined with a single photon emission computed tomography (SPECT) or positron emission tomography (PET) scan. The problem is to relate function or function defects to anatomical structures.

For ultrasound, multi-modality imaging could be very useful for combination of detailed anatomy, say from MRI, with a live ultrasound display. This would be particularly valuable in some types of invasive ultrasound, where one might be looking for a small lesion at surgery, identified from MRI. Having registered the live ultrasound image with the MRI, a combined display allows one to home in on the site of the lesion with the localizing ultrasound probe, guiding surgery quickly to the target.

ACQUISITION METHODS FOR THREE-DIMENSIONAL ULTRASOUND

There are several possible ways to record the three-dimensional echo pattern from a block of real tissue which we now examine briefly.

TWO-DIMENSIONAL ARRAY TRANSDUCERS

One of these possibilities is to build a two-dimensional array of transducer elements, thus extending the idea of a linear array, to produce a solid beam. This technically difficult approach has been studied by a number of groups over many years; see, for example, the recent work of von Ramm and his group.[5,6] Their devices are being developed with electronic steering and dynamic focus on receive. However, an important intrinsic limitation with these is the requirement for a large area of skin contact, with the consequent difficulty of mechanical beam steering, dealing with irregular surfaces and viewing through small spaces such as ribs.

SWEPT LINEAR ARRAYS

Alternatively we might use a standard two-dimensional system, adding an extra dimension by sweeping the transducer, in combination with sensing the position and orientation of the transducer. There are several ways to do this:

1. Hand-operated mechanical gantry system, as used in the older B-scanners.[7]
2. Mechanically driven scanning gantry. This has been used to scan the carotid artery,[8] and is also useful in laboratory studies.
3. Mechanically scanned linear arrays or sector scanners within a single hand-piece. In this way Sohn et al[9] used a rotational motion to sweep a region of three-dimensional space. Some commercial systems[10] sweep out various shaped regions using this technology. This approach provides a neat way of scanning uniformly a solid volume. However, it is subject to certain limitations. Firstly, the transducer tends to be rather bulky. Secondly, it requires the operator to hold the probe steady during the acquisition. Thirdly, and most importantly from our perspective, this requires an expensive scanning probe for each organ or scanning mode required.

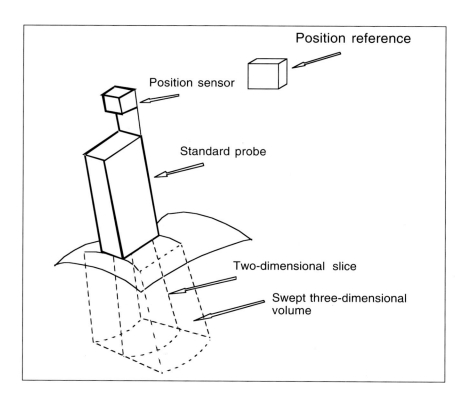

Figure 15.3 *Acquisition methods: manually swept probe with electromagnetic position-sensing*

4. An alternative approach is to use a standard probe and to record its position in space using a non-mechanical sensing technique. Several such techniques have been developed to date. Firstly, one can use an acoustic method.[11] Another possibility is to use optical techniques. A system of emitters may be sensed by a system of detectors, the relative position and orientation being determined using geometric techniques. A limitation of both this and the acoustic approach is the need to keep the optical path clear. Another sensing method which has received considerable attention depends on electromagnetic fields.

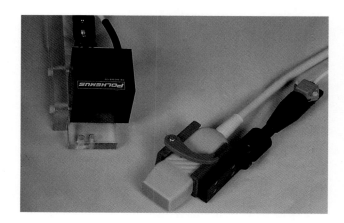

Figure 15.4 *A magnetic position sensor attached to a small linear array. The sensor is kept a small distance from the transducer to avoid electromagnetic distortion.*

ELECTROMAGNETIC POSITION-SENSING WITH LINEAR ARRAYS

The technique used by a number of groups, including ourselves, relies on commercial electromagnetic sensing systems. In these, the coupling between transmitter and sensor coil systems is used to determine their relative position and orientation (Fig. 15.3).

This technique can provide an accuracy of about 1 mm in positional location and down to the order of 0.1° in orientation over an active volume of about 1 m³. Accuracy decreases with distance, but it provides an adequate means of locating the transducer for the purpose of three-dimensional ultrasound techniques. There is of course potential interference from magnetic or electrically conductive objects and it is recommended by these manufacturers that the sensing coil is kept at some small distance from the probe itself, typically a few inches (Fig. 15.4). In this way, following a calibration for the probe tip position relative to the sensor, we can record the position and orientation of each two-dimensional image in relation to the entire scan. It is necessary, then, to calibrate the scaling and offset for pixels within the two-dimensional image, so that on reconstruction we can determine the relative position in space of each picture element or pixel of the sampled ultrasound image.

Image Information

Using a position-sensing technique we can record three-dimensional images from existing clinical scanners provided only that we can gain access to the image information. There are currently few, if any, commercial ultrasound scanners which provide digital access to digital information. However, it is perfectly feasible to extract the picture from the scanner by means of digitizing the video output. This is not particularly efficient, since the machine invariably stores the data digitally; it is converted to analogue form and then reconverted back into digital form at the acquisition system. However, we notice little, if any, extra noise in the system from this source. What this then provides is a system for acquisition of three-dimensional information from a standard scanner using standard probes.

Other Benefits from Position-Sensing

We have so far talked purely in terms of the acquisition of a three-dimensional data set. However, for ultrasound there are several significant benefits in having three-dimensional geometric information associated with the scan, other than to produce a full three-dimensional image. These include the simple labelling of two-dimensional slices with the position reference, and use of the position in space for guidance of biopsy and laser procedures, discussed below.

EXAMPLE OF A CLINICAL THREE-DIMENSIONAL ULTRASOUND SYSTEM

Producing systems to record three-dimensional images from clinical scanners is relatively straightforward, although making a system capable of clinically

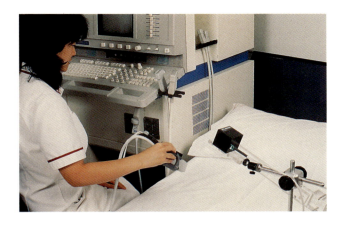

Figure 15.5 *Scanning using a manual, electromagnetically sensed system. The electromagnetic source is fixed above the patient.*

convenient operation is more challenging. With our own system[12] the position sensor is mounted on the probe and any routine clinical scanning carried out as normal. When required, three-dimensional acquisition is initiated by a combination of the control keyboard and a footswitch. The probe is moved at a steady rate over the volume to be scanned, the acquisition taking typically from 2–10 s. The speed of acquisition is determined by the rate at which the scanner can update frames. In the case of colour Doppler this is slower than for unprocessed displays, requiring slower scan speed. Since too rapid a scan speed can lead to gaps in the three-dimensional image, an audible warning is given by the acquisition system if the sample interval is too large. Fig. 15.5 illustrates how the electromagnetic sensor is attached and how the system is used.

RECONSTRUCTION

It will be useful to describe briefly the process of reconstruction of three-dimensional ultrasound images, although this has so far been studied in only a rather preliminary way, with little in the way of published results. This brief review will serve to highlight the relevance of reconstruction problems to the value of the resulting images. A detailed discussion of the technical problems is outside the scope of this text.

If we take the three-dimensional image (or data set if preferred) to consist of a rectangular array of basic elements (known as voxels), then reconstruction consists of the problem of using the component two-dimensional sample slices to assign values to the three-dimensional voxels. In the simplest case the sample slices contain elements of the width and height of a voxel, are separated by exactly the voxel depth and are sampled parallel with the desired image. Reconstruction then consists of a trivial 1 to 1 placing of two-dimensional samples into three-dimensional image voxels. If either of the dimensions do not match there are simple procedures to resample the data onto the desired three-dimensional array.

In the more general case, the two-dimensional sample slices will cross the three-dimensional image space at some oblique angle making reconstruction more difficult in principle as well as practice. In CT, by comparison, two-dimensional slices are reconstructed from one-dimensional samples on a regular though oblique grid. In this case the samples are isotropic projection values, which are of equal weight. There are well-defined reconstruction procedures which transform from the linear projections to the tomogram.

In the case of manual three-dimensional ultrasound scan reconstruction, the samples will not be uniform and they may be anisotropic in the sense that a voxel sampled from different directions may give different values. Extreme cases will result in voxels either (1) having no samples, i.e. having data gaps, or (2) having multiple samples.

Gaps cause visually distracting artifacts in the resulting displays, and the best solution is to not allow any, by means of adequate sampling. However, this may not always be either feasible or necessary. It is possible to fill gaps by interpolation from nearest samples.

In the case where the voxel has been sampled more than once there is the problem of how to assign a value. Maximum, mean and various other possibilities, such as a measure of anisotropy, may be used. It may be that the different values obtained are useful in different ways; for example, the anisotropy of back-scattering would be of significance to imaging of muscle, where the level of echoes is normally highly anisotropic. In diseases such as muscular dystrophy this order is lost. In such a case suitable reconstruction could produce a map of the anisotropy of the tissue. There is clearly a case for using several different types of reconstruction, depending on the characteristics being sought.

RAPID RECONSTRUCTIONS

In some cases it is useful to reconstruct using simple rapid methods, e.g. if there is no accurate position information or a very rapid image is required. In the case of three-dimensional IVUS, for example, there is currently no way of providing directional information about the transducer. Rapid reconstruction assumes that successive planes are approximately parallel, and a three-dimensional image is obtained simply by stacking these together. This procedure clearly does not provide geometric accuracy, but is often useful in making an assessment, prior to making a full reconstruction, which is currently fairly time-consuming.

ACCURACY OF RECONSTRUCTION

The magnetic position sensor operates with surprisingly good accuracy, considering the complicated nature of the magnetic field from a coil and its decrease with distance. However, with present systems errors can show up in angle measurements, particularly at larger distances from the transmitter source. The accuracy is also made worse by the need to calibrate the setting up of the sensor relative to the probe tip. This can be a practical problem of some difficulty. Another problem with current scanners is the calibration of the image geometry, since errors in the two-dimensional image scale and offset cause position errors in reconstruction. The effect of all these is most noticeable when attempts are made to do precise reconstructions from widely different angles, as in compound scanning.

We have so far tried to avoid large compounding, preferring to use almost parallel samples wherever possible, unless there are no overlapping scans, as for example, in transrectal and transvaginal scanning, where the reconstructions do not overlie each other.

IMAGE PROCESSING

Image processing in the present context includes such procedures as segmentation, speckle reduction and intensity remapping. It is important to recognize that any processing can at best preserve the initial information content. Most processes, particularly smoothing, decrease the information. This may be desirable in some cases. If there is an image cluttered with noise, the observer's visual perception 'channel' may be overloaded, and detail may consequently be missed. Smoothing may therefore be appropriate to match the image information to a subsequent stage of processing (observation in this case), where there is a limitation in capacity.

The loss of information may not be apparent at first. It may turn out, however, that after smoothing there are details missing, or that geometric accuracy is reduced. It is always essential to display unprocessed images together with processed, in order that misinterpretations do not occur as a result of image processing.

SPECKLE IN THREE-DIMENSIONAL IMAGES

The phenomenon of speckle is very apparent in most two-dimensional ultrasound images. It is not yet generally agreed to what extent speckle can be used to characterize tissue, or whether on the contrary it is entirely useless and to be removed. Speckle characteristics depend on the existence of tissue structures below the resolution limit of the system, the signal characteristics of the particular probe and detection system, and the effects of overlying tissues. These effects result in apparent fine image texture which bears little or no relation to identifiable physical structures. The speckle pattern is sometimes found to be different for different tissue types, e.g. between tumour and normal tissue. However, the question as to whether the speckle pattern can serve to make reliable quantitative differentiation has not yet been resolved. Currently, one approach is to use speckle reduction of some form in order to replace the speckle structure by some smoother representation.

SPECKLE REDUCTION

It would appear that in three-dimensions we have extra information available as to whether a given image texture element is due to a real physical structure or due to three-dimensional speckle. Speckle formation is always a three-dimensional process, so that in analysing it either visually or quantitatively, the availability of the full context of each voxel ought to be important. So far there appear to have been few attempts to study speckle structures from three-dimensional image data sets, although two-dimensional speckle smoothing, using a statistical method due to Bamber and Cook-Martin,[13] has been applied

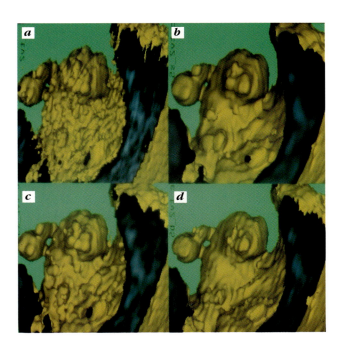

Figure 15.6 *Effects of speckle smoothing on surface views. (a) The effect of speckle interference causes artifactually roughened surfaces. Effects of various smoothing algorithms are seen in (b – d).*

in producing three-dimensional surface views by our own group.

The effect of speckle on surface smoothness is often very noticeable (Fig. 15.6). It is clear that there can be a strong motivation to remove this structure, from a subjective point of view. Analytically, the removal of speckle will remove information from the image, and unless very special conditions are used this information could be of clinical significance. Improvement results from the reduction in the distracting 'clutter' of high-frequency noise through the visual pathway, which tends to depress the signal visibility of real structures. However, in performing any type of signal or image processing, one should always present the viewer with the raw as well as the processed data sets, in order to be sure that vital information is not lost.

We have had good results from applying the Bamber speckle smoothing technique, in spite of the fact that this method was developed with the aim of leaving boundaries intact. In many cases this produces quite a striking improvement in the apparent surface smoothness. An example of the effect of different degrees of speckle smoothing on surfaces can be seen in Figs. 15.6a–d. The images become cleaner but some information may be lost.

TISSUE CHARACTERIZATION

There has been a major body of work carried out since the early 1970s directed towards the use of ultrasound techniques for characterizing tissues. Many sonologists make assessments of tissue types on the basis of the speckle structure in two-dimensional images. How valid this subjective procedure is still remains to be seen.

Quantitative tissue characterization covers an area which is too broad to survey here. Measured parameters include: speckle statistics from two-dimensional processed images; frequency spectral analysis of radio-frequency data; velocity variations; attenuation mapping; and other means of parameterization.

In general these methods have not yet produced reliable clinically useful information. This is because the signals received for analysis are subject to various interfering processes, including: (1) instrumental limitations 'colouring the signal'; (2) overlying tissues similarly masking the characteristics sought; (3) inadequate bandwidth; and (4) inadequate sampling of tissues. And, of course there is the possibility that the sought tissue differences are simply not reflected in acoustic parameters.

Several of these important restrictions are potentially reduced using invasive methods, particularly when applied with three-dimensional imaging. As remarked earlier, the probes are generally higher bandwidth, there is minimal overlying tissue, and three-dimensional acquisitions and processing should allow better discrimination of large- and small-scale structures. The potential benefit will be in providing a real-time local tissue assessment, with the possibility of better outlining of diseased anatomy.

COMPUTED TOMOGRAPHY WITH ULTRASOUND (UCT)

The use of tomographic reconstruction methods forms a natural extension to the problem of reconstruction of a discrete set of samples from compound acquisitions in three dimensions. This was first demonstrated by Greenleaf et al.[14] It is natural to expect that when hardware becomes more readily and cheaply available, it will be possible for the entire three-dimensional image to be acquired in radio-frequency format, allowing full three-dimensional processing and reconstruction, including synthetic aperture methods to generate optimum image quality.

In UCT the reconstruction may be made in principle either from transmission or back-scatter information. In the case of transmission, there is a close analogy with the principles of conventional X-ray CT. There are, however, some important special problems. In tissue, both propagation velocity and attenuation vary across the scanned object. Therefore, both attenuation maps and velocity maps could be generated, offering different diagnostic information. The variability of velocity, however, turns both types of reconstruction into mathematically 'ill-posed' problems. That is to say, there is usually not a unique solution to the problem of reconstruction by inversion of the data. Sound may take different (curved) paths between source and detector, depending on local elastic properties. Determining which paths, and the distribution of attenuation along these paths, may not be possible from the limited amount of numerical information acquired from measurements which are remote from the regions themselves. In extreme cases, problems with bone and air will preclude transmission tomography from imaging correctly in many regions. For a detailed review of these methods see Wade.[15]

In conventional back-scatter imaging there may equally be lack of information about the distribution of velocities. The effect of lack of information in this case will be to distort geometrically the back-scatter image. This is much less severe than the ambiguities introduced into transmission CT reconstruction.

In back-scatter tomography, by comparison, there is the possibility of reconstruction using a map of velocity to correct the geometry. Jago and Whittingham[16] have produced some excellent images by this means (Fig. 15.7). Results such as these suggest that compound reconstructions from three-dimensional acquired data could allow significant improvements to the three-dimensional image on post-processing, by fitting velocity and attenuation maps during reconstruction.

ULTRASOUND CONTRAST AGENTS

Use of ultrasound contrast agents, based on stabilized microbubbles, greatly enhances the reflections from vascular, ductal and cystic spaces. This can be used to generate much more sensitive colour Doppler

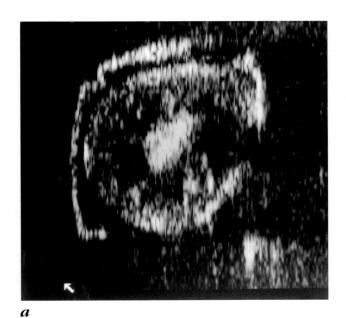 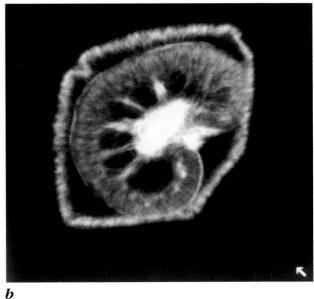

a   *b*

Figure 15.7 *(a) B-scan of ox kidney in saline. (b) A reconstruction of a kidney imaged using pulse-echo UCT methods. A velocity map was used to correct the echo positions obtained from scanning from many different angles (from Jago and Whittingham[16] with permission).*

images. When used with three-dimensional imaging, there is benefit from increased Doppler signal, e.g. in prostate studies, as will be described later. There is also benefit in filling cavities such as the uterus with contrast, in order to permit their rendering as positive rather than as negative spaces.

In addition to simple direct use of contrast agents, some preliminary work has been reported on harmonic imaging. In this, a dual-frequency method is employed, with the received signal being selected at a harmonic of the transmitted signal. The scattering of acoustic pulses from microbubbles is very non-linear, so that significant amounts of energy are generated at harmonic frequencies. This results in images which have a very high signal to noise ratio for blood containing contrast.

CLINICAL APPLICATIONS

In the following sections we try to show that although there is much still to be done in developing three-

dimensional ultrasound techniques, there is good reason to believe that this work will be justified by the results to be obtained. Not all these examples are taken from invasive ultrasound, since in some cases noninvasive material is needed to illustrate better the potential.

THREE-DIMENSIONAL INTRAVASCULAR ULTRASOUND

The new technique of IVUS has been described in more detail in an earlier chapter. There are good reasons for believing that extending this to three dimensions will greatly enhance the clinical value.

In order to record a three-dimensional image using this endoluminal scanner, the catheter is withdrawn steadily so that the two-dimensional cross-sections sweep through the volume of interest. The volume is sampled at fixed axial distances by recording two-dimensional cross-sectional images at these known positions. Kitney[17], Rosenfeld et al[18] and Chong et al[19] amongst others, have used variants of this method.

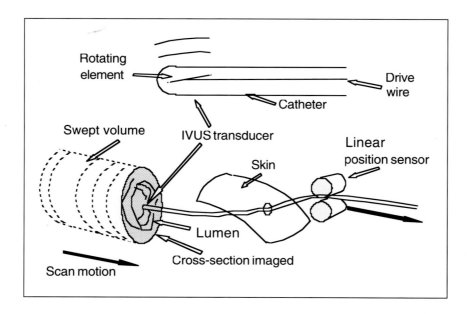

Figure 15.8 *Intravascular ultrasound: three-dimensional image acquisition. The probe axial position is recorded during withdrawal. Radial position and orientation are not available.*

Both single-element rotating transducers and radial arrays have been used in three-dimensional IVUS. Currently the rotating element is more commonly used, although development work is still proceeding on the array approach. Sensing the position of the transmitting element is more of a problem than in the case of a large external transducer. Ideally one wishes to know the absolute position of each individual echo from the three-dimensional set. In fact this is difficult and is not achieved currently because the available position coordinates are only (1) the azimuthal rotation angle of the catheter drive wire, which may differ from the azimuthal position of the transducer element, due to the rotational compliance of the wire, and (2) the axial position of the guiding catheter measured externally to the patient. This is indirectly related to the axial position of the transducer, due to the flexure of the catheter. The compliance effect of (1) causes azimuthal distortions of the three-dimensional image, and errors in (2) cause distortions in the linear spacing of sections.

The missing angular and position coordinates require that the reconstructed three-dimensional image be constrained to an assumed straight line set. The net effect of these distortions may not be important unless accurate measurements are being sought.

Azimuthal positions are taken implicitly from the two-dimensional images; the axial position may be recorded as shown in Fig. 15.8. A position encoder is used to sense the rotation of a pair of guide rollers, through which the IVUS catheter is drawn. Although this is technically adequate, the use of the sensing system adjacent to the introducer is clumsy. In fact, if accurate axial positional information is not required, e.g. in obtaining only the relative topography, a satisfactory alternative is simply to withdraw the catheter a fixed distance in a measured time at uniform speed. In view of the other position uncertainties this is in many cases adequate for good qualitative three-dimensional images. The long-term solution to the position-sensing will be to use an electromagnetic sensing scheme, similar to that described earlier. In view of the necessarily very small size of the probe tip, this electromagnetic system would be technically difficult, requiring the use of a large or extended set of transmitter coils. Such a technique has been demonstrated for tracking endoscopes in the body.

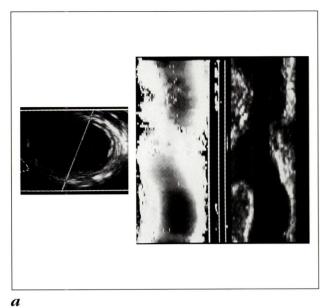

a

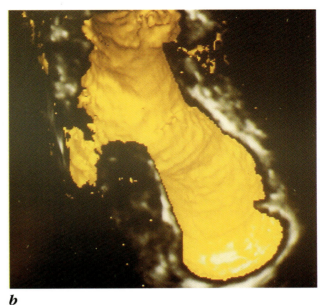

b

Figure 15.9 *(a) Coronal reformat of intravascular ultrasound data (common femoral artery bifurcation). (b) A three-dimensional view of (a), surface rendered.*

Reconstruction of the data consists of simple stacking of the recorded sections, together with any required interpolation, e.g. speckle smoothing or other three-dimensional image conditioning. Display is again by one of the methods already described.

Application of three-dimensional techniques to endoluminal ultrasound offers a number of important advantages:

- Since endovascular examinations typically involve diseased vessels, repeated passes of the probe up and down the vessel pose a serious risk of dissection or other damage. Use of three-dimensional acquisitions to record the entire structure from a single pass, taking a few seconds, followed by off-line study minimizes this risk.
- The three-dimensional image set shows considerably more coherent structure from within the lumen and from within the vessel wall.
- Since the rotating element IVUS probe is longer than it is wide, there is potentially better resolution axially than transversely. This is clearly seen in three-dimensional images.

Fig. 15.9a shows the transverse and coronal sections and the interior surface of the common femoral artery, including the bifurcation. Surface-rendered images such as that of Fig. 15.9b show the disposition of atherosclerotic plaque on the vessel wall. There are several important features to be seen here. The bifurcation is visible. However, although it appears possible to 'see into' the branch vessel, the short range of the 20-MHz ultrasound restricts the depth of this view. More importantly in this case evidence is seen of a spiral band of plaque deposited on the wall immediately above the bifurcation. In this study, the plaque was not severe. However, this illustrates a possible application of the visualization of plaque structures prior to interventional procedures. Current developments of combined angioplasty–IVUS systems are clearly relevant to this problem. The potential also for studying the wall structure following interventions, with a view to assessment and planning of further treatment, is also apparent.

The surface views do not give any guide to the internal structure of the vessel wall. As we stressed earlier, in order to see all the information in the three-dimensional image it is necessary to view several different types of display. The longitudinal layered structure of the vessel wall is much more apparent from longitudinal MPR views (Fig. 15.9a) than from the transverse sections. The use of three dimensions gives a much better guide to which components of apparent structure are real and which are artifactual. In the still images shown here we see this less obviously than when using an interactive workstation, when the entire volume can be presented rapidly in this way to give a much more vivid impression of the 'real' structure.

Some groups have thought it desirable to employ some form of tissue characterization, combined with colour coding to segment surfaces according to some automatic interpretation of tissue type.[20] The 'modelled' images produced by this means should, of course, always be shown together with images containing the maximum amount of unprocessed information. This is because the tissue typing can never be precise using ultrasound, and will usually result in a significant amount of misclassification. The best this type of processing can achieve is to draw attention to possible areas of interest, which must then be examined using unprocessed image data.

OBSTETRICS AND FETAL IMAGING

Some of the most useful applications of three-dimensional ultrasound lie in the traditional ultrasound applications in obstetrics, where early detection of abnormalities by visualization and measurement is most important. Fetal movement is always a potential problem. We have found that it may be minimized by the facility for rapid and easy acquisitions, allowing multiple repeats.

Several three-dimensional studies of the fetus and embryo have been reported at various stages of development.[21–23] The image quality of these early studies is enhanced by means of the use of transvaginal (TV) scanning where appropriate.

We have obtained images of embryos and fetuses of all ages from a few weeks to term. In seeking surface views of the head, trunk and limbs, scanning transabdominally at 16–20 weeks gives very good results. The fetus is well developed at this stage, yet is normally immersed in sufficient amniotic fluid to provide for clear separation from the uterine wall and placenta. Figure 15.10 shows two views of a 12-week fetus. Details of the face, trunk and limbs are clearly seen from these surface views. Using MPR in

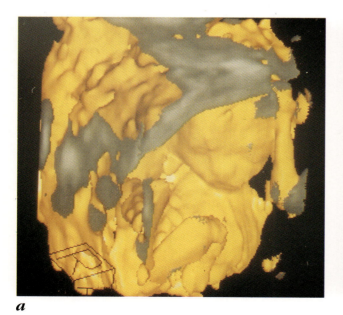
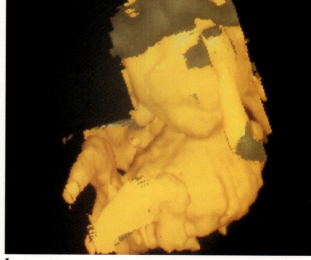

a *b*

Figure 15.10 *Two views of a 12-week fetus.*

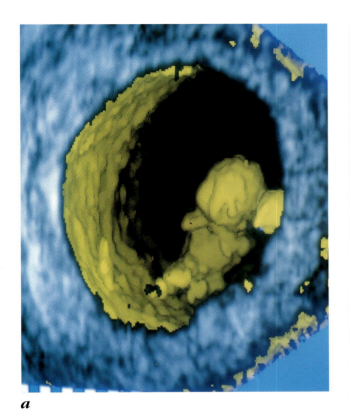

a

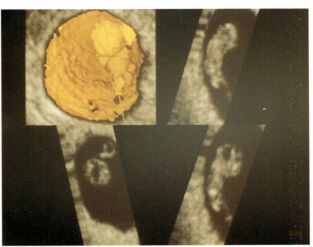

b

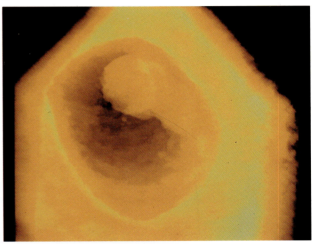

c

Figure 15.11 *(a) A 20-mm embryo (8 weeks gestation). Full three-dimensional surface-rendered view. (b) Simultaneous multiplanar reformatted view of (a). The sections are moved in real time by a pointing device. (c) A summed voxel (pseudo-radiographic) projection of (a). Rotation gives a translucent impression of internal structures.*

registration with these surface views, the internal anatomy can also be clearly seen post-scan.

By surgically editing the skull, detailed surface-rendered views of intracranial features may be seen. These images are best seen dynamically, using the interactive workstation display, when the three-dimensional anatomical relationships are more clearly manifest.

At greater gestational age there may be parts of the fetus in close proximity to the walls and placenta, making segmentation impossible for surface views using our present methods. Development of segmentation based on local texture, required to separate out tissues in contact, may prove possible. However, in

this case the surface position will be based on some statistical texture measure, necessarily derived from an extended spatial region. The resolution would not be expected to be good in this case.

It is important to note that it is only the striking surface views which are lost in this case. Displaying fetal anatomy by means of multiplanar reformatting, or rendering of internal structures, is likely to provide much more clinically useful information in any case. The MPR will allow both visualization and measurement of selected anatomical features.

For very young fetuses and embryos, the use of TV scanning provides access to some remarkably good early detail. The embryo of Fig. 15.11 is about 20 mm long (8 weeks gestational age). It was imaged with an Acuson 128 (5-MHz TV probe). Details of the anatomy which can be clearly seen include: the forebrain and hindbrain; the open neural groove; incompletely formed limb buds; and the bulge in the umbilicus due to the gut, which is at this stage migrating into the abdomen. These three images illustrate different display methods, although the interactive viewing facility of the workstation is highly important in conveying fully the different features shown in each. Fig. 15.11a shows the uterine wall, partly cut away, in grey scale cross-section as described earlier, in addition to the surface view of the fetal anatomy. Fig. 15.11b illustrates the visualization using MPR in conjunction with the surface image.

There is a clear advantage in scanning using the TV probe at this age, since transabdominal scans generally show much poorer quality images, due to the problems of beam distortion described earlier. Figs. 15.12 and 15.13 show embryos of 3 mm and 10 mm obtained using the TV probe.

MULTIDIMENSIONAL ECHOCARDIOGRAPHY

Owing to the problems of its motion, accessibility and specialized problems, imaging of the heart is usually treated separately from other clinical applications. To record all the information requires a four-dimensional scan, a procedure which is quite straightforward in principle, though technically difficult, using ECG gating. Assuming the heart moves only as a result of its own regular cycle (i.e. no respiration or patient movements), the acquisition of two-dimensional sections from a set of samples of chosen cardiac phases at each slice position may be used to reconstruct a four-dimensional image. Notice how this use of the term image naturally extends the usage of 'three-dimensional imaging' as defined earlier. Note also the important caveat about the need for strictly cyclic motion. Any beat-to-beat motion irregularity will cause blurring and other problems and may not be readily detectable from the image. In performing this type of acquisition it is necessary to use some independent means of assessing regularity, e.g. beat regularity from the ECG, and of respiratory motion, by some form of monitoring.

Reconstruction presents problems which require sophisticated solutions. For example the cardiac motion, even when regular, includes rotations, so that a section fixed in space will not be fixed in the heart. Display of the results of such a four-dimensional scan could include, for example, the M-mode traces in any chosen plane in addition to the planar sections at each selected phase, together with all the

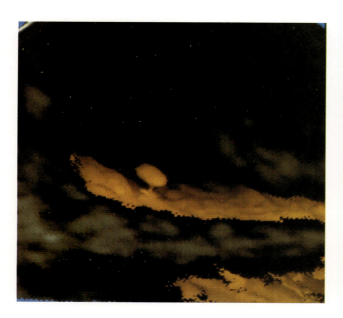

Figure 15.12 *A 3-mm embryo.*

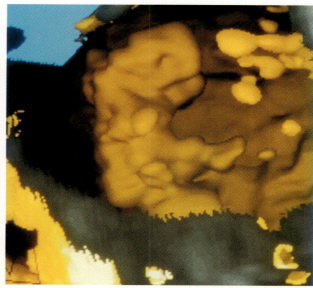

Figure 15.13 *A 10-mm embryo.*

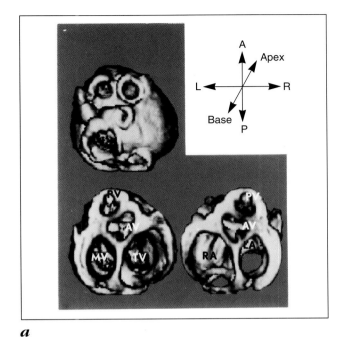

a

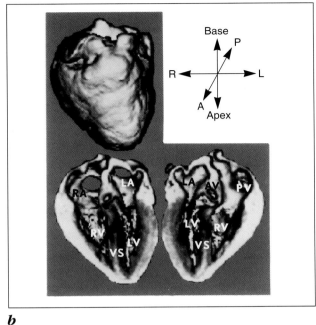

b

Figure 15.14 *Three-dimensional images of a canine heart, compound scanned, in vitro. (From Beloblavek et al,[26] by courtesy Mayo Clinic Publications.)*

two-dimensional representations of three-dimensional structures already described, now at each of the heart phases. These also offer the potential for making analytical displays, e.g. of wall motion abnormalities, in terms of phase and amplitude of local motion. There is clearly a great deal of information to be conveyed to the viewer.

Significant studies of the motion of the chambers of the heart have been made by a number of workers over many years, notably Greenleaf and co-workers.[24] King et al[11] used a transabdominal system for recording sections of the left ventricle (LV) using an acoustic position sensor. In their case the display required manual outlining of the walls in each plane, producing a wire-frame type of display. Moritz et al[25] used similar techniques in studies measuring the chamber volume of the LV, reporting accuracies of about 1 per cent on excised bovine hearts.

More recently it has been possible to scan the heart using more invasive transoesophageal methods. Here the much superior acoustic window achieved invasively allows use of higher frequencies and there is freedom from the restrictions imposed by overlying ribs and fat. Greenleaf and co-workers[24] have been developing techniques for recording, segmentation and display of the adult heart in three and four dimensions. Fig. 15.14 shows one of their recent images, obtained by compound scanning a canine heart in vitro. This represents a standard against which other images must be judged. A more complete review of three-dimensional echocardiography is given in Beloblavek et al.[26]

FETAL ECHOCARDIOGRAPHY

There are more difficult problems facing attempts to acquire three- and four-dimensional fetal echocardiograms. The fetal ECG is not readily accessible for monitoring the heart phase without invasive attachment of ECG electrodes. Fetal motion is unpredictable and not easily monitored independently of the scan being performed, so that certain types of subtle non-cardiac motion may go undetected and distort the scan. Also, the motion in combination with the small size makes reconstruction into a coherent image very difficult.

Nevertheless there are motivations for attempting to do this. The acquisition of a good three-dimensional image from any direction would allow reconstruction of a four-chamber view to be made from the image after scanning. It would also be very useful to be able to estimate various size parameters in cases of suspected anomaly. Measurements of gross heart size and chamber volumes might be possible and would provide important information for diagnosis and clinical monitoring. There are, however, serious problems to be overcome even after the gating problem has been solved. The outer border may not be well defined in relation to adjacent tissues. The positions of the internal ventricular borders will be subject to large relative errors by virtue of the small size. Progress in this depends on the development of suitable segmentation methods.

COLOUR FLOW DOPPLER IN THREE-DIMENSIONS

The simplest example of segmentation can be obtained from colour Doppler images. Given position-sensing using one of the methods described, we require to visualize the shape of the lumen of a vessel. By digitizing the video from one of the colour channels (usually red or blue) associated with the Doppler coding, we have a simple structure based on the blood flow, segmented already by the ultrasound machine; see, for example, Picot et al.[8]

However, there are problems and limitations associated with this technique. The segmented edge is not well defined, for several reasons. The resolution of the colour flow border is usually fairly low intrinsically. The effect of cardiac modulation causes regular changes in border position, which will produce a rippled surface unless cardiac gating is applied. In short these will only produce useful images when the pathology is relatively gross.

COLOUR DOPPLER AMPLITUDE IMAGING

New variants of colour flow imaging are becoming available, using Doppler flow parameters not previously used. It is possible, for example, to display either the amplitude or the power of the signal from moving scatterers in the blood. This mode is known by various terms including 'power Doppler', or 'colour Doppler energy' (CDE) (as used by Acuson). The image intensity derives from the number of scatterers moving above some threshold velocity and is largely independent of the angle of insonation. Not being sensitive to flow direction, these images are useful for imaging low flow rates and turbulence, and are effective for collections of small vessels not seen under normal colour mapping due to the 'averaging out' of forward and reverse flows over small volumes.

PROSTATE IMAGING

The most important requirement of prostate imaging is to detect and delineate the distribution of tumour. Prostate carcinomas usually have an abnormal blood supply which can be easily rendered visible by contrast-enhanced colour Doppler or latterly by Doppler amplitude imaging. Using real-time techniques it can be difficult to visualize the pattern of blood flow, which is a most important feature in

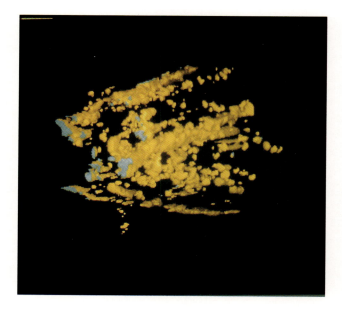

Figure 15.15 *Prostatic blood flow, using contrast agent. This type of image is much more informative when rotated interactively on a workstation.*

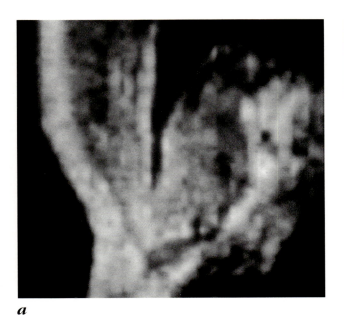
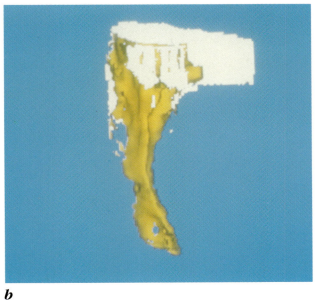

a   *b*

Figure 15.16 *(a) Sagittal reformat of an interactive prostate and urethra during micturition. (b) A three-dimensional model of urethral lumen from (a).*

cancer diagnosis. Using three-dimensional techniques such as segmentation and surface rendering, the networks of supplying vessels may be readily visualized. Fig. 15.15 shows a typical example. Here the complete networks are visible together, rather than restricted sections. The static image reproduced here does not of course provide the clear three-dimensional structure seen from an interactive three-dimensional workstation, when there is access to real-time rotation.

URETHRA

The urethra may be imaged using an endoluminal probe although, as already noted, the position can only be recorded as axial translations for these devices. The proximal urethra may also be imaged in three-dimensional using a transrectal probe during micturition. Although there is the possibility of using contrast agent to aid visualization, good images are readily obtained using simply the negative contrast

of urine flow and inverting the image intensities, as seen in Fig. 15.16. This shows how the surface-rendered view and the interactively positioned sagittal section may be used to display the anatomical information.

Another interesting potential application is in the measurement of dimension and position of urethral stents (Fig. 15.17). This image illustrates the use of geometric modelling as a means of displaying solid structures. The transrectal three-dimensional image allowed identification of the stent structure which has been segmented and rendered separately from the surrounding tissue. This allows measurement of dimensions to be made from selected directions. The oval cut section visible is a section through a lobe of the prostate protruding into the bladder.

RECTUM AND ANAL SCANNING

In scanning the rectum and anal region, typical questions will relate to the degree of penetration of

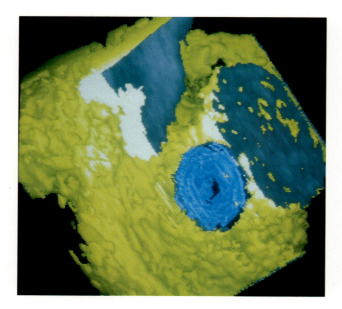

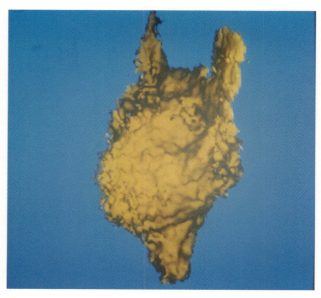

Figure 15.17 *A view from the inside of the bladder looking into the end of a urethral stent which protrudes into the bladder slightly.*

Figure 15.18 *Surface-rendered view of the endometrial cavity flattened and distorted by a large fibroid.*

tumours through the wall, damage to the anal sphincter and so forth. These will generally require images of internal tissue structures, sometimes in 'inaccessible' scan planes, which may be generated with MPR of three-dimensional images.

GYNAECOLOGY

In these studies the uterine cavity and tubes are outlined by both positive (Echovist, Schering, Berlin) and negative (saline) contrast media. Of particular interest are the precise relationships of masses such as fibroids and polyps to the endometrial cavity, when new therapies such as transendometrial resection or laser ablation are being considered.[27] Fig. 15.18 shows a typical study of a fibroid within the endometrial cavity using these methods.

Other gynaecological applications include attempts to detect and localize breast tumours using three-dimensional ultrasound.[28]

TREATMENT GUIDANCE

GUIDANCE OF BIOPSY AND LASER ABLATION

The use of three-dimensional position-sensing associated with three-dimensional ultrasound imaging provides important new techniques for guidance of biopsy needles, laser ablation and similar procedures. If the planar ultrasound images are registered using some type of position sensor then the use of a second position sensor, attached to the invasive tool enables exact registration in relation to the image.

The potential advantages attached to the use of the technique are considerable. In normal guided biopsy, the position of the needle tip is detected in the ultrasound beam from a guiding device on the probe. The needle is inserted along the same axis as the ultrasound beam. If the beam axis and the needle axis can be the same, this is a convenient technique.

However, this is frequently not the case. It is, for example, convenient to visualize through the gall bladder, but this is not an ideal route for needle puncture. If the needle can be guided by a free-hand method, then the ultrasound image can be used to locate the tool relative to the anatomy. However, to guide the tool free-hand is a considerable skill, usually possessed by experts who will usually not be available for routine procedures.

The critical guidance steps are in:

1. making the first trajectory, since steering a needle, for example, is not easy;
2. guarding against needle bending on route to the target;
3. detecting the depth of penetration.

There are several potential problems attached to the use of the technique. These relate to the various effects which could cause unexpected misregistration of the tool with the image. These include patient movement, failure to calibrate the position-sensing mechanism, distortion of the sensing device (e.g. electromagnetic, acoustic) or optical effects relevant to the position-sensing technique in operation.

We are developing the use of a patient positioning sensor, together with three-dimensional ultrasound scanning, based on the electromagnetic device already described. The sensor system in use allows up to four individual sensors, which allow the measuring of:

1. ultrasound probe;
2. tool position;
3. patient position changes;
4. electromagnetic field changes.

Although the sensing of patient gross motion allows for correction or relocation of the image, we would feel that this should be used simply as a warning mechanism. Patient movement should signal the need to restart the procedure, using new images. There is also the possibility that respiratory movements could be sensed in the same manner.

Likewise, the use of the 'spare' sensor element to detect changes in the field would only be for detecting that some unexpected environmental change had occurred, requiring restarting the whole procedure. The sensitivity to accidental distortions depends on the ability to place the distortion sensor close to the tool axis on some rigid support. It is not yet clear whether this can be done in a convenient and practical manner.

The reliable use of electromagnetic sensing techniques depends on the absence of field distortions, which is a significant uncertainty in the case where large amounts of conductive material are to be placed near the patient.

The preliminary application of this method in laboratory studies is very encouraging. In these studies a biopsy needle was guided to a target using the electromagnetic position sensor. The accuracy was such that a 5-mm target was hit 96 per cent of the time.

HEAD-UP DISPLAYS AND VIRTUAL REALITY

Systems allowing 'head-up' image displays suitable for medical image presentation are being developed commercially as well as in research laboratories. These systems provide a projected image on a semi-translucent screen or headset, such that the wearer can 'see through' the projected image. This arrangement has been exploited for head-up instrument displays in aircraft for some time.

What can be readily envisaged is a scheme whereby an image of internal anatomy, produced from some type of scanner, either before or during surgery, is projected onto a direct view of the anatomical surface. This could be kept in registration with the motion of the operator and the patient by means of motion sensors of the form already described. In this way an invasive procedure could proceed with the operator having a continuous view of the target internal anatomy, correctly registered and projected on the overlying structure, whilst carrying out the procedure. Suitable displays would include three-dimensional ultrasound images generated before and during the procedure.

Ohbuchi et al[29] reported the development of a system for viewing ultrasound images projected onto the abdomen of obstetric patients. In initial demonstrations the system was limited by the speed of updating the image, which caused a noticeable lag-induced distortion. This is a temporary technical limitation, soluble with developing technology, should the method prove useful.

LASER-GENERATED ULTRASOUND

One of the limitations associated with intravascular ultrasound, discussed earlier, is that there is currently no forward view. This is quite a disadvantage, particularly in relation to interventional approaches to unblocking arteries. IVUS cannot see the problem stenosis if it is too severe to fit through.

In a novel approach being used in conjunction with laser recanalization of arteries, Beard et al[30] are developing optical methods to generate and receive ultrasound pulses along the vessel axis. The laser generates an acoustic pulse by very rapidly heating an absorbing fluid at the end of the delivery fibre. This thermo-acoustic pulse propagates forward, generating reflections at interfaces. The low-level returning echoes are detected using an interferometric method, via the same fibre link. This method is currently only one-dimensional, but the tissue interrogated is that which is directly in line for laser ablation. Ideally the method will enable assessment of how much plaque, and of what type, lies ahead of the laser. Perforation of arterial wall is a serious problem for laser recanalization, and might be prevented by use of this technique.

OTHER DEVELOPMENTS

ACOUSTIC MICROSCOPY

The term acoustic microscopy can refer to a variety of techniques, the most common being the scanning acoustic microscope, in which a high-frequency acoustic beam is brought to a sharp focus by a large f-number lens. The sample is mechanically scanned in a raster pattern over the thin section defined by the focal zone. Then either transmission is recorded by means of an identical lens behind the sample, or reflection is measured at the transmitter.

The frequency used can vary from tens of megahertz to several gigahertz, thus overlapping the high-resolution end of pulse-echo imaging. Images based on velocity/phase differences or attenuation can be obtained for a wide range of different materials. To date the principal applications have been in semiconductor technology; no routine medical applications appear to have been developed in spite of considerable early interest. The obvious application to invasive procedures would be in performing histological examination of samples of tissue. The advantages would include the rapid availability of results, without the requirement of tissue staining.

Foster et al[31] have reviewed the possibilities for ultrasound back-scatter microscopy, using a variety of high-frequency transducers, including those associated with intravascular imaging. Clearly there is little qualitative difference between most of this and conventional two-dimensional section imaging. Foster shows some C-scan images of a tumour nodule, which bear an obvious relationship to conventional microscope images. These could themselves be generated from three-dimensional techniques similar to those described above.

It is conceivable that the development of very high-frequency, catheter-based probes, operated in conjunction with three-dimensional scanning, could allow real-time microscopic biopsy analyses before, during and after interventions.

TEACHING

As we have mentioned already, a major advantage of the technique of storing ultrasound in three-dimensional format is that the stored information may be interrogated by means of a pseudo-scan. That is, if the stored echographic information is located at some virtual position in space, then scanning using a virtual probe attached to a position sensor allows the generation of realistic two-dimensional ultrasound images. This has a number of uses, teaching being particularly important, where hands-on experience of abnormalities is essential.

Teaching in obstetrics, for example, will ideally involve presenting the student with a wide range of cases of abnormal fetal development. Even when the suitable case is available, the procedure of calling in students to scan a mother who has just been informed of an abnormality is highly undesirable. What is now possible is for a database of abnormalities to be acquired using three-dimensional acquisition techniques. These studies will need to be scanned carefully in order to allow reconstruction with good resolution from a range of different orientations, i.e. to provide a nearly isotropic data set. The teaching sessions can then allow the student to scan in two-dimensional, using the three-dimensional data set to produce two-dimensional sections in real time. There are practical difficulties in simulating the patient's physical surface in registration with the images; however, this need not be important, compared with the real problem of choosing the correct views.

The availability of teaching facilities in invasive and guided procedures will also be a considerable advantage. These new techniques provide an apparently much easier way of performing complex and risky procedures. It is therefore vital that training and evaluation of operator performance is provided in a readily accessible manner. This appears to be readily possible for most of the techniques described in this chapter.

ACKNOWLEDGEMENTS

The images presented here, unless otherwise acknowledged, were produced on workstations developed by the MGI group, Medical Physics Department, University College London. Clinical material was provided by colleagues in the Radiology Department, The Middlesex Hospital, London, under the direction of Dr W. R. Lees.

REFERENCES

1. Baum G, Greenwood I, Orbital lesion localisation by three-dimensional ultrasonography, *NY State J Med* (1961) **61**:4149–57.

2. Greenleaf JF, Three-dimensional imaging in ultrasound, J Med Syst (1982) **6**:579–89.

3. Udupa JK, Herman G, *3D Imaging in Medicine* (CRC Press: Florida, 1991).

4. Tan AC, Richards R, Developing the MGI (Medical Graphics Imaging) workstation: a multi-transputer based medical graphics system. *Transputer* (1991) **2**:801–12.

5. von Ramm OT, Smith SW, Pavy HG, High-speed ultrasound volumetric imaging system. Part II: Parallel processing and image display, *IEEE Trans Ultrasonics* (1991) **38**:109–15.

6. Smith SW, Pavy HG, von Ramm OT, High-speed ultrasound volumetric imaging system. Part I: Transducer design and beam steering, *IEEE Trans Ultrasonics* (1991) **38**:100–8.

7. Baba K, Satoh K, Sakamoto S et al, Development of an ultrasonic system for three-dimensional reconstruction of the fetus, *J Perinat Med* (1989) **17**:19–24.

8. Picot PA, Rickey DW, Mitchell R et al, Three-dimensional colour Doppler imaging of the carotid artery, *SPIE* (1991) **1444**:206–13.

9. Sohn Ch, Grotepass J, Swobodnik W, MoglichKeiten der 3dimensionalen Ultraschalldarstellung, *Ultraschall* (1989) **10**:307–13.

10. Kirbach D, Whittingham TA, 3D ultrasound – the Kretztechnik Voluson approach, *Eur J Ultrasound* (1994) **1**:85–9.

11. King DL, King DL, Shao MY, Three dimensional spatial registration and interactive display of position and orientation of real-time ultrasound images, *J Ultrasound Med* (1990) **9**:525–32.

12. Gardener JE, Three-dimensional imaging of soft tissues using ultrasound. *In 3D Imaging for Medicine: IEE Colloquium Digest 91/083* (Institute of Electrical Engineers: London, 1991).

13. Bamber JC, Cook-Martin G, Texture analysis and speckle reduction in medical echography, *SPIE International Symposium on Pattern Recognition and Acoustical Imaging* (1987) **768**:120–7.

14. Greenleaf JF, Johnson SA, Lee SL et al, Algebraic reconstruction of spatial distributions of acoustic absorption within tissues from their two-dimensional acoustic projections, *Acoust Hologr* (1974) **5**:591–603.

15. Wade G, Ultrasonic imaging by reconstructive tomography, *Acoust Imag* (1980) **9**:379–431.

16. Jago JR, Whittingham TA, The use of measured acoustic speed distributions in reflection ultrasound CT, *Phys Med Biol* (1992) **37**:2139–42.

17. Kitney R, Moura L, Straughan K, 3-D visualisation of arterial structures using ultrasound and voxel modelling, *Int J Cardiac Imag* (1989) **4**:135–43.

18. Rosenfeld K, Losordo DW, Ramaswamy K et al, Three-dimensional reconstruction of human coronary and peripheral arteries from images recorded during two-dimensional intravascular ultrasound examination, *Circulation* (1991) **84**:1938–56.

19. Chong WK, Lawrence R, Gardener J, Lees WR, The appearance of normal and abnormal arterial morphology on intravascular ultrasound, *Clin Radiol* (1993) **48**:301–6.

20. Burrell CJ, Kitney RI, Rothman MT et al, Intravascular ultrasound imaging and three-dimensional modelling of arteries, *Echocardiography* (1990) **7**:475-84.

21. Kelly IMG, Lees WR, Gardener JE, Three-dimensional foetal ultrasound, *Lancet* (1992) **339**:1062–4.

22. Pretorius DH, Jaffe JS, Nelson TR, Three-dimensional sonography of the fetus, *Radiology* (1990) **177**:194.

23. Nelson TR, Jaffe JS, Pretorius DH, 3D Ultrasound of the fetus, *J Gynaecol Obstet* (1992) **2**:166–74.

24. McCann HA, Sharp JC, Kinter TM et al, Multidimensional imaging for cardiology, *Proc IEEE* (1988) **76**:1063–71.

25. Moritz WE, Pearlman AS, McCabe DH et al, An ultrasonic technique for imaging the ventricle in three dimensions and calculating its volume, *IEEE Trans Biomed Eng* (1983) **30**:482–92.

26. Belohlavek M, Foley DA, Gerber TC et al, Three- and four-dimensional cardiovascular imaging: a new era for echocardiography, *Mayo Clin Proc* (1993) **68**:221–40.

27. Balen F, Allen CM, Gardener J et al, 3-Dimensional reconstruction of the uterine cavity, *Br J Radiol* (1993) **66**:592–9.

28. Rotten D, Levaillant JM, Constancis E et al, Three-dimensional imaging of solid breast tumours with ultrasound: preliminary data and analysis of its possible contribution to the understanding of the standard two-dimensional sonographic images, *Ultrasound Obstet. Gynaecol* (1991) **1**:384–90.

29. Ohbuchi R, Chen D, Fuchs H, Incremental volume reconstruction and rendering for 3D ultrasound imaging, *SPIE Proc Visualisation in Biomedical Computing* (1992) **1808**:312.

30. Beard PC, Cornforth RJ, Essenpreis M, Mills TN, Photoacoustic response of post mortem human aorta to 10 ns laser pulses, *Lasers in Medicine – Proceedings of the 11th International Congress, Munich* (Springer-Verlag: Berlin, 1993) 148–51.

31. Foster FS, Pavlin CJ, Lockwood GR et al, Principles and applications of ultrasound backscatter microscopy, *IEEE Trans Ultrasonics* (1993) **40**:608–16.

Index

WITHDRAWN